Applied Epidemiology

Applied Epidemiology

Theory to Practice

Edited by
ROSS C. BROWNSON
DIANA B. PETITTI

New York   Oxford
OXFORD UNIVERSITY PRESS
1998

Oxford University Press

Oxford   New York
Athens   Auckland   Bangkok   Bogota   Bombay
Buenos Aires   Calcutta   Cape Town   Dar es Salaam
Delhi   Florence   Hong Kong   Istanbul   Karachi
Kuala Lumpur   Madras   Madrid   Melbourne
Mexico City   Nairobi   Paris   Singapore
Taipei   Tokyo   Toronto   Warsaw

and associated companies in
Berlin   Ibadan

Copyright © 1998 by Oxford University Press, Inc.

Published by Oxford University Press, Inc.
198 Madison Avenue, New York, New York 10016

Oxford is a registered trademark of Oxford University Press

Library of Congress Cataloging-in-Publication Data
Applied epidemiology : theory to practice /
edited by Ross C. Brownson, Diana B. Petitti.
p.   cm.   Includes bibliographical references and index.
ISBN 0–19–511190–7
1. Epidemiology—Research—Methodology.
I. Brownson, Ross C.   II. Petitti, Diana B.
[DNLM: 1. Epidemiology.
2. Epidemiologic Methods.
3. Quality of Health Care.
4. Health Policy.
WA 105 A652 1998]
RA652.4.A278   1998
614.4'072—dc21   DNLM/DLC   for Library of Congress   97–16894

9 8 7 6 5 4 3

Printed in the United States of America
on acid-free paper

To Carol and Selene

Foreword

In 1949, the Epidemiology Section of the American Public Health Association celebrated its twentieth anniversary in a session on "The History of American Epidemiology." John Gordon, chairman of the Department of Epidemiology at the Harvard University School of Public Health, spoke on "The Future in Epidemiology." He defined the province and promise of epidemiology in succinct and comprehensive terms:

> As the diagnostic discipline of public health, epidemiology should find increasing usefulness in the definition of health problems, in determining principles to guide programs for control, and in evaluation of accomplishment. The promise of a more scientific and a more statesmanlike public health has a close relationship with operational epidemiology.*

More than 30 years later, in an article on "Epidemiology and the Public Health Movement: A Historical Perspective," Abraham and David Lilienfeld noted that:

> During the past two decades, the discipline of epidemiology has become increasingly divorced from those activities in the real world that result in the improvement of public health. Public health administration was at one time intimately associated with epidemiology. . . . Our excursions in the historical development of epidemiology have led us to realize that epidemiology is closely interwoven with the public health movement, and our study of the evolution of the public health movement has indicated that its roots must be firmly implanted in an epidemiologic base. In order to continue with the past successes of both movements, they must be constantly nourished by each other.†

The great need for a textbook that teaches epidemiology as "the diagnostic discipline of public health," a textbook that is concerned with "usefulness in the definition of health problems, with determining principles to guide programs for control, and with evaluation of accomplishment," becomes abundantly clear when one reviews the content of leading textbooks in the field.

*Winslow, C.-E. A., Smillie, W. G., Doull, J. A., and Gordon, J. E., edited by Top, F. H. *The History of American Epidemiology*. St. Louis: C. V. Mosby, 1952.
†Lilienfeld, A. M., and Lilienfeld, D. E. "Epidemiology and the Public Health Movement: A Historical Perspective," *J. Public Health Policy* 3 (1982): 140–49.

For example, the third (1994) edition of *Foundations of Epidemiology*, revised by David Lilienfeld and Paul Stolley, resembles its previous editions in that it provides practically no discussion of the use of epidemiology in public health practice. On the other hand, as the authors state, "a new chapter on the use of epidemiologic information in clinical settings has been added to this edition." The new chapter has two sections: (1) Clinical Decision Making and (2) Reading and Interpreting Scientific Literature.

In sharp contrast, *Applied Epidemiology: Theory to Practice* considers epidemiology to be, as John Gordon said, "the diagnostic discipline of public health." Its 12 chapters provide a thorough and comprehensive analysis of problems, issues, and methods, and describes the advantages and disadvantages of various alternative approaches. In addition, the case studies of actual programs which conclude each chapter emphasize the authors' orientation to the real world of public health practice.

Applied Epidemiology: Theory to Practice is the book that the public health movement has been waiting for. It will be treasured by every public health worker who needs state-of-the-art information and guidance in defining health problems and attempting to solve them. It needs to be studied by policy-makers in all levels of government, in the schools of public health, and in the state and national public health associations. There has been no recognition of the crucial need for a large-scale program of federal aid to remedy the severe shortage of trained epidemiologists in state and local health departments, and to finance the development of a truly adequate information system that will provide health departments with the data required for effective planning and monitoring of programs and services. Commitment and leadership by the public health movement are essential to convince federal administrators and the Congress of the rich promise of epidemiology so clearly demonstrated by this landmark volume.

Milton Terris, MD, MPH

Preface

These are exciting times for epidemiology. Because of the increasingly large demand for epidemiologic expertise and the many advances in epidemiologic methods, both the opportunities and challenges in this field have never been greater. The advances in epidemiologic methods afford more sophisticated ways to evaluate the health risks associated with many exposures and with environmental contaminants in modern society. New information technologies, including powerful microcomputers, software, and the Internet, offer exciting opportunities for the conduct of a broader array of studies. Changes in how health care is delivered, particularly the growth of organized systems of care, open new chances for epidemiologists to become involved in population-based medicine and the assessment of health care utilization and quality. Despite the vast potential of epidemiology, decisions are frequently made and policy is often formed in the absence of sound epidemiologic data and scientific reasoning.

The need for this book became clear as a result of the authors' day-to-day work in public health and health care, experiences in the classroom, and discussions with colleagues. Individual epidemiologists and several expert advisory bodies have called for stronger links between educational institutions and public health practice: One link may include a curriculum in epidemiology that more closely reflects the day-to-day practice of public health.

In our view, applied epidemiology synthesizes and applies the results of etiologic studies to set priorities for intervention; it evaluates public health interventions and policies; it measures the quality and outcome of medical care; and it effectively communicates epidemiologic findings to health professionals and the public. Within this broad framework, the chapters in this book were chosen to emphasize some of the areas of public health practice in which systematic application of epidemiologic methods can have a large and positive impact. A major goal is to extend the scope of more traditional epidemiology books that tend to focus only on methods for determining disease etiology (e.g., study design, sources of bias, causal reasoning).

Following an introductory chapter, three overview chapters deal with study design and interpretation, methods in outbreak and cluster investigations, and principles of public health surveillance. The remaining eight chapters cover important contemporary topics that have strong conceptual or methodologic linkages with epidemiology. The chapters are designed to highlight key issues and to provide practical recommendations. Case studies at the end of each chapter illustrate major points and provide a basis for teaching exercises. Each case study follows a standard format (i.e., background, key questions, and implications for practice).

Topics covered in this book underline the multidisciplinary nature of epidemiology. Even within the overall science of epidemiology, there are a number of subdisciplines, such as clinical epidemiology, behavioral epidemiology, occupational epidemiology, chronic disease epidemiology, infectious disease epidemiology, and environmental epidemiology. In this regard, our book is intended to complement other recent Oxford texts in epidemiology and biostatistics.

The target audience for this text includes practicing epidemiologists, students in epidemiology, and practitioners and students in related disciplines that rely heavily on epidemiologic methods and reasoning. We hope the book will be useful in academic institutions, state and local health agencies, federal agencies with significant training missions, and health care organizations. Although the book is intended primarily for a North American audience, examples are drawn from all parts of the world and we believe that much of the information will be applicable in any developed or developing country. If used in course work, the students should already be familiar with the basic concepts in epidemiology.

Epidemiologic reasoning and methods inevitably will move beyond the boundaries of etiologic research and become integral to the practice of public health and the delivery of health care. We believe this book will be a useful resource.

August, 1997   R. C. B.
                                                                 D. B. P.

Acknowledgments

We are grateful to have chapters contributed by some of the top researchers and practitioners in the fields of epidemiology and public health: Andy Amster, Thomas A. Burke, Jennifer L. Kelsey, Abby C. King, Thomas D. Koepsell, Patrick L. Remington, Jonathan M. Samet, Donna F. Stroup, Steven M. Teutsch, Stephen B. Thacker, and Benedict I. Truman.

Many others contributed to the development of this book or reviewed earlier drafts of chapters. Our thanks to: Elena M. Andresen, James R. Davis, Ronald M. Davis, Kathleen N. Gillespie, Richard A. Goodman, Richard F. Hamman, Garland Land, James S. Marks, Raymond R. Neutra, Charles Poole, Kenneth J. Rothman, Mervyn Susser, and Fredric D. Wolinsky.

Finally, special thanks to Jeffrey House, Oxford University Press, who provided valuable advice and ideas throughout the genesis and production of this book.

Contents

Contributors

ANDY AMSTER, MSPH
Care Assessment and Improvement
Kaiser Permanente Medical Care
  Program
Southern California Region
Pasadena, California

ROSS C. BROWNSON, PhD
Prevention Research Center and
  Department of Community Health
School of Public Health
Saint Louis University
St. Louis, Missouri

THOMAS A. BURKE, PhD
Department of Health Policy and
  Management
School of Hygiene and Public Health
The Johns Hopkins University
Baltimore, Maryland

JENNIFER L. KELSEY, PhD
Division of Epidemiology
Stanford University School of Medicine
Palo Alto, California

ABBY C. KING, PhD
Department of Health Research and
  Policy
Stanford University School of Medicine
Palo Alto, California

THOMAS D. KOEPSELL, MD, MPH
Departments of Epidemiology, Health
  Services and Medicine
School of Public Health
University of Washington
Seattle, Washington

DIANA B. PETITTI, MD, MPH
Research and Evaluation
Kaiser Permanente Medical Care
  Program
Southern California Region
Pasadena, California

PATRICK L. REMINGTON, MD, MPH
Department of Preventive Medicine
University of Wisconsin Medical School
Madison, Wisconsin

JONATHAN M. SAMET, MD, MS
Department of Epidemiology
School of Hygiene and Public Health
The Johns Hopkins University
Baltimore, Maryland

DONNA F. STROUP, PhD, MSc
Epidemiology Program Office
Centers for Disease Control and
  Prevention
Atlanta, Georgia

MILTON TERRIS, MD, MPH
Journal of Public Health Policy
Burlington, Vermont

STEVEN M. TEUTSCH, MD, MPH
Epidemiology Program Office
Centers for Disease Control and
    Prevention
Atlanta, Georgia

STEPHEN B. THACKER, MD, MSc
Epidemiology Program Office
Centers for Disease Control and
    Prevention
Atlanta, Georgia

BENEDICT I. TRUMAN, MD, MPH
Epidemiology Program Office
Centers for Disease Control and
    Prevention
Atlanta, Georgia

Applied Epidemiology

1

Epidemiology:
The Foundation of Public Health

ROSS C. BROWNSON

Epidemiology has a rich, yet relatively brief history in determining the underlying causes of numerous health conditions and in assessing the effectiveness of preventive strategies and technologies. In part because it is such a new science, epidemologists have focused much of their attention over the past few decades on the development and refinement of research methods; less emphasis has been placed on how to effectively apply epidemiologic principles to public health and health care.

This chapter briefly reviews some of the historical contributions of epidemiology and some of the most pressing current issues encountered in the application of epidemiologic methods. Many of the topics discussed here are covered in more detail in later chapters.

Scope and Definitions of Epidemiology

Epidemiology is often considered the basic science of public health. This pivotal role was emphasized by the Institute of Medicine in its definition of public health as "organized community efforts aimed at the prevention of disease and promotion of health. It links many disciplines and rests upon the scientific core of epidemiology" (Committee for the Study of the Future of Public Health 1988).

Since the 1920s, several dozen definitions of epidemiology have been advanced (Lilienfeld 1978). A widely accepted version is "the study of the distribution and determinants of health-related states or events in specified populations, and the application of this study to control of health problems." (Last 1995). Perhaps the most comprehensive definition, and the one most relevant to public health practice, was crafted by Terris (1992):

Epidemiology is the study of the health of human populations. Its functions are:

1. To discover the agent, host, and environmental factors which affect health, in order to provide the scientific basis for the prevention of disease and injury and the promotion of health.
2. To determine the relative importance of causes of illness, disability, and death, in order to establish priorities for research and action.
3. To identify those sections of the population which have the greatest risk from specific causes of ill health, in order that the indicated action may be directed appropriately.
4. To evaluate the effectiveness of health programs and services in improving the health of the population.

Each of these four functions directly applies to improving the overall health of the population. Recognition of epidemiology's role in improving the overall health of the public was not consistently present in earlier definitions (Lilienfeld 1978).

Many in epidemiology and public health may view the linkage between etiologic research and public health intervention as implicit. However, it has been observed that "the discipline of epidemiology has become increasingly divorced from those activities in the real world that result in the improvement of public health" (Lilienfeld and Lilienfeld 1982). Expressing a similar concern, Pearce (1996) noted that epidemiology "has become a set of generic methods of measuring associations of exposure and disease in individuals, rather than functioning as part of a multidisciplinary approach to understanding the causation of disease in populations." Although epidemiologists need not be health promotion activists, they should work closely with communities, public health agencies, and health care providers to ensure the sound application of epidemiologic research (Wynder 1985).

Historical Aspects

Table 1-1 provides an abbreviated summary of key events in the evolution of epidemiology. The underpinnings of epidemiology and its relationship to health promotion and disease prevention go back as far as ancient Greek civilization. In his work *On Airs, Waters, and Places*, Hippocrates recommended that physicians attend to "the mode in which the inhabitants live and what are their pursuits, whether they are fond of drinking and eating to excess, and given to indolence, or are fond of exercise and labor, and not given to excess in eating and drinking" (Hippocrates 1938). During the next 2,000 years, causes of disease were considered without much emphasis on measuring their impact (Hennekens and Buring 1987). John Graunt's analysis of weekly births and deaths in London is one of the earliest examples of a descriptive epidemiologic study. William Farr was the superintendent

Table 1-1. Selected Milestones in the Historical Development of Epidemiology

Year	Event
400 B.C.	Hippocrates suggested that the development of human disease might be related to lifestyle factors and the external environment
1600s	Bacon and others developed principles of inductive logic, forming a philosophical basis for epidemiology
1662	Graunt analyzed births and deaths in London and quantified disease in a population
1747	Lind conducted a study of treatments for scurvy—one of the first experimental trials
1839	Farr set up a system for routine summaries of causes of death
1849–1854	Snow formed and tested a hypothesis on the origins of cholera in London—one of the first studies in analytic epidemiology
1920	Goldberger published a descriptive field study showing the dietary origins of pellagra
1949	The Framingham Heart Study was begun—among the first cohort studies
1950	Doll and Hill, Levin et al., Schreck et al., and Wynder and Graham published the first case-control studies of cigarette smoking and lung cancer
1954	Field trial of the Salk polio vaccine was conducted—the largest formal human experiment
1959	Mantel and Haenszel developed a statistical procedure for stratified analysis of case-control studies
1960	MacMahon published the first epidemiology text with a systematic focus on study design
1964	The US Surgeon General's Advisory Committee on Smoking and Health establish criteria for evaluation of causality
1971–1972	North Karelia Project and Stanford Three Community studies are launched—the first community-based cardiovascular disease prevention programs
1970s	New multivariate statistical methods developed, such as log-linear and logistic analysis
1970s–present	Invention and continuing evolution of microcomputer technologies allowing linkage and analysis of large databases
1990s	Development and application of techniques in molecular biology to large populations

of the Statistical Department of the Registrar General's Office of England and Wales from 1839 to 1879 and is considered the founder of the modern disease surveillance due to his work in collecting and reporting vital statistics (Thacker and Berkelman 1988).

The evolution of modern epidemiology, marked by many of the milestones noted in Table 1-1, has been broadly divided into three stages: sanitary statistics, infectious disease epidemiology, and chronic disease epidemiology (Susser and Susser 1996). The era of sanitary statistics was the first half of the 19th century, when the prevailing etiologic theory was "miasma" (i.e., poisoning by foul emanations from soil, air, and water). Methods focused on assessing the clustering of morbidity and mortality and on preventive measures such as drainage, sewage, and sanitation. In the era of infectious disease epidemiology (the late 19th century through the first half of the 20th century), the germ theory prevailed, in which single agents are related, one to one, to specific diseases. Others (Lilienfeld and Stolley 1994) have called this the period of bacteriology. The prevalent analytic approach was laboratory isolation and culture of infectious agents (e.g., bacteria) from disease sites. The overriding preventive approach was to interrupt transmission of the infectious agent. The era of chronic disease epidemiology has prevailed since World War II. The underlying paradigm of many studies in this era has been termed the "black box" approach, in which exposures are related to outcomes without always understanding the intervening factors or pathogenesis (Susser and Susser 1996). One of the primary analytic methods involves the use of risk ratios to relate exposures to outcomes. Preventive measures have emphasized the control of risk factors by modifying the environment or human behavior (e.g., smoking, physical inactivity).

The field of epidemiology is continually adapting and evolving, particularly as advances in other fields open up new opportunities. Epidemiology is interdisciplinary, a fertile and complex science that draws on many other fields including molecular biology, medicine, environmental sciences, statistics, sociology, demography, and economics (Terris 1979; Lilienfeld and Stolley 1994). During the post–World War II years in the United States, new tools in epidemiology (e.g., statistical methods using microcomputers) have proliferated at a rapid rate. Similarly, advances in molecular biology in recent decades have led to increasingly sophisticated and sensitive methods of exposure assessment. As epidemiology developed into an academic discipline in the United States, it was institutionalized in schools of public health and medicine (Oppenheimer 1995).

The Importance of Applied Epidemiology

Throughout its history, epidemiology has provided a basis for understanding the underlying causes of many diseases and health conditions. A variety of analytic tools and statistical methods have been developed (Kelsey et al. 1996), resulting in a better understanding of etiology. This knowledge of causes has fostered the development of applied epidemiology, which can be defined as the application and evaluation of epidemiologic discoveries and methods in public health and health care settings. Often the most important research issue in this context is not the efficacy of the technology itself but the effectiveness of its application to the general population and of its adaptation to population subgroups at highest risk (Taylor et al. 1993). Research in this area reflects the need to increase the benefits from prevention by bringing it into more widespread use in the community and in the health care system. Epidemiologists must continue to move from developing the science base of etiology to implementing and evaluating public health interventions.

Successes of Epidemiology and Public Health

The accomplishments of epidemiology, public health, and related social changes have changed the pattern of death and disease in modern society. Infant mortality in the United States has fallen from 150 per 1,000 live births in 1900 to 8.5 per 1,000 in 1992 (Taylor et al. 1993; National Center for Health Statistics 1996a). Life expectancy from birth has risen from 47 years in 1900 to more than 75 years in 1992 (National Center for Health Statistics 1996a). This represents an increase of over 2 days of life expectancy for every week since the beginning of this century. Only about 5 of the additional 30 years gained in life expectancy can be attributed to the work of the medical care system (Bunker et al. 1994). It is likely that the majority of the gain in life expectancy can be attributed to provision of safe water and food, sewage disposal, control of infectious diseases through immunization, and other population-based, public health activities (Centers for Disease Control and Prevention [CDC] 1993a).

A few examples illustrate the progression from epidemiologic research to public health action. Since the earliest links between smoking and lung cancer were established at the beginning of the 1950s (Doll and Hill 1950; Wynder and Graham 1950; Levin et al. 1950; Schreck et al. 1950), thousands of studies have documented cigarette smoking as a cause of numerous diseases. Epidemiologic studies were the basis for the 1964 report of US surgeon general's advisory committee on smoking and health (US Dept of Health, Education, and Welfare [US DHEW] 1964) that declared the relationship between smoking and lung cancer to be causal. The relationship was described as consistent, strong, specific, temporally appropriate, and coherent. This report marked the beginning of a long series of public health efforts to control tobacco use. These have included policy changes (e.g., advertising restrictions, clean indoor air policies), clinical interventions (e.g., physician advice to patients on smoking cessation), and smoking prevention programs in schools (e.g., curricula that focus on effective prevention strategies). As a marker of the success of tobacco control efforts, the overall rate of cigarette smoking among US adults declined from 42% in 1965 to 25% in 1993 (National Center for Health Statistics 1996a) (Figure 1-1).

Epidemiology can also take some credit for reducing the incidence of cardiovascular diseases in recent decades, particularly coronary heart disease (CHD). CHD has been the leading cause of death in the United States for most of the 20th century. US death rates from CHD peaked in 1963 (Figure 1-2). Since 1968, the decline in CHD mortality has been consistent and nearly uniform across race and sex groups. The decline has been steeper in younger than in older age groups (Higgins and Luepker 1988). By 1993, the age-adjusted mortality rate for CHD was 95 per 100,000 (National Center for Health Statistics 1996a), representing a decline of about 60% since 1968 (Figure 1-2). This decline in CHD mortality is not fully understood. A major contributor has probably been change in lifestyle risk factors (e.g., cigarette smoking, hypertension, physical inactivity, nutrition) (Fielding 1978; Goldman and Cook 1988). In the United States, these modifiable risk factors were identified through large-scale epidemiologic studies such as the Framingham Study (Dawber 1980). These epidemiologic investigations and subsequent public health programs (e.g., the National High Blood Pressure Education Program begun in 1972 (Roccella and Horan 1988)) heightened awareness of the modifiable nature of many CHD risk factors among health professionals

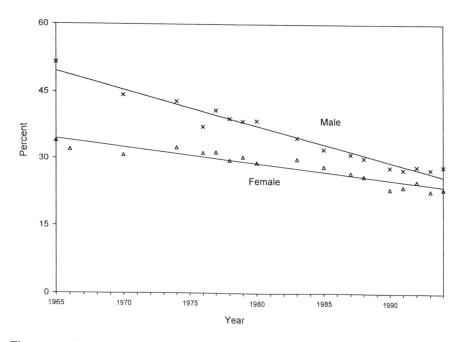

Figure 1-1. Age-adjusted prevalence of current smokers among adults (aged 18 years and older), with least-squares trend line, by gender, United States, 1965–1994

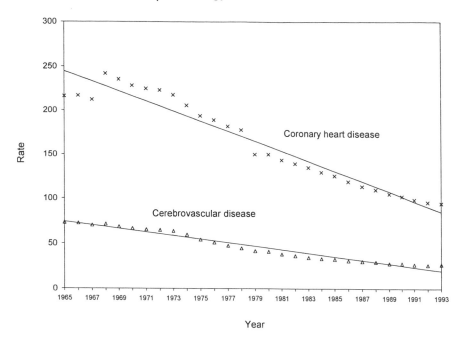

Figure 1-2. Age-adjusted cardiovascular disease death per 100,000, with least-squares trend line, United States, 1965–1993

and the general public (Kannel 1995). Improvements in medical care and treatment of CHD are also likely contributors to the overall decline (Goldman and Cook 1988).

Current Challenges and Opportunities in Epidemiology

The historical contributions of epidemiology provide a backdrop against which we may consider current challenges and opportunities that confront its application. This section highlights 11 key areas—not an exhaustive list—(Table 1-2) where epidemiology will very likely play an increasing role. The issues outlined generally follow the sequence of Terris's definition (1992), moving from etiologic research, to priority setting, to the evaluation of health programs, policies, and service delivery.

Applying Advances from Molecular Biology

The recent scientific approach of combining principles of population-based epidemiology with those of the basic laboratory is the basis for "molecular epidemiology" (Schulte and Perera 1993). Molecular epidemiology should not be viewed as a subdiscipline in itself; rather, it should be seen as the use of

Table 1-2. Summary of Modern Challenges and Opportunities in Epidemiology

- Applying advances from molecular biology
- Increasing attention to ethical issues
- Measuring and communicating weak associations
- Measuring outcomes and quality of health care
- Setting priorities and measuring progress
- Investigating public health outbreaks
- Preventing chronic diseases and other "modern epidemics"
- Measuring the effects of public health interventions
- Informing public health policies
- Applying new computer and information technologies
- Increasing epidemiologic capacity in applied settings

methods in molecular biology to enhance measurement of exposure, effect, or susceptibility (McMichael 1994). Techniques such as DNA typing have proven useful in identifying molecular structures that may be damaged by disease or environmental exposures that define susceptibility to disease. In particular, molecular epidemiology has revealed substantial variability in biologic response to carcinogens, which suggests that certain subgroups (e.g., the young, those with predisposing genetic traits) are at greater risk of disease (Perera 1996). Such advances may lead to new approaches to risk assessment, in which susceptible groups are identified, necessitating new regulatory policies or different intervention programs. In the realm of field investigations, molecular typing of viruses and bacteria has led to clearer definition of common source outbreaks.

While advances in molecular epidemiology may lead to new and innovative opportunities in prevention, early detection, and treatment, they also raise profound ethical questions. For example, the presence of a mutation in a gene (BRCA1) on chromosome 17q12-21 (Hill et al. 1990) has been shown to greatly increase the risk of breast cancer in women. Women with germline mutations to BRCA1 are estimated to have an 80–90% lifetime risk of developing breast cancer (Easton et al. 1993). Although techniques to assess mutations in the BRCA1 gene are currently limited to a few families for research purposes, tests are likely to be available for population-based screening in the next few years. A few of the ethical considerations relevant to use of new genetic markers include:

- How should information be provided to participants of a research study when there are enormous health consequences (Biesecker et al. 1993)?
- How can confidentiality be maintained?
- Would identification of a strong genetic predisposition toward a particular cancer affect an individual's ability to be employed and/or insured?
- How should such tests enter the clinical and public health marketplace?
- Who should control the availability of such tests?

Increasing Attention on Ethical Issues

The preceding section and other chapters in this book highlight the need to carefully consider ethical principles when conducting epidemiologic research and applying the results of epidemiologic studies. In the late 1980s and the early 1990s, there was a surge in interest in the application of ethics in epidemiologic research and practice (Coughlin and Beauchamp 1996). The interrelationships between ethics and epidemiology are vast and comprehensive coverage is beyond the scope of this chapter. Readers are referred to the Council for International Organizations of Medical Sciences (1991) and Coughlin and Beauchamp (1996) for a full coverage of ethical issues.

In epidemiological studies, subjects should be adequately informed and protected from undue risks, and the potential societal benefits of epidemiology should be maximized (Coughlin and Beauchamp 1996). In the United States, a growing interest in applying ethical principles has been fostered by several outrageous events. For example, the Tuskegee Syphilis Study (1932–1972) breeched ethical principles by studying the natural history of untreated syphilis among poor black men who lacked informed consent. Widespread distrust can develop between vulnerable populations and researchers if formal safeguards are not in place.

The growing role of ethics in epidemiology has led to the development of an explicit list of professional responsibilities (Coughlin and Beauchamp 1996) organized under four major headings:

Responsibilities to Research Subjects
- Welfare protection
- Informed consent
- Privacy
- Confidentiality
- Committee review

Responsibilities to Society
- Provide benefits
- Public trust
- Avoid conflict of interest
- Impartiality

Responsibilities to Employers and Funding Sources
- Formulate responsibilities
- Protect privileged information

Responsibilities to Professional Colleagues
- Report methods and results
- Report unacceptable behavior and conditions

Measuring and Communicating Weak Associations

Quantitatively, a weak epidemiologic association is one in which the estimate of relative risk (often in the form of an odds ratio) is less than 3 (Wynder

1987). The abilities to assess weak associations with validity and to appropriately communicate epidemiologic findings to the public are continuing challenges for modern epidemiology. Epidemiology has had great success in identifying the origins (and magnitude) of many public health epidemics. Examples include cigarette smoking/lung cancer, asbestos/mesothelioma, and alcoholism/cirrhosis of the liver. Relative risk estimates for many of these risk factors range from 5 to 20, making their identification and inferences about causation relatively easy. In contrast, for many risk factors currently being studied, it is increasingly difficult to find overwhelming evidence for causality (Gordis 1988). The closer a relative risk estimate comes to unity, the more likely that it can be explained by methodologic difficulties such as confounding or misclassification, or other sources of bias. New techniques in molecular epidemiology (noted earlier) may prove extremely beneficial in identifying biological markers of exposure when assessing weak associations.

Among the most challenging of weak associations are those that are made in an attempt to measure the relationship between environmental chemicals and health outcomes. Evaluating the independent and combined effects of chemical mixtures on disease risk is one of the most demanding tasks in epidemiology (Samet 1995). Application of knowledge gained from epidemiologic and from other studies of possible environmental hazards requires a combination of research skills and an understanding of the policy-making process.

The accurate communication of the results of epidemiologic studies to the general public and to policy-makers is an on-going challenge (Taubes 1995). At times, it seems the public is subjected to a "health scare a week." Often, provocative studies are published in leading scientific journals and result in considerable media coverage. There is a tendency for the media and researchers to overstate the importance of findings from one or a small number of studies. Such overstatement may explicitly or implicitly result in a public health recommendation for the general population.

A single risk factor may also have both negative and positive effects on health. For example, moderate alcohol use may increase the risk of breast cancer (Kelsey and Bernstein 1996) but may decrease the risk of CHD (Marmot and Brunner 1991). Should a physician or public health expert recommend that middle-aged women consume moderate amounts of alcohol or that they refrain from consumption? If a medical or public health professional is educated in a systematic approach (Fischhoff et al. 1993) to risk communication, the individuals he or she counsels will be able to make informed decisions about their health. The risk communication process consists largely of quantitative assessment (e.g., Do people know how large the risk is?) and qualitative assessment (e.g., Are health professions and laypersons unwittingly using different terms?) (Fischhoff et al. 1993).

Measuring Outcomes and Quality of Health Care

The United States spends more per capita on health care than any other country in the world—14% of our gross domestic product in 1994. Primarily due to concern about rising costs, the US health care system is currently undergoing profound changes that will influence the practice of epidemiology in the coming decade. Health maintenance organizations (HMOs) have grown from enrollments of 6 million people in 1976 to 46 million in 1995 (National Center for Health Statistics 1996a). Sometime within the next decade (the first decade of the next millenium), 80–90% of the insured US population will receive its health care through various forms of managed care (Pew Health Professions Commission 1995).

Principles of epidemiology are increasingly used to shape and evaluate the changing health care system. Managers of health care systems are recognizing that the most cost-effective strategies will be achieved through a population-based perspective, which places epidemiology in a pivotal role (Oleske 1993). Measures of how well health care services are being delivered now are being demanded as evidence of both quality and outcome of care. One example of such a measure is the Health Plan Employer Data and Information Set (HEDIS) (National Committee for Quality Assurance 1993). Many of the indicators within HEDIS (e.g., infant low birth weight, mammography screening) provide a basis for measuring the delivery of preventive services.

Applications of epidemiology in a modern health care organization encompass a wide range of activities, including (1) linking national or regional policy initiatives with institutional efforts, (2) strategically developing new services or planning changes in existing ones, (3) projecting the human resources to provide care to a population, (4) monitoring system performance with respect to patient outcomes, and (5) measuring the success of institutional linkages and/or system configurations to effect changes in the health status of the population (Lerner 1995).

This enhanced role of epidemiology is evident within various models of health care delivery. For example, the Expanded Behavioral Model predicts health services utilization (Aday 1980) according to numerous factors (Figure 1-3). Within this model, epidemiology can play a key role at several different points because of the need for measurement and expertise in measurement.

The changing health care system will call for new skills and competencies among health care providers (Pew Health Professions Commission 1995). Among the necessary skills are the abilities to assess the health care needs of the population; develop intervention programs; and evaluate cost, efficacy, and effectiveness of interventions. These skills relate closely to the intellectual discipline of epidemiology. New opportunities abound to train epidemiologists to meet the needs of health care organizations and to retrain clinicians in

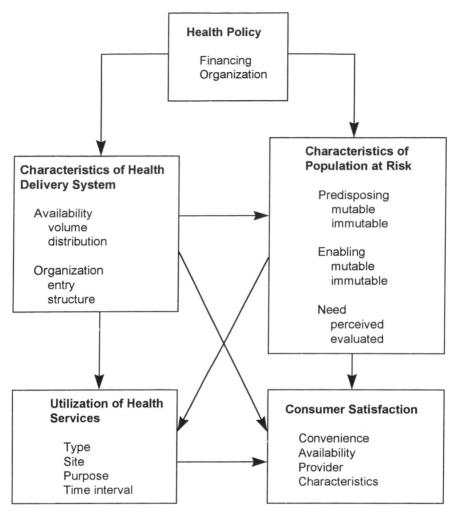

Figure 1-3. The Expanded Behavioral Model of health services utilization. *Source:* Aday (1980)

areas such as managerial epidemiology (Pew Health Professions Commission 1995).

Setting Priorities and Measuring Progress

Establishing public health and health care priorities in an era of limited resources is a demanding task. Epidemiologic tools and approaches can make important contributions to priority setting. Measuring progress toward explicit goals has become an essential feature of goal setting.

Public health leaders began to formulate concrete public health objectives as a basis for action in the years following World War II. This was a clear shift from earlier efforts in that emphasis was placed on quantifiable objectives and explicit time limits (Breslow 1990). A few key examples illustrate the use of epidemiologic data in setting and measuring progress toward health objectives.

In 1966, the World Health Organization established a goal of eliminating smallpox by interrupting its transmission throughout the world by the end of 1976 (World Health Organization 1971). The last known smallpox cases were observed very close to the 1976 goal—a case in Somalia in October 1977 and two laboratory infections in England in 1978 (Breslow 1990).

A paper by the Institute of Medicine (Nightingale et al. 1978) sparked a US movement to set objectives for public health (Breslow 1990). These initial actions by the Institute of Medicine led to the 1979 *Surgeon General's Report on Health Promotion and Disease Prevention,* which set five national goals—one each for the principal life stages of infancy, childhood, adolescence and young adulthood, adulthood, and older adulthood (US DHEW 1979).

Most recently, the US Public Health Service established three overarching health goals for the year 2000 (called the *Healthy People 2000* objectives): increase the span of healthy life for Americans, reduce health disparities among Americans, and provide access to preventive services for all Americans. To achieve these three goals, a comprehensive set of 300 unduplicated main health objectives were established in 22 priority areas (Table 1-3). There are 223 unduplicated special population targets (i.e., for persons with low incomes, with disabilities, or who are members of a racial/ethnic minority group). The core of the year-2000 objectives is based on decades of epidemiologic research showing modifiable risk factors that could substantially influence the disease burden in the United States (US Dept of Health and Human Services [US DHHS] 1990). Progress toward the year-2000 objectives is being measured in annual reports (National Center for Health Statistics 1996b). Establishment of national, quantifiable objectives has stimulated state and local efforts in program and organizational planning. For example, an estimated 70% of all US local health agencies (from a total of about 3,000) have used Healthy People 2000 objectives (National Association of County and City Health Officials 1995). Presently, efforts are underway to update *Healthy People 2000* objectives for the year 2010, which are slated for release in January 2000.

Investigating Public Health Outbreaks

Persons working in public health are frequently called upon to investigate potential outbreaks of acute diseases and to assess potential exposure to envi-

Table 1-3. Priority Areas in Healthy People 2000

Major Category	Priority Area
Health promotion	Physical activity and fitness
	Nutrition
	Tobacco
	Alcohol and other drugs
	Family planning
	Mental health and mental disorders
	Violent and abusive behaviors
	Educational and community-based programs
Health protection	Unintentional injuries
	Occupational safety and health
	Environmental health
	Food and drug safety
	Oral health
Preventive services	Maternal and infant health
	Heart disease and stroke
	Cancer
	Diabetes and chronic disabling conditions
	HIV infection
	Sexually transmitted diseases
	Immunization and infectious diseases
	Clinical preventive services
Surveillance and data systems	Surveillance and data systems

Source: Healthy People 2000 (US DHHS 1990).

ronmental or occupational hazards. Such studies one called "field investigations" (Goodman et al. 1990; Gregg et al. 1996). Public health agencies have the primary responsibility for conducting field investigations of outbreaks (Dwyer et al. 1994).

These epidemiologic events can be characterized as outbreaks (i.e., the occurrence of more cases of an adverse health event than expected in a given geographic area over a particular period of time, CDC 1993b) or clusters (i.e., the aggregation of events in space and time, Rothenberg et al. 1990). "Outbreaks" usually refer to (the investigation of) acute health effects—such as an epidemic of foodborne disease due to the *Salmonella* bacterium. "Clusters" have tended to focus on longer-term, chronic conditions such as (the investigation of whether living near a radiation tailing site increases the risk of) childhood leukemia.

Field investigations present special challenges and opportunities for public health professionals. Unlike most studies in analytic epidemiology (which are carefully planned, rely on controlled data collection, and are carried out over a period of years), field studies frequently rely on data that are less controlled and protocols that may change with each successive hour or day (Goodman et al. 1990). Field investigations may be based on a relatively small number of persons and collection of biological specimens (e.g., the suspected food in a foodborne outbreak) may not always be possible (Gregg et al. 1996). The substantial media attention commonly surrounding acute disease outbreaks can be a mixed blessing—on the one hand, it may assist investigators in finding disease cases, but on the other, it may introduce bias if affected persons form preconceived notions of their illness after hearing press coverage (Gregg et al. 1996). Field epidemiologic studies present unique opportunities because they are "natural experiments" (Goodman et al. 1990). Within a short period of time, field studies can lead to new discoveries and policy recommendations that will improve the health of the public.

Preventing Chronic Diseases and Other "Modern Epidemics"

During the past century, the United States has experienced a dramatic shift in the leading causes of death and disability and in the costs of disease: The chronic have supplanted the infectious. In 1900, pneumonia, tuberculosis, and gastritis were the three leading causes of death, accounting for 31% of all deaths (Table 1-4). Today, heart disease, cancer, and cerebrovascular diseases (stroke) are the three leading causes of death, accounting for 63% of deaths (Table 1-5). It is estimated that chronic diseases accounted for three-fourths of US health care expenditures in 1990 ($425 billion in direct health care costs and $235 billion in indirect costs that year) (Hoffman et al. 1996). Reflecting these changes in the leading causes of mortality, public health priorities have shifted from a primary emphasis on microbiologic investigation of communicable diseases to emphasis on the etiologic role of behavioral and environmental risk factors and methods for preventing disease, disability, and death in a population (Table 1-3). Terris (1983) has termed the focus in chronic disease epidemiology the "second epidemiologic revolution."

When considering the epidemiology and control of chronic diseases, it may be useful to review and extend the concepts of "epidemics" and "endemics." An epidemic can be described as the "occurrence in a community or region of cases of an illness, specific health-related behavior, or other health-related events clearly in excess of normal expectancy" (Last 1995). In contrast, an endemic is the "constant presence of a disease or infectious agent within a geographic area or population group" (Last 1995). The shift in burden discussed earlier has served to broaden the meaning of "epidemic." Because chronic diseases may develop over many years and remain relatively constant in incidence over long periods, they may therefore be considered endemic—implying a less urgent need for public health action. However,

Table 1-4. Death Rates and Percent of Total Deaths for the 10 Leading Causes of Death in the United States, 1900

Cause of Death	Death Rate per 100,000	Percent of Total Deaths
All causes	1,719	100.0
Pneumonia and influenza	202	11.8
Tuberculosis	194	11.3
Gastritis, enteritis, colitis	143	8.3
Diseases of heart	137	8.0
Symptoms, senility, ill-defined conditions	118	6.8
Vascular lesions affecting central nerve system	107	6.2
Chronic nephritis and renal sclerosis	81	4.7
Unintentional injuries	72	4.2
Malignant neoplasms	64	3.7
Diphtheria	40	2.3
All other causes	—	32.6

Source: National Office of Vital Statistics (1954).

such a consideration is not prudent in many cases, since risk factors are well known and a chronic disease may be almost entirely preventable (e.g., cigarette smoking and lung cancer). Public health leaders must recognize that certain conditions at endemic levels deserve urgent attention.

Chronic disease epidemiology may also call for a more complicated definition of a public health "burden." Surveillance data can estimate burden for infectious diseases simply in terms of case numbers or rates. For many chronic diseases, a simple measure of burden might be reflected in mortality rates. However, this may be a misleading figure because successful preventive strategies and technologies may lead to an increase in disease-free life (i.e., the absence of disability) without a large reduction in mortality (Thacker et al. 1995).

Other modern public health epidemics include intentional injuries (e.g., homicide and other acts of violence) and infection with the human immunodeficiency virus (HIV) resulting in acquired immune deficiency syndrome (AIDS). The problem of violence in modern society illustrates the complexity of certain epidemics. Analysis of public health statistics shows that violence in US society has increased in frequency and severity over the past few decades. Epidemiologic data show the disproportionate impact of violence on young men, women, and children, African-Americans, and the poor (Mercy et al.

1993). It is clear that a complex array of factors must be addressed to prevent violence: individual knowledge and attitudes, in the social environment (e.g., economic circumstances), and the physical environment (e.g., safe structures for walking or transportation) (Mercy et al. 1993) all must be changed. A public health model has been proposed (Figure 1-4) for prevention of violence and other public health problems. Applied epidemiology plays a key role in this model in defining the problem, assessing risk factors, and evaluating intervention effectiveness.

Measuring the Effects of Public Health Interventions

Increasingly, researchers are recognizing the community as the proper and most effective focus for public health interventions (Green and Kreuter 1990). The "community" might be a county, town, neighborhood, school, work site, or a health plan. A level of collective decision-making and some sense of urgency must exist regarding a health issue for this to work (Green and Kreuter 1990).

A public health intervention may encompass a wide range of activities. Large community-based prevention projects have demonstrated the effectiveness of combined interventions that address both individual behavior change

Table 1-5. Death Rates and Percent of Total Deaths for the 10 Leading Causes of Death in the United States, 1995

Cause of Death	Death Rate per 100,000	Percent of Total Deaths
All causes	880	100.0
Diseases of heart	281	32.0
Malignant neoplasms	205	23.3
Cerebrovascular diseases	60	6.8
Chronic obstructive pulmonary diseases	40	4.5
Accidents and adverse effects	34	3.9
Pneumonia and influenza	32	3.6
Diabetes mellitus	23	2.6
Human immunodeficiency virus infection	16	1.8
Suicide	12	1.3
Homicide and legal intervention	10	1.1
All other causes	168	19.1

Source: Rosenberg et al. (1996).

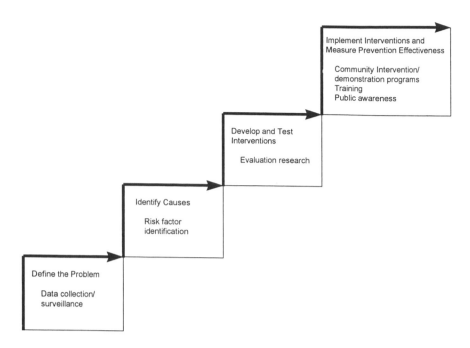

Figure 1-4. Public health model of a scientific approach to prevention. *Source:* Mercy (1993)

and system-level change. Large-scale disease prevention initiatives include well-designed and -implemented community-based projects such as the North Karelia Project in Finland (Puska 1984), the Stanford Five-City Project (Farquhar et al. 1985), the Pawtucket Heart Health Program (Carleton et al. 1987), and the Minnesota Heart Health Program (Blackburn et al. 1984). In these projects, interventions were delivered via mass media, health professionals, education professionals, community leaders, co-workers, neighbors, friends, family members, and other individuals in the community.

Measuring the effects of community-level interventions can be challenging, in part because evaluation data are typically collected at the individual level (Koepsell et al. 1991). Epidemiologic evaluations of community interventions need to account for a specific theoretical model, accounting for intraclass correlations when the community is the unit of assignment, and the validity of self-reported health characteristics (Koepsell et al. 1991, 1992), among others.

Evaluating community-based interventions presents an ideal opportunity to create productive partnerships between health agencies and universities. Each entity brings unique abilities to the table. In general, health agencies have greater access to populations at risk and have more experience working at the community level. University researchers can add epidemiologic expertise and information on relevant intervention theories and strategies.

Informing Public Health Policies

Others (Stallones 1982; Terris 1980) have written convincingly about the critical linkage between epidemiology and public health policies. Indeed, Terris (1980) has suggested that health policies should be *based* on epidemiology. Some would argue that policy-related interventions can best improve overall health (Schmid et al. 1995). As health resources are stretched at the federal, state, and local levels, policy interventions are likely to grow in prominence.

Several methods, based on epidemiologic principles, help inform policy decisions—meta-analysis, decision analysis, and cost-effectiveness analysis (Petitti 1994). Basing policy on objective assessment of evidence (evidence-based policy) is likely to assume increasing prominence in the policy-making area.

Development of rational health policies takes into account efficiency, safety, and cost. The primary goal, however, is to improve health status at a reasonable cost, not simply to contain cost (Thacker et al. 1994). Table 1-6 describes several examples where the burden of the condition, effectiveness of the prevention method, cost, and population coverage have been taken into account in setting prevention policies.

In summary, epidemiologists can play a key role in policy-related interventions. First, through etiologic studies, epidemiologists can identify potential interventions based on causal criteria (US DHEW 1964; Hill 1965; Susser 1973) and their likely impact on disease burden based on the population attributable risk (Lilienfeld and Stolley 1994). Second, epidemiologists can work closely with behavioral scientists in designing interventions and evaluation protocols. And third, following implementation of a particular intervention, epidemiologists can assist policy-makers in evaluating the effects of the intervention and in formulating broader policies related to the intervention.

Applying New Computer and Information Technologies

The proliferation of computer and information technologies will continue to provide exciting opportunities and challenges for epidemiologists. Changes are occurring in three general areas: (1) expanded use of the information "superhighway," enabling expanded transmission of information relevant to epidemiology, (2) increased analysis of "secondary" data, and (3) enhanced information systems in public health and health care (Friede et al. 1995).

Table 1-6. Selected Examples of Prevention Effectiveness

Prevention Type[a]	Undesired Outcome	Annual US Incidence Without Intervention	Prevention Method	% Effectiveness	Economic Analysis	% of Persons at Risk Covered by Method
Primary	Measles	4,000,000	Vaccination	95–98	$16.85 per case prevented	By age 2, 50–80%; by age 6, 98%
Secondary	Breast cancer deaths	50,000	Mammography screening women >40 years	20–70	$45,000–$165,000 per year of life saved	15–38
Tertiary	Blindness from diabetes	24,000	Retinal screening, treatment	50	$100 per year of vision saved	60–80

[a]Primary prevention = directed at susceptible persons before they develop a particular disease (risk factor reduction); secondary prevention = directed at persons who are asymptomatic but who have developed biologic changes (early detection and treatment); tertiary prevention = directed at preventing disability in persons who have symptomatic disease (prevent complications and rehabilitation).

Source: Thacker et al. (1994).

The information superhighway offers numerous possibilities due to its ability to rapidly transfer electronic information. Opportunities include networking of public health professionals, monitoring of disease patterns on a global basis, on-line access to vital statistics, monitoring of environmental determinants of disease on a global basis, e-mail searches, access to distance education, and on-line access to journals and other epidemiologic resources (Laporte et al. 1994). Several web sites may be particularly useful for epidemiologists (CDC 1997a,b; University of California San Francisco 1997; US Dept of Energy 1997).

One of the most important opportunities created by the explosion in information and surveillance systems is the analysis of "secondary" data sets. Today's microcomputers are of sufficient size and speed to allow sophisticated statistical analysis of extremely large data sets (e.g., records representing millions of person-years). Along with new opportunities, researchers and practitioners should be aware of the limitations of secondary data analysis. Several key factors are summarized in Table 1-7. In addition to these factors, concerns about confidentiality may limit use of secondary data (Sørensen et al. 1996).

An information system has been defined as "a combination of vital and health statistical data from multiple sources, used to derive information about the health needs, health resources, costs, use of health services, and outcomes of use by the population of a specified jurisdiction" (Last 1995). There are a number of similarities between public health surveillance systems and systems used by health care providers (i.e., clinical information systems). The transformation of clinical information systems to build systems that focus on the entire population at risk, not just the person who presents

Table 1-7. Factors and Methods Affecting the Use of Secondary Data in Epidemiologic Research

1. Completeness of registration of individuals
   a. Case by case comparison of the data source with one or more independent reference sources
   b. Comprehensive records review to assess misclassification
   c. Aggregated methods to compare the total number of cases in the data source with other sources
2. The accuracy and degree of completeness of variables
   a. Precision
   b. Validity
3. The size of the data sources
4. Registration period
5. Data accessibility, availability, and cost
6. Data format
7. Record linkage

Source: Sørensen et al. (1996).

for health care services, is an important turning point in information availability.

Recommendations to improve data systems (Lasker 1995) include:

- Data from management information systems as well as traditional public health surveys
- A balanced approach to data collection, including information about health and functional status; behavioral, environmental, occupational, and infectious risks to health; the capacity and functioning of the medical and public health systems; and the costs, utilization, and financing of individuals and population-based health services
- The capacity to link different types of data together and to aggregate them geographically and temporally
- Comparable health-related information at national, state, and local levels
- Meaningful and reliable data to support program measurement and performance measurement
- Federal/state and public/private partnerships to develop data strategies and to collect information

Increasing Epidemiologic Capacity in Applied Settings

Epidemiologic research in the public health agency setting is likely to evolve in the next decade. Public health departments have traditionally focused on the provision of health care services to populations at risk, with relatively little emphasis on epidemiologic research. However, the public health role of providing clinical preventive services is changing and is likely to evolve further. Largely due to the growth of managed care, fewer health departments will provide direct services to clients as underserved populations are increasingly moved to managed-care settings. Epidemiologic capacity in the public health setting can be defined in relation to three general areas: need, staffing patterns, and training.

Survey data support the importance of epidemiology in the public health setting. A recent survey of 40 state health agency directors found that among 11 key areas, epidemiology was rated as having the highest importance to respondents (a mean of 9.5 on a 10-point scale) (Morris et al. 1994). In contrast, the percentage of respondents who believed that research needs in epidemiology were being met by universities was much lower (a mean of 4.4 on a 10-point scale).

Although obtaining accurate estimates of research personnel needs is difficult (Winkelstein and French 1977) and relatively little empirical data exist, it is widely accepted that a shortage of trained epidemiologists has existed in public health agencies for several decades (Detels 1979; Williams et al. 1988). It is also likely that the continually growing demand for quality health care will increase the need for epidemiologists in the private and nonprofit sectors. The shortage of master's- and doctoral-trained epidemiologists may be most acute for non–infectious disease epidemiologists (Boss and Foster 1994). For example, in a 1994 survey of state health agencies, 10 states and the District of Columbia did not have at least one full-time equivalent chronic disease epidemiologist on staff (personal communication, Dr. Leonard Palozzi, CDC, August 31, 1995).

Training of epidemiologists occurs through a variety of mechanisms. Many epidemiologists at the master's and doctoral levels are trained by schools of public health (Williams et al. 1988). Other important sources include schools of medicine and the Epidemic Intelligence Service of the Centers for Disease Control and Prevention (Thacker et al. 1990). Survey data and expert groups have also shown the need for expanded and perhaps different formal training in epidemiology (Committee for the Study of the Future of Public Health 1988; Pew Health Professions Commission 1995). In general, the curricula and internship opportunities in schools of public health have not consistently reflected the needs of practitioners. Successful educational programs need to maintain close contact with public health practice (Committee for the Study of the Future of Public Health 1988).

Summary

This chapter has briefly summarized several substantial historical contributions of epidemiology and some of the most important opportunities and challenges facing epidemiology. The current epidemiologic and technologic advances provide unprecedented opportunities for practicing health professionals. To take full advantage of these, continued skill enhancement will be necessary. Training programs must account for the needs in public health practice, and practicing professionals should develop at least a basic understanding of epidemiologic methods and ways of accurately interpreting the large body of scientific literature. Many of the issues introduced in this chapter can aid in this understanding—these will be covered in more detail in subsequent chapters.

As early as the 19th century, Pasteur emphasized not only the discovery of new knowledge but the application of research. In many cases, the discovery of the factors responsible for disease causation is easier than changing environmental conditions or behaviors to reduce exposure to such factors (Wynder 1985). If findings from etiologic research are not put into practice, the epidemiologic puzzle is incomplete and the ultimate goal of epidemiology—to improve human health—will not be achieved.

CASE STUDIES

The Epidemiology of Hantavirus Pulmonary Syndrome in the United States

Background

The hantavirus is a lipid-enveloped, trisegmented, RNA virus. It is named for the protype virus, Hantaan, which was isolated from a striped field mouse caught near the Hantaan River, South Korea, in 1976 (Lee et al. 1978). The virus is transmitted to humans primarily by the inhalation of aerosols generated from rodent saliva, urine, and feces (Khan et al. 1996). In the United States, at least three types of hantaviruses are known to cause hantavirus pulmonary syndrome (HPS), which is a severe cardiopulmonary illness first identified in 1993. The principal host of hantavirus in the United States is the deer mouse.

Public health surveillance for HPS was established by the CDC after an outbreak of acute pulmonary failure in the southwestern United States in May–August 1993. This surveillance system was based on cooperation between private providers of health care and local, state, and federal governmental health agencies. A comprehensive case definition was developed and a telephone hot line was established to report suspected cases (Khan et al. 1996). Laboratory verification of cases was ascertained through use of state-of-the-art techniques in molecular biology. Serologic testing was conducted for IgM and IgG by the enzyme-linked immunosorbent assay (ELISA) method. In addition, polymerase chain reaction was used to test tissue samples for hantaviral RNA.

Key Questions

1. What is the distribution of HPS in the United States in terms of the common epidemiologic categories of person, place, and time?

The epidemiologic description of the first 100 US cases of HPS showed that the cases were distributed in 21 states and that the condition had gone unrecognized since 1959 (Khan et al. 1996). The condition had a distinct spring–early summer seasonality. Among cases, 54% were male, 63% were Caucasian, and 35% were Native American. The average age of cases was 35 years and the case-fatality rate was 52% (Figure 1-5).

2. Using HPS as an example, how can methods in molecular biology be used to enhance public health surveillance efforts?

Within weeks after cases emerged in spring 1993, public health workers had characterized the clinical illness, etiologic agent, and rodent host (Khan et al. 1996). The ability to conduct rapid and accurate laboratory tests was a direct benefit in the HPS outbreak. There was a 91% concordance between serologic, immunohistochemical, and molecular results (Khan et al. 1996).

3. Based on these data, what were the recommendations for prevention of HPS?

Recommendations to reduce the risk of exposure to hantavirus include precautions for persons involved in activities associated with exposure to rodents, rodent excreta, and contaminated dust.

Implications for Practice

The "emergence" of HPS as a new disease in 1993 and the subsequent field investigations provide excellent examples of rapid characterization of a modern epidemic using traditional principles in epidemiology and new methods in molecular biology. Collaborative reporting of potential cases of HPS to the CDC from health care providers

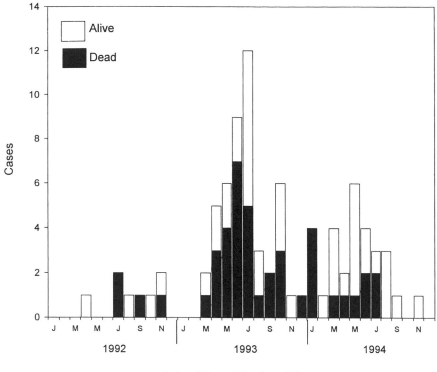

Figure 1-5. Hantavirus pulmonary syndrome by outcome, United States, January 1993–December 1994. *Source:* Khan et al. (1996)

and public health agencies was essential for characterizing the clinical spectrum of disease, refining the diagnostic criteria for HPS, identifying additional hantaviruses and rodent hosts, and identifying additional risk factors for hantavirus infection (CDC 1996).

Estimating the Burden of Excess Chronic Diseases

Background

As noted earlier in this chapter, many of today's populations have seen a large shift in the major causes of death and disability from infectious to chronic diseases. Thousands of epidemiologic studies have demonstrated that the burden of chronic diseases can be greatly reduced by elimination of behavioral risk factors such as cigarette smoking, physical inactivity, or lack of mammography utilization (Brownson et al. 1993).

Using this premise of preventability, Hahn et al. (1990) examined differences in state mortality rates for nine chronic diseases (i.e., breast cancer, uterine cervical cancer, lung cancer, colorectal cancer, coronary heart disease, stroke, diabetes, chronic obstructive pulmonary disease, and chronic liver disease/cirrhosis) in the United States and calculated excess (preventable) mortality based on the lowest state rates for each disease. Three lowest achievable mortality rates were calculated: (1) the rate in that state that had the lowest overall age-adjusted mortality rate for the composite nine chronic diseases, (2) the rate constructed by using the sum of the lowest age-adjusted rate for each disease found in any state, and (3) a "risk-eliminated mortality rate" that was based on population attributable risk estimates (see Chapter 2) and the elimination of one key risk factor for each of the nine chronic diseases (Hahn et al. 1990).

Key Questions

1. What is the distribution of the excess chronic disease burden in the United States?

Hahn et al. (1990) found the overall, age-adjusted US mortality rate for nine chronic diseases was 427.4 per 100,000. Michigan had the highest rate (483.1 per 100,000) and Hawaii had the lowest rate (304.7 per 100,000). Using the sum of the lowest state rates for each chronic disease, the lowest achievable rate was 284.1/100,000. The risk-eliminated mortality rate was 224.5 per 100,000. Excess mortality rates were calculated using each of the three minima. Regional mapping of excess mortality showed the highest rates in the upper Midwest and eastern coast of the United States.

2. Based on this distribution, which risk reduction strategies are warranted?

Risk reduction strategies of greatest benefit are those focusing on primary prevention (e.g., smoking prevention, increasing physical activity) and secondary prevention (e.g., Pap testing, mammography screening). Strategies that have been proven effective by well-conducted research studies should receive priority.

3. If one risk factor were eliminated for each of nine chronic diseases, how much could the life expectancy of the US population be increased?

Using a linear regression model, the authors estimated that elimination of a single risk factor for each of nine chronic diseases would increase life expectancy in the population by almost 4 years.

4. How can a public health agency use similar data at the local level to plan chronic disease prevention and control programs?

State health departments in Missouri (Hoffarth et al. 1993) and Wisconsin (McGown et al. 1993) have used a similar approach to that taken by Hahn et al. (1990) to map excess chronic disease at the county level. As noted in Chapter 12, local area data can be extremely valuable for public health agencies.

Implications for Practice

Analyses such as that conducted by Hahn et al. can provide the basis for planning chronic disease control programs and help in setting priorities when public health resources are limited. Along with these benefits, careful consideration must be paid to the estimation of disease rates at the local levels when small numbers may make estimates imprecise.

SUGGESTED READINGS

Coughlin SS, Beauchamp TL, eds. Ethics and Epidemiology. New York: Oxford University Press; 1996.

Gordis L. Challenges to epidemiology in the next decade. Am J Epidemiol 1988; 128:1–9.

Green LW, Kreuter MW. Health promotion as a public health strategy for the 1990s. Annu Rev Public Health 1990;11:319–334.

Oleske DM. Linking the delivery of health care to service population needs: the role of the epidemiologist on the health care management team. J Health Admin Educ 1993;11:531–539.

Pearce N. Traditional epidemiology, modern epidemiology, and public health. Am J Public Health 1996;86:678–683.

Susser M. Epidemiology in the United States after World War II: the evolution of technique. Epidemiol Rev 1985;7:147–177.

Susser M, Susser E. Choosing a future for epidemiology: I. Eras and paradigms. Am J Public Health 1996;86:668–673.

REFERENCES

Aday LA, Andersen R, Fleming GV. Health Care in the U.S.: Equitable for Whom? Beverly Hills, CA: Sage; 1980.

Biesecker BB, Boehnke M, Calzone K, et al. Genetic counseling for families with inherited susceptibility to breast and ovarian cancer. JAMA 1993;269:1970–1974.

Blackburn H, Luepker RV, Kline FG, et al. The Minnesota Heart Health Program: A research and demonstration project in cardiovascular disease prevention. In: Matarazzo JD, Weiss SM, Herd JA, Miller NE, Weiss SM, eds. Behavioral Health: A Handbook of Health Enhancement and Disease Prevention. New York: Wiley-Interscience; 1984.

Boss LP, Foster LR. Survey of state health agencies' staff who practice the epidemiology of noninfectious diseases and conditions. Public Health Rep 1994;109:112–117.

Breslow L. The future of public health: prospects in the United States for the 1990s. Annu Rev Public Health 1990;11:1–28.

Brownson RC, Remington PW, Davis JR, eds. Chronic Disease Epidemiology and Control. Washington, DC: American Public Health Association; 1993.

Bunker JP, Frazier HS, Mosteller F. Improving health: measuring effects of medical care. Milbank Q 1994;72:225–258.

Carleton RA, Lasater TM, Assaf AR, Lefebvre RC, McKinlay SM. The Pawtucket Heart Health Program: an experiment in population-based disease prevention. RI Med J. 1987;70:533–538.

Centers for Disease Control and Prevention. Public Health in the New American Health System. Discussion Paper. Atlanta, GA: Centers for Disease Control and Prevention; March 1993a.

Centers for Disease Control and Prevention. Investigating an outbreak. In: Principles of Epidemiology: An Introduction to Applied Epidemiology and Biostatistics. Atlanta, GA; Centers for Disease Control and Prevention, Epidemiology Program Office;1993b:435–525.

Centers for Disease Control and Prevention. CDC Wonder home page. [on-line]. 1997a. Available: http://wonder.cdc.gov.

Centers for Disease Control and Prevention. Data warehouse. [on-line]. 1997b. Available: http://wonder.cdc.gov/nchswww/datawh.

Centers for Disease Control and Prevention. Hantavirus pulmonary syndrome—United States, 1995 and 1996. Morb Mortal Wkly Rep 1996;45:291–295.

Committee for the Study of the Future of Public Health. Institute of Medicine. The Future of Public Health. Washington, DC: National Academy Press, 1988.

Coughlin SS, Beauchamp TL, eds. Ethics and Epidemiology. New York: Oxford University Press; 1996.

Council for International Organizations of Medical Sciences. International guidelines for ethical review of epidemiological studies. Law Med Health Care 1991;19:247–258.

Dawber TR. The Framingham Study: The Epidemiology of Coronary Heart Disease. Cambridge, MA: Harvard University Press; 1980.

Detels R. The need for epidemiologists. JAMA 1979;242:1644–1646.

Doll R, Hill AB. Smoking and carcinoma of the lung: preliminary report. Br Med J 1950;2:1225–1236.

Dwyer DM, Strickler H, Goodman RA, Armenian HK. Use of case-control studies in outbreak investigations. Epidemiol Rev 1994;16:109–123.

Easton DF, Bishop DT, Ford D, et al. Genetic linkage analysis in familial breast and ovarian cancer: results from 214 families. Am J Hum Genet 1993;52:678–701.

Farquhar JW, Fortmann SP, Maccoby N, et al. The Stanford Five-City Project: design and methods. Am J Epidemiol 1985;122:323–334.

Fielding JE. Successes of prevention. Milbank Memorial Fund Q 1978;56:274–302.

Fischhoff B, Bostrom A, Quandrel MJ. Risk perception and communication. Annu Rev Public Health 1993;14:183–203.

Friede A, Blum HL, McDonald M. Public health informatics: how information-age technology can strengthen public health. Annu Rev Public Health 1995;16:239–252.

Goldman L, Cook EF. Reasons for the decline in coronary heart disease mortality: medical interventions versus life-style changes. In: Higgins MW, Luepker RV, eds. Trends in Coronary Heart Disease Mortality: The Influence of Medical Care. New York: Oxford University Press; 1988:67–75.

Goodman RA, Buehler JW, Koplan JP. The epidemiologic field investigation: science and judgement in public health practice. Am J Epidemiol 1990;132:9–16.

Gordis L. Challenges to epidemiology in the next decade. Am J Epidemiol 1988;128:1–9.

Green LW, Kreuter MW. Health promotion as a public health strategy for the 1990s. Annu Rev Public Health 1990;11:319–334.

Gregg MB, Dicker RC, Goodman RA, eds. Field Epidemiology. New York: Oxford University Press; 1996.

Hahn RA, Teutsch SM, Rothenberg RB, Marks JS. Excess deaths from nine chronic diseases in the United States, 1986. JAMA 1990;264:2654–2659.

Hennekens CH, Buring JE. Epidemiology in Medicine. Boston, MA: Little, Brown; 1987.

Higgins MW, Luepker RV. Appendix: mortality from coronary heart disease and related causes of death in the United States, 1950–85. In: Higgins MW, Luepker RV, eds. Trends in Coronary Heart Disease Mortality: The Influence of Medical Care. New York, NY: Oxford University Press; 1988.

Hill AB. The environment and disease: association or causation? Proc R Soc Med 1965;58:295–300.

Hill JM, Lee MK, Newman B, et al. Linkage of early onset breast cancer to chromosome 17q21. Science 1990;250:1684–1689.

Hippocrates. On airs, waters, and places. Med Classics 1938;3:19.

Hoffarth S, Brownson RC, Gibson BB, Sharp DJ, Schramm W, Kivlahan C. Preventable mortality in Missouri: excess deaths from nine chronic diseases, 1979–1991. Mo Med 1993;90:279–282.

Hoffman C, Rice D, Sung H-Y. Persons with chronic conditions. Their prevalence and costs. JAMA 1996;276:1473–1479.

Kannel WB. Clinical misconceptions dispelled by epidemiological research [review]. Circulation 1995;92:3350–3360.

Kelsey JL, Whittemore AS, Evans AS, Thompson WD. Methods in Observational Epidemiology. Second Edition. New York: Oxford University Press; 1996.

Kelsey JL, Bernstein L. Epidemiology and prevention of breast cancer. Annu Rev Public Health 1996;17:47–67.

Khan AS, Khabbaz RF, Armstrong LR, et al. Hantavirus pulmonary syndrome: the first 100 US cases. J Infect Dis 1996;173:1297–1303.

Koepsell TD, Martin DC, Diehr PH, et al. Data analysis and sample size issues in evaluations of community-based health promotion and disease prevention programs: a mixed-model analysis of variance. J Clin Epidemiol 1991;44:701–713.

Koepsell TD, Wagner EH, Cheadle AC, Patrick DL, Martin DC, Diehr PH, Perrin EB. Selected methodological issues in evaluating community-based health promotion and disease prevention issues. Annu Rev Public Health 1992;13:31–57.

Laporte RE, Akazawa S, Hellmonds P, et al. Global public health and the information superhighway. Br Med J 1994;308:1651–1652.

Lasker RD. The Quintessential Role of Information in Public Health. Keynote Address. Washington, DC: Public Health Conference on Records and Statistics; July 17, 1995.

Last JM, ed. A Dictionary of Epidemiology. Third Edition. New York: Oxford University Press; 1995.

Lee HW, Lee PW, Johnson KM. Isolation of the etiologic agent of Korean hemorrhagic fever. J Infect Dis 1978;137:298–308.

Lerner WM. Managing health care systems from an epidemiologic perspective. In: Oleske DM, ed. Epidemiology and the Delivery of Health Care Services. New York: Plenum Press; 1995:171–185.

Levin ML, Goldstein H, Gerhardt PR. Cancer and tobacco smoking: a preliminary report. JAMA 1950;143:336–338.

Lilienfeld DE. Definitions of epidemiology. Am J Epidemiol 1978;107:87–90.

Lilienfeld AM, Lilienfeld DE. Epidemiology and the public health movement: a historical perspective. J Public Health Policy 1982; vol. 3, June:140–149.

Lilienfeld DE, Stolley PD. Foundations of Epidemiology. Third Edition. New York: Oxford University Press; 1994.

Marmot M, Brunner E. Alcohol and cardiovascular disease: the status of the U shaped curve. Br Med J 1991;303:565–568.

McGown R, Remington PL, Chudy N. Deaths from nine chronic diseases, Wisconsin, 1979–1988. WI Med J 1993;92:524, 526–529.

McMichael AJ. Invited commentary—"molecular epidemiology": new pathway or new travelling companion. Am J Epidemiol 1994;140:1–11.

Mercy JA, Rosenberg ML, Powell KE, Broome CV, Roper WL. Public health for preventing violence. Health Affairs 1993; vol. 12, Winter:7–29.

Morris J, Schneider D, Greenberg MR. Universities as resources to state health agencies. Public Health Rep 1994;109:761–766.

National Association of County and City Health Officials. 1992–1993 National Profile of Local Health Departments. National Surveillance Series. Washington, DC: National Association of County and City Health Officials; 1995.

National Center for Health Statistics. Health, United States, 1995. Hyattsville, MD: Public Health Service; DHHS publication no. (PHS) 96-1232; 1996a.

National Center for Health Statistics. Healthy People 2000 Review, 1995–96. Hyattsville, MD: US Dept of Health and Human Services publication no. (PHS) 96-1256; 1996b.

National Committee for Quality Assurance. Health Plan Employer Data and Information Set and User's Manual, Version 2.0. Washington, DC: National Committee for Quality Assurance; 1993.

National Office of Vital Statistics. Vital Statistics—Special Reports, National Summaries, 1950. Washington, DC: US Dept of Health, Education, and Welfare; 1954.

Nightingale EO, Cureton M, Kamar V, Trudeau MB. Perspectives on Health Promotion and Disease Prevention in the United States. [staff paper]. Washington, DC: Institute of Medicine, National Academy of Sciences; 1978.

Oleske DM. Linking the delivery of health care to service population needs: the role of the epidemiologist on the health care management team. J Health Admin Educ 1993;11:531–539.

Oppenheimer GM. Comment: epidemiology and the liberal arts—toward a new paradigm? Am J Public Health 1995;85:918–920.

Pearce N. Traditional epidemiology, modern epidemiology, and public health. Am J Public Health 1996;86:678–683.

Perera FP. Molecular epidemiology: insights into cancer susceptibility, risk assessment, and prevention. J Natl Cancer Inst 1996;88:496–509.

Petitti DB. Meta-Analysis, Decision Analysis, and Cost-Effectiveness Analysis. Methods for Quantitative Synthesis in Medicine. New York: Oxford University Press; 1994.

Pew Health Professions Commission. Critical Challenges: Revitalizing the Health Professions for the Twenty-First Century. The Third Report of the Pew Health Commission. San Francisco, CA: UCSF Center for the Health Professions; November 1995.

Puska P. Community based prevention of cardiovascular disease: the North Karelia Project. In: Matarazzo JD, Weiss SM, Herd JA, Miller NE, Weiss SM, eds. Behavioral Health: A Handbook of Health Enhancement and Disease Prevention. New York, NY: Wiley-Interscience; 1984.

Roccella EJ, Horan MJ. The National High Blood Pressure Education Program: measuring progress and assessing its impact. Health Psychol 1988;7(Suppl): 297–303.

Rosenberg HM, Ventura SJ, Maurer JD, Heuser RL, Freedman MA. Births and Deaths: United States, 1995. Monthly Vital Statistics Report; Vol 45, No 3, Suppl 2. Hyattsville, MD: National Center for Health Statistics; October 4, 1996.

Rothenberg RB, Steinberg KK, Thacker SB. The public health importance of clusters: a note from the Centers for Disease Control. Am J Epidemiol 1990;132 (Suppl 1):S3–S5.

Samet JM. What can we expect from epidemiologic studies of chemical mixtures? Toxicology 1995;105:307–314.

Schmid TL, Pratt M, Howze E. Policy as intervention: environmental and policy approaches to the prevention of cardiovascular disease. Am J Public Health 1995;85:1207–1211.

Schreck R, Baker LA, Ballad G, et al. Tobacco smoking as an etiological factor of cancer. Cancer Res 1950;10:49–58.

Schulte PA, Perera FP. Molecular Epidemiology. Principles and Practice. Orlando, FL: Academic Press; 1993.

Sørensen HT, Sabroe S, Olsen J. A framework for evaluation of secondary data sources for epidemiological research. Int J Epidemiol 1996;25:435–442.

Stallones RA. Epidemiology and public policy: pro- and anti-biotic. Am J Epidemiol 1982;115:485–491.

Susser M. Causal Thinking in the Health Sciences: Concepts and Strategies in Epidemiology. New York: Oxford University Press; 1973.

Susser M, Susser E. Choosing a future for epidemiology: I. Eras and paradigms. Am J Public Health 1996;86:668–673.

Taylor WR, Marks JS, Livengood JR, Koplan JR. Current issues and challenges in chronic disease control. In: Brownson RC, Remington PL, Davis JR, eds. Chronic Disease Epidemiology and Control. Washington, DC: American Public Health Association; 1993:1–18.

Taubes G. Epidemiology faces its limits. Science 1995;269:164–169.

Terris M. The epidemiologic tradition. The Wade Hampton Frost Lecture. Public Health Rep 1979;94:203–209.

Terris M. Epidemiology as a guide to health policy. Annu Rev Public Health 1980;1:323–344.

Terris M. The complex tasks of the second epidemiologic revolution: the Joseph W. Mountin Lecture. J Public Health Policy 1983;4:8–24.

Terris M. The Society for Epidemiologic Research (SER) and the future of epidemiology. Am J Epidemiol 1992;136:909–915.

Thacker SB, Berkelman RL. Public health surveillance in the United States. Epidemiol Rev 1988;10:164–190.

Thacker SB, Goodman RA, Dicker RC. Training and service in public health practice, 1951–90—CDC's Epidemic Intelligence Service. Public Health Rep 1990; 105:599–604.

Thacker SB, Koplan JP, Taylor WR, Hinman AR, Katz MF, Roper WL. Assessing prevention effectiveness using data to drive program decisions. Public Health Rep 1994;109:187–194.

Thacker SB, Stroup DF, Rothenberg RB, Brownson RC. Public health surveillance for chronic conditions: a scientific basis for decisions. Stat Med 1995;14:629–641.

University of California San Francisco. Epidemiology. [on-line]. 1997. Available: http://www.epibiostat.ucsf.edu/epidem.

US Dept of Energy. Office of Environment, Safety and Health. Comprehensive epidemiologic data resource. [on-line]. 1997. Available: http://cedr.lbl.gov.

US Dept of Health, Education, and Welfare. US Public Health Service. Smoking and Health. Report of the Advisory Committee to the Surgeon General of the Public Health Service. Washington, DC: Center for Disease Control; Publication (PHS) 1103; 1964.

US Dept of Health, Education, and Welfare. Healthy People. The Surgeon General's Report on Health Promotion and Disease Prevention. 1979. Washington, DC:

US Dept of Health, Education, and Welfare (PHS) Publication no. 79-55071; 1979.

US Dept of Health and Human Services. Healthy People 2000: National Health Promotion and Disease Prevention. Washington, DC: US Govt Printing Office; Publication no. 017-001-00473-1;1990.

Williams SJ, Tyler CW Jr, Clark L, Coleman L, Curran P. Epidemiologists in the United States: an assessment of the current supply and the anticipated need. Am J Prev Med 1988;4:231–238.

Winkelstein W Jr, French FE. Biostatistics and epidemiology programs in schools of public health. In: Work TH, ed. Tracing the Patterns of Disease: The Role of Epidemiology and Biometry. Washington, DC: US Dept of Health, Education, and Welfare; DHEW Publication no. (NIH) 77-1285; 1977.

World Health Organization. Handbook of Resolutions and Decisions of the World Health Assembly and the Executive Board. Geneva: WHO; 1971.

Wynder EL, Graham EA. Tobacco smoking as a possible etiological factor in bronchogenic carcinoma: a study of 684 proved cases. JAMA 1950;143:329–336.

Wynder EL. Applied epidemiology. Am J Epidemiol 1985;121:781–782.

Wynder EL. Workshop on guidelines to the epidemiology of weak associations. Introduction. Prev Med 1987;16:139–141.

2

Key Methodologic Concepts and Issues

JENNIFER L. KELSEY
DIANA B. PETITTI
ABBY C. KING

As described in Chapter 1, epidemiology is used for many purposes. One is to determine the magnitude and impact of diseases or other conditions in populations or in certain segments of populations. This information can help to set priorities for investigation and control, to decide which subgroups of the population should be the focus of investigation, and to determine what types of treatment facilities are needed. Epidemiologic studies can also be used to ascertain the natural history, clinical course, and pathogenesis of disease. They can be used to evaluate disease prevention programs and preventive and therapeutic interventions. Most often, epidemiology is used to learn about the etiology of disease.

This chapter addresses methodologic concepts and issues that are most pertinent to epidemiology as it is used in public health settings and health care organizations. The intent is to give the reader an overview of key topics. The chapter assumes knowledge of the basics of epidemiology—the calculation of incidence and prevalence and the estimation of measures of association (relative risk and odds ratios). It does not cover statistical analysis of epidemiologic data or the mechanics of estimating sample size and statistical power. Instead it focuses on these concepts as they affect the design and interpretation of epidemiologic studies. Some of the material is adapted from other sources (Friedman 1994; Kelsey et al. 1996; Kelsey and Sowers 1996; Kelsey and Parker 1993), to which the reader is referred for more detail.

Study Designs

Epidemiologic studies can be broadly categorized as either *observational* or *experimental*. In observational studies, relationships are studied as they occur in nature. In experimental studies, the investigator intervenes and studies the effects of the intervention.

Observational studies have two fundamental objectives—to *describe* the occurrence of disease or disease-related phenomena and to *explain* them. Studies attempting to identify the causes of disease are generally called analytic epidemiologic studies. Analytic studies address the question of *why* diseases are distributed the way they are.

Most analytic epidemiologic studies are observational; that is, the investigator observes what is occurring in the study populations of interest and does not interfere with what he or she observes. Case-control, cohort, experimental, and some hybrid study designs are discussed in this chapter as analytic study designs. The distinction between descriptive and analytic studies is not, however, clear-cut (Friedman 1994). Thus, a descriptive study may provide data that give a clear answer to a specific question.

Cross-sectional study designs are regularly used both descriptively and analytically. The distinction between description and analysis is frequently blurred in cross-sectional studies. Cross-sectional studies have a particularly important role in planning and evaluating public health programs. For this reasons, cross-sectional studies are discussed in detail in a separate section.

Descriptive Studies

Descriptive studies provide information on the frequency of occurrence of a particular condition and on patterns of occurrence according to such attributes as person, place, and time. Routinely collected statistics from such sources as mortality data, hospital discharge records, general health surveys, and disease surveillance programs are used for most descriptive studies (see Chapter 4). Characteristics related to "person" often include age, gender, race, ethnicity, marital status, socioeconomic class, and occupation. Studies that focus on person can provide information about the magnitude of a problem in different segments of the population, suggest leads about causation, and identify quality-of-care problems. Knowledge that high blood pressure occurs most frequently among blacks, for instance, indicates that it is important that programs to detect hypertension and provide treatment include black populations. Knowledge that osteoporosis occurs most frequently in postmenopausal women led to the hypothesis that declining estrogen levels were a cause and hence that estrogen replacement therapy might be used as a prophylactic agent. The observation that mortality following coronary artery bypass surgery is high in hospitals with low surgical volumes suggested that quality of care in these institutions needed to be examined (Hannan et al. 1991; Showstack et al. 1987; Luft et al. 1990).

Descriptive studies of the occurrence of conditions according to "place" might involve examining their frequency within or between natural or political boundaries, in urban versus rural localities, or by latitude. For example, maps of cancer mortality rates in the United States according to county of residence were first published in 1975 (Mason et al. 1975). These atlases called attention to certain geographic areas with unusually high cancer mortality rates. This led to further research into the reasons for high rates in areas such as New Jersey and the Louisiana Gulf Coast. Similarly, a 1975 descriptive study of geographic variation in surgery rates (Wennberg and Gittelson 1975) was instrumental in initiating formal, critical examination of the reasons for these differences that continue to the present.

Examination of "time" relationships can both identify and evaluate hypotheses related to the causes of changes in conditions. The recent decrease in mortality rates for coronary heart disease in many western countries, for instance, has led to hypotheses about the roles of better diets, decreasing cigarette consumption, better control of hypertension, more physical activity, and improved methods of detection and treatment of coronary heart disease that have become the subject of further research. The decline in the incidence of Reye syndrome in the time period following a Public Health Service and American Academy of Pediatrics recommendation to avoid use of aspirin to treat children with respiratory illness, chickenpox, and fever provided evidence that aspirin use and Reye syndrome are causally linked.

Descriptive studies often combine assessment of trends in relation to both time and place. Figure 2-1 shows time trends in the incidence of advanced HIV disease from 1991 through 1995 in two areas of Los Angeles County that have been heavily burdened by the epidemic. It shows that incidence rates are declining in all of the affected areas. Availability of effective treatments for HIV disease (AIDS) is considered a major contributor to the decline in advanced HIV disease, since other data suggest that there have not been dramatic changes in the incidence of new HIV infections in LA County over the same time period (Los Angeles Department of Health Services 1996).

Analytic Studies

Case-Control Studies

Case-control studies are those in which persons with a specified condition (the cases) and persons without the condition (the controls) are selected for study. The proportion of cases and of controls with certain characteristics or who have had the exposure of interest is then measured and compared (For a

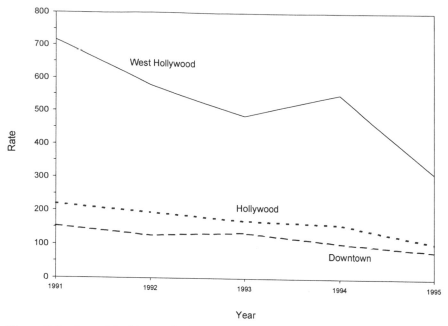

Figure 2-1. Annual incidence of advanced HIV disease (AIDS) per 100,000 population in three Los Angeles communities, 1991–1995; *Source:* Los Angeles Department of Health Services (1996)

numerical characteristic such as blood pressure, the mean level in the cases may be compared to the mean level in the controls.).

Newly occurring cases are preferred in order to maximize the likelihood that the exposure of interest preceded the condition rather than occurred as a consequence of the disease, and to make sure that rapidly fatal cases and cases of short duration are not underrepresented in the case group. Controls are most commonly selected from the general population from which the cases came, from people who live in the same neighborhood as the cases, or from among patients seeking medical care for other diseases at the same facilities as the cases.

Case-control studies have been extensively used in etiologic research. Their use to assess the adverse effects of drugs and other therapies is also common. Studies of the case-control design have been used with increasing frequency to evaluate the efficacy of preventive interventions (Selby et al. 1992; Weiss 1994), including vaccines (Comstock 1994).

Case-control studies can be carried out relatively quickly, usually do not require as large a sample size as cohort studies (to be described later), and are less expensive as a result. For a rare event, they are usually the only practical type of hypothesis-testing study. Table 2-1 summarizes the results of four

Table 2-1. Efficacy of Pneumococcal Vaccine in Adults: Selected Case-Control Studies From the United States

Author (year)	Location	Age of Population Studied (years)	Total N		N Vaccinated		Efficacy[a] (95% Confidence Intervals)
			Cases	Controls	Cases	Controls	
Shapiro and Clemens (1984)	Connecticut	>18	90	90	6	16	0.67 (0.13, 0.87)
Forrester et al. (1987)	Denver	>30	89	89	26	21	−0.2 (−2.2, 0.55)
Sims et al. (1988)	Pennsylvania	>55	122	244	10	51	0.7 (0.36, 0.86)
Shapiro et al. (1991)	Connecticut	>18	983	983	123	195	0.56 (0.42, 0.67)

[a] Defined as one minus the odds ratio for use of the vaccine (Mills and Rhoads 1996).

case-control studies that have evaluated the efficacy of the pneumococcal vaccine in adults (Mills and Rhoads 1996). It would be very costly and probably impossible to conduct four different cohort studies of vaccine efficacy because of the rarity of pneumococcal illness. The data from these three of the four case-control studies find a lower odds ratio for pneumococcal illness in persons who had been vaccinated, providing strong evidence for a benefit of pneumococcal vaccination in adults.

Case-control studies are subject to certain limitations, which have been described in detail by Sackett (1979) and Austin et al. (1994). Among the common concerns: Accurate information on the exposure may not be available either from a person's memory or from records. Accurate information on other relevant variables (such as confounders and effect modifiers, to be discussed below) may not be available. Patients may search for a cause for their condition and therefore be more likely to report an exposure than controls (a form of recall bias, to be described below). It may be impossible to determine with complete certainty whether the exposure of interest caused the condition or whether the condition caused the person to have the exposure. Assembling a case group representative of all cases may be difficult. Finally, the appropriate control group may be difficult to define. Each case-control study should be evaluated individually to determine the extent to which these problems affect its credibility, since some studies are affected by these and other problems to a large extent, whereas others are affected very little.

In addition to the general limitations of case-control studies mentioned above, in any observational study evaluating interventions there is a major concern that, in the absence of randomization, persons who choose or who are told to use a particular intervention are already on average at different risk for the outcome compared with those who are not assigned or who do not choose to use the intervention (Selby 1994). For preventive interventions, there is particular concern that people who are especially health conscious may participate in the intervention program (e.g., an exercise program) or comply with a recommendation (e.g., to have a mammogram). In studies of therapies, the possibility exists that persons with a disease who are prescribed a particular drug or treatment may have a different severity of illness than those not prescribed the drug or treatment. For example, patients with hypertension who are prescribed calcium-channel blockers may also be more likely to have severe hypertension than those prescribed diuretics. A case-control comparing use of calcium-channel blockers and diuretics in hypertensive patients who have died of acute myocardial infarction finds that the odds ratio for acute myocardial infarction is higher than in users of diuretics because they have more severe hypertension. Sometimes case-control studies of interventions can largely overcome these problems. For instance, a case-control study to evaluate the efficacy of screening sigmoidoscopy in reducing mortality from colon cancer was particularly convincing because the protective effect was limited to the part of the colon where lesions can be seen by the sigmoidoscope (Selby et al. 1992).

Notwithstanding their limitations, policy decisions regarding preventive and therapeutic interventions based on information from case-control studies may be necessary because results from observational cohort studies will not be available for many years and/or because randomized trials are too small to detect true associations with rare events. For example, FDA approval to market diethylstilbestrol (DES) as an agent to prevent miscarriage was rescinded after case-control studies showed that DES exposure during pregnancy was associated with a markedly elevated risk of cancer of the vagina in the offspring of mothers who took it during pregnancy (Herbst et al. 1971; Greenwald et al. 1974).

Cohort Studies

In the typical *prospective cohort study*, persons free of the condition of interest at the time the study begins are classified according to their level of exposure. The cohort is then followed for a period of time (which may be many years) and incidence rates (number of new cases of the condition of interest per population at risk per unit time), mortality rates (number of deaths per population at risk per unit time), or other outcomes (e.g., changes in symptoms, changes in blood pressure or lipids) among those with different exposures are compared. For example, an observational cohort study to address the question of whether screening for prostate cancer prevents death from invasive disease would involve assembling a cohort of men free of prostate cancer and determining whether they were screened for prostate cancer. These individuals could be followed for several years, and mortality from prostate cancer examined in relation to screening history.

Cohorts are sometimes chosen to be representative of the general population, (e.g., the Framingham Heart Study). Subjects more often are selected to facilitate recruitment and follow-up, thus reducing cost, and to maximize the validity and/or reliability of exposure and outcome information. A cohort that has provided a great deal of information about various exposures and disease risk in recent years is the Nurses' Health Study cohort (Hennekens et al. 1979). Nurses were selected, not because of any particular occupational exposure, but because it was believed that their level of cooperation would be high and they could report exposures and disease occurrence with a high degree of accuracy. Although one may question the generalizability of results from such select cohorts, the ability to obtain high-quality data and the efficiency of using a cohort that is cooperative and can be followed over time generally outweighs concerns about generalizability.

Cohort studies have a major advantage over case-control studies: The exposures of interest are measured before the condition of interest has developed, thus making it easier to differentiate cause from effect. However, prospective cohort studies generally require large sample sizes, long periods of follow-up, large monetary expense, and complex administrative and organizational arrangements. Therefore, prospective cohort studies are usually launched when either sufficient (but not definitive) evidence has already been obtained from less expensive studies to warrant a more expensive approach or the exposure (e.g., a widely used medication) may affect risk for several conditions.

As mentioned above in regard to case-control studies, a particular problem with observational cohort studies for evaluation of preventive or therapeutic interventions is that the persons choosing (or prescribed) the particular intervention may differ from those who do not choose (or are not prescribed) the intervention. For instance, although an apparent protective effect of estrogen replacement therapy against coronary heart disease has been noted in many observational cohort studies, this association is not universally accepted as causal because it has not been tested in randomized trials. Users of replacement estrogen tend to be more physically active and healthy than women who do not use estrogen. These characteristics would be expected to result in a lower incidence of coronary heart disease regardless of estrogen use.

In *a retrospective cohort study* (also sometimes called a *historical cohort study*), a cohort is assembled by reviewing records to identify exposures in the past (often decades ago). Based on the recorded exposure histories, cohort members are divided into exposed and nonexposed groups, or according to level of exposure. The investigator then reconstructs health experience subsequent to exposure, up to some defined point in the more recent past or up to the present time. A common application of the retrospective cohort design is to assess the effects on disease of occupational exposures, such as prostate cancer in farmers exposed to herbicides and other agents (Morrison et al. 1993) and silicosis in gold miners exposed to silica (Steenland and Brown 1995). Other cohorts assembled retrospectively have included college students with certain attributes and armed forces veterans (Bullman and Kang 1996).

Retrospective cohort studies have many of the advantages of prospective cohort studies but can be completed much more quickly and often with less expense. However, retrospective cohort studies depend on the availability of accurate information on past exposures. If this information is not available, a retrospective cohort study is not feasible. Also, it must be possible to trace the members of the study population in order to determine whether they have developed the conditions of interest. If information on potential confounders is not available, it may be difficult to interpret the results. Retrospective cohort studies, like prospective cohort studies, can usually only be carried out when the outcome of interest is relatively common, or a prohibitively large study population will be needed.

As with other observational studies, retrospective cohort studies can be undertaken to evaluate preventive or therapeutic interventions, but there is again concern that those who had the intervention may differ in other ways from those who did not. A retrospective cohort study to determine whether calcium consumption reduces the risk for hip fracture illustrates the problem. People examined in the first National Health and Nutrition Examination Survey (NHANES I) of 1971–1975 had answered an extensive dietary questionnaire. Looker et al. (1993) related this information to the subsequent occurrence of hip fracture and found that higher calcium consumption was related to a lower hip fracture risk in women who were at least 6 years past menopause and who did not use hormone replacement therapy. However, the possibility remains that the women with higher calcium consumption differed from women with lower calcium in other ways that the investigators could not take into account because they had not been measured in NHANES I.

Hybrid Study Designs

It is sometimes expedient to include a case-control design within a retrospective or a prospective cohort study. Suppose that an investigator is interested in whether serum beta carotene affects the risk of colon cancer. In a traditional prospective cohort study, beta carotene levels would be measured in blood samples from all the cohort members, and subsequent disease incidence would be determined according to the level of beta carotene. In a *nested case-control study*, blood samples from all of the (say, 10,000) cohort members would be frozen and stored without measuring beta carotene. Suppose that after 10 years, 200 cohort members had been diagnosed with colon cancer and 9,800 are free of colon cancer. All of the cases and a sample of, for example, 400 controls without the disease could be selected and beta carotene could be measured in the stored serum. The cases and controls could then be compared according to beta carotene level, as in a traditional case-control study. Controls are usually selected from unaffected cohort members who are still alive and under surveillance at the time the cases developed the disease. Typically the controls are matched to the cases according to age, gender, and time of entry into the cohort. Sampling nondiseased individuals greatly reduces the cost compared with measurement of beta carotene levels of all 10,000 cohort members but assures that beta carotene measures represent levels before the diagnosis of the disease. The availability of a variety of banks of stored blood and the current interest in serologic and genetic predictors of disease make nested case-control studies an attractive approach, as long as the marker of interest does not undergo degradation over time and the specimens have been processed in a way that allows the marker to be determined in the sample.

A *case-cohort study* is another method of increasing efficiency compared to traditional cohort studies. Like the nested case-control study, all cases and a sample of controls are included, but the controls are sampled from the entire cohort, not just those free of disease, and are not matched to the cases. Instead, other relevant variables are taken into account in the statistical analysis. A case-cohort design is particularly useful when the associations between an exposure (e.g., serum beta carotene) and several diseases (e.g., cancers of the colon, lung, and pancreas) are of interest.

Nested case-control and case-cohort designs are also particularly useful when collecting information about confounders from a cohort involves review of medical records or a survey. In these instances, data can be collected from all of the cases and a sample of controls, greatly reducing the cost of data collection.

Experimental Studies

In general, experimental studies provide the strongest evidence that a given exposure is the cause of a disease or other condition or that a preventive or therapeutic intervention is effective. In experimental studies, the investigator randomly assigns individuals or another unit (e.g., community, school, clinic) either to be exposed or not exposed to an intervention and then follows them through time to determine the outcomes of interest. Randomization attempts to create comparability on factors other than exposure between those who are and are not assigned to the exposure or intervention.

Experimental studies are typically expensive and challenging to conduct. They are generally used when sufficient evidence already exists from observational studies or small-scale experimental studies to merit a large-scale, formal test of a question. The Lipid Research Clinics Coronary Primary Prevention Trial (LRC-CPPT) was a multicenter, randomized, double-blind clinical trial that evaluated the efficacy of lowering blood cholesterol in reducing risk of coronary heart disease in asymptomatic middle-aged men with primary hypercholesterolemia (Lipid Research Clinics Program 1984). The treatment group received cholestyramine resin, a bile acid sequestrant, and the control group received a placebo for an average of 7.4 years. Both groups followed a moderate cholesterol-lowering diet. At the end of the intervention period, the treatment group experienced a significant reduction in coronary events relative to the placebo group. This study provided convincing evidence for a benefit of cholesterol-lowering treatment in the prevention of coronary artery disease in men with high cholesterol, and important recommendations for cholesterol screening and treatment were made based on the study results.

Experimental studies are usually *not* undertaken when the outcome of interest is rare or when the efficacy of the intervention is well established. In the latter circumstance, it may be unethical to assign subjects to no treatment or to a placebo.

In order to optimize the amount of information gained from these resource-intensive efforts, recent randomized clinical trials have been initiated to investigate the effects of multiple therapies on a broader set of outcomes. The largest and most expensive research study ever sponsored by the National Institutes of Health is the ongoing Women's Health Initiative (Buring and Hennekens 1992), which is using randomized trials to test (as primary hypotheses) whether a low-fat dietary pattern protects against breast cancer and colon cancer, whether hormone replacement therapy reduces risk for coronary heart disease, and whether calcium/vitamin D supplementation protects against hip fracture.

While randomized clinical trials and other experimental approaches are generally considered to be the strongest type of research design available to ascertain causal relationships, a number of issues must be considered in designing and carrying out these trials. The recruitment of subjects may be difficult and expensive. For example, in the LRC-CPPT described earlier, approximately 480,000 age-eligible men had to be screened over a 3-year period to recruit the 3,806 men who were eventually entered into the trial. Because of the difficulties in identifying persons who meet all of the often-rigorous eligibility criteria demanded by many clinical trial protocols and securing their willingness to participate fully in the trial procedures, recruitment is often much more time consuming than anticipated, making the cost of such trials and the time to results long.

The choice of the most relevant or useful control condition against which to compare the intervention of interest can present a number of challenges. Investigators need to determine the type of control condition that will provide study subjects with sufficient motivation to remain in the trial for the duration of the study but that will not have a significant impact on the primary outcomes of interest. Control conditions that may appear in some situations to be ideal from a scientific perspective may be unethical or impractical to use. Although placebo-controlled trials may be theoretically ideal, for many interventions, including a number of lifestyle interventions, appropriate and/or acceptable placebos do not exist.

Ongoing promotion and accurate monitoring of subject adherence to the target intervention(s) for the duration of the study can be difficult to achieve, especially when the intervention involves complicated lifestyle changes. For instance, experimental studies of physical activity promotion have often reported participant drop-out rates at 6 months of 50% or greater (King et al. 1992).

In order to accrue a sufficiently large sample size and to enhance generalizability, experimental studies often require that several investigative sites be involved. Issues related to standardization of both intervention and measurement protocols then become particularly critical. For instance, in the LRC-CPPT, the original plan was to use measurement of HDL-cholesterol levels at the second screening visit as the baseline measurement for the trial. However, the second screening measurement was not performed according to protocol at several of the study clinics, and measurements made at the first screening visit had to be used (Lipid Research Clinics Program 1984).

Cross-Sectional Studies

Overview. *Prevalence* is the number of cases of a condition per population at risk at one time or in a relatively short period of time. In a cross-sectional study, prevalence rates of disease among those with varying levels of exposure are measured and sometimes compared between groups. Cross-sectional studies can be used descriptively, to describe differences in prevalence between groups, or analytically, to test hypotheses. Cross-sectional study designs are generally less useful in studying disease causation but are very important in public health planning and evaluation.

Limitations in Etiologic Research. The main problem with cross-sectional study designs in etiologic research is the difficulty of sorting out temporal relationships. For example, a cross-sectional study of the relationship between calcium consumption and osteoporosis might find that those with high calcium consumption were more likely to have osteoporosis than those without, but this finding might be because people who know that they have osteoporosis increase their calcium consumption when told of this diagnosis. Interpretation of cross-sectional studies in terms of etiology is clear only for potential risk factors that will not change as a result of the disease, such as ABO blood groups or HLA antigens.

A second limitation of cross-sectional studies in etiologic research occurs because cross-sectional studies include both new and old cases. Accordingly, the case group will have more than its fair share of individuals with disease of long duration, because those who die or recover quickly will not be included. If the etiologic exposure affects disease duration or the likelihood of dying, relationships between exposure and disease will be distorted. In the most extreme instance, which is both hypothetical and unlikely, those with the disease who are exposed all die immediately upon developing the disease but those developing the disease who are not exposed live for a long time. No cases included in a cross-sectional study that assesses disease and exposure will be exposed (they are all dead) and, the exposure will appear to protect against the disease.

Uses in Public Health Planning and Evaluation. Cross-sectional studies are very important in public health planning and evaluation. They are widely used in these settings for a variety of purposes. For example, if a public health administrator wants to obtain an idea of how many and what sort of facilities are needed to treat people with a certain disease at a given point in time, knowledge of the prevalence of the disease in the community is important. Often prevalence rates are needed for specific segments of the population or according to the severity of the disease, since different methods of treatment and types of facilities may be needed for people with various stages of the disease. Cross-sectional studies are also used to help set research priorities based on consideration of the burden of the disease. For example, a study of the prevalence of chronic gynecologic conditions among US women of reproductive age found that the most common conditions are menstrual disorders, adnexal conditions, and uterine fibroids. This information suggests that not only are more effective treatments for these disorders needed, but also that more research on their causation would be highly desirable (Kjerulff et al. 1996).

Sampling Issues in Cross-Sectional Study Design. Determining the prevalence of a disease (or other condition) in a community often involves sampling people in the community and measuring the occurrence of disease by questionnaire, physical examination, or other method. When taking a sample of the population, it is important to use scientifically sound sampling methods. One may be tempted, for instance, to save money by asking for volunteers to be in a study (e.g., convenience sampling). Volunteers, however, almost always have different characteristics from the population as a whole. Volunteers for health surveys tend to be overrepresented with the "worried well" and with people who believe they will benefit from participation. One should also avoid the temptation to save money by letting study personnel choose the people to be included in a survey. These personnel may select the most accessible people or those who they think are most likely to benefit from participation.

When deciding which of several scientifically sound sampling methods to employ in a given situation, it is important to keep in mind that the basic purpose of sampling, rather than making measurements on an entire population, is to save time and money. Sampling may also result in greater accuracy of measurements, since more effort can be spent on ensuring that the measurements are of high quality if a manageable number of people is included.

Perhaps the most familiar method of sampling is *simple random sampling*, in which each member of the population has an equal chance of being included in the sample. Although simple random sampling is simple to carry out and easy to understand, it may not be the most efficient method of sampling in many instances.

Another type of sampling is *systematic sampling*, in which the units are sampled at equal intervals; for instance, every 10th person on a list may be selected for the sample, or every fourth house on the block may be included. Systematic sampling is often simpler to administer under field conditions than simple random sampling, and it also does not require a list of the entire population in advance.

In *stratified sampling*, the population is divided into strata, or groups of units having certain characteristics in common (such as males and females, or geographic areas within a city), and a simple random sample is then taken from each stratum. Stratified sampling, which is frequently used in practice, offers several advantages over simple random sampling. With stratified sampling, one can be certain that members of each stratum are represented in the overall sample. If the strata are more homogenous than the population as a whole, then more precise overall estimates for the entire sample can be made. Finally, the strata can be constructed so that those that are least expensive to include, or in which there is the most variability, can be sampled more heavily, simultaneously reducing cost and increasing precision.

In *cluster sampling*, clusters (e.g., schools) rather than individuals (e.g., children) are sampled and then measurements are made on all children within the school. Cluster sampling can offer two major advantages. First, it is not necessary to enumerate the entire population, only the individuals in the clusters that are selected. Second, cluster sampling can allow the inclusion of larger numbers of individuals for a given cost, because once one has access to the unit (e.g., the school), one can efficiently make measurements on all of individuals in the unit.

In *multistage sampling*, combinations of these methods are used within the same survey. Stratified sampling might be used to ensure that schools representing different socioeconomic areas of a large city are represented in the sample, and cluster sampling of classrooms within the selected schools might then be employed for efficiency.

The different methods of sampling require different statistical procedures in order to obtain estimates of measures that are applicable to the population from which the sample was taken and to provide the correct estimates error associated with these measures. Estimates made on the basis of cluster sampling must take into account that the individuals sampled within a cluster tend to be more alike than individuals from different clusters. Estimates made from stratified sampling involve combining in an appropriate way the estimates made from the individual strata. The reader is referred to sampling textbooks (e.g., Levy and Lemeshow 1991) and specialized software programs (e.g., SUDAAN 1991) for descriptions of methods of estimation when various sampling schemes have been used and for more detailed descriptions of the sampling methods described above.

Confounding, Effect Modification, Bias

Confounding

A variable that is a known or suspected cause of the outcome under study (or is a surrogate for cause) and is also statistically associated with the exposure of interest is a confounding variable. Formally, a confounding variable may be defined as a variable that is causally related to the condition under study independently of the exposure of primary interest, and is associated with the exposure of primary interest in the study population, but is not a consequence of the exposure. Because of confounding (among other issues), a statistical association between an exposure and a condition does not necessarily mean that the exposure is causally related to the condition. For instance, a statistical association between coffee drinking during pregnancy and an increased likelihood of giving birth to an infant of low birth weight might occur because women who drink coffee are more likely to smoke than non–coffee drinkers. It is possible that cigarette smoking, not coffee drinking, is the factor that increases the risk for delivery of a low-birth-weight infant.

Confounding is common in observational studies. Rarely are exposures distributed without regard to some aspect of person. In observational studies of the effects of drugs and other therapies, confounding by indication and confounding by severity of illness are particular concerns. Confounding by indication occurs when the provision of a drug or therapy is determined by another factor that is causally related to the outcome of interest, thus distorting the relationship between the therapy and outcome. For example, diuretics are prescribed to treat hypertension. In a study that reported an increased risk of renal cancer in users of diuretics, the possibility that hypertension, the indication for diuretic use, rather than diuretics themselves might be the true risk factor for renal cancer must be considered. Confounding by severity of illness is discussed in Chapter 8.

Confounding variables may be taken into account in the study design by matching study subjects on them. Alternatively, confounding variables may be taken into account in data analysis using various statistical procedures. Both matching in the study design and controlling in the analysis are valid ways of taking confounding variables into account. In some instances one can match variables roughly in the study design and then control for them more finely in the analysis.

Careful measurement of confounding variables is important. Unmeasured variables cannot be controlled for in the analysis. Mismeasured variables cannot be adequately controlled. The effects of mismeasurement of confounders is discussed in more detail in a later section.

Effect Modification

Effect modification, sometimes called statistical interaction, also needs to be considered when studies are designed, analyzed, and interpreted. Effect modification is said to occur when the magnitude of the association between one variable and another differs according to the level of a third variable. For instance, obesity increases the risk for breast cancer in postmenopausal but not premenopausal women; thus, menopausal status is a modifier of the effect of obesity on breast cancer. Asbestos appears to be a stronger risk factor for lung cancer among smokers than among nonsmokers; in other words, smoking modifies the effect of asbestos on lung cancer risk. Detecting effect modification is an important component of the analysis of epidemiologic data.

Bias

Bias refers to the tendency of a measurement or a statistic to deviate from the true value of the measure or statistic. Bias can arise from many sources and is a common concern in epidemiologic studies. Biases can affect estimates of outcome, of exposure frequency, and of the magnitude of the association between a risk factor and a disease and an intervention or an outcome. As described above, uncontrolled or inadequately controlled confounding can lead to misleading estimates of measures of association. Mismeasurement also has the potential to cause bias, as discussed in detail in a later section of this chapter. Table 2-2 describes the other common sources of bias that are of

Table 2-2. Most Common Sources of Bias in Epidemiologic Studies

- Information bias
    - Interviewer bias
    - Recall bias
    - Reporting bias
- Selection bias
    - Ascertainment bias
    - Detection bias
    - Response bias
- Uncontrolled confounding
- Mismeasurement

concern in epidemiologic studies (see also Last 1995; Hennekens and Buring 1987).

Information bias is systematic error in measuring the exposure or outcome such that information is more accurate or more complete in one group than another. Examples of information bias include interviewer bias, recall bias, and reporting bias.

- Interviewer bias is systematic error occurring because an interviewer does not gather information in a similar manner in groups being compared. For example, if an interviewer believes, either subconsciously or consciously, that oral contraceptives cause breast cancer, the interviewer might probe more deeply into the oral contraceptive history of cases than of controls.
- Recall bias is systematic error resulting from differences in the accuracy or completeness of recall of past events between groups. For example, mothers of infants whose children are born with a congenital malformation may remember events during the pregnancy to a greater extent than mothers of apparently healthy infants.
- Reporting bias is a systematic error resulting from the tendency of people in one group to be more or less likely to report information than others. Cases with certain diseases might be more likely to deny that they had used alcohol than controls.

Selection bias is systematic error occurring because of differences between those who are and are not selected for a study or selected to be in a certain group within a study. Ascertainment bias, detection bias, and response bias are generally considered to be types of selection bias.

- Ascertainment bias is systematic error resulting from failure to identify equally all categories of individuals who are supposed to be represented in a group. For instance, a specialty hospital may provide only the sickest of cases to a study and not a representative sample of cases for comparison with controls.
- Detection bias is systematic error resulting from greater likelihood of some cases being identified, diagnosed, or verified than others. For example, pulmonary embolism may be more likely to be detected in women using oral contraceptives than in those not using oral contraceptives because of a greater likelihood of doing a lung scan in oral contraceptive users with chest pain Thus, an association between use of oral contraceptives and pulmonary embolism might result from the greater likelihood of disease detection in oral contraceptive users rather than from the oral contraceptives themselves.
- Response bias is systematic error occurring because of differences between those who do and do not choose to participate in a study. It also arises because of differences between those who remain in a study and those who are lost-to-follow-up. In a cross-sectional study, even when a sample is scientifically selected, if a substantial proportion of those selected decline to participate, the sample is still likely to give biased results. Respondents and nonrespondents almost always differ in important ways. If one is trying to learn about the prevalence of a disease, those with serious disease may not be well enough to participate, and those who feel healthy may have little motivation to partici-

pate. If very ill people are unable to come to a clinic to participate in a study, very ill people will be underrepresented as cases in a study. If busy people are less likely than others to be willing to participate as controls in a case-control study, the controls will not be representative of the general population. Similarly, if persons who are sicker are less likely to return for follow-up in a randomized trial, outcome information based on those who return will not be representative of outcomes in all persons who entered the study.

Other Measurement Issues in Epidemiologic Studies

The possibility of measurement error is of concern for all variables of interest. Some exposures, such as diet and physical activity, are almost always measured by questionnaire and can be associated with a great deal of measurement error. Measurement of some diseases such as arthritic disorders and psychiatric disorders is very difficult because of the absence of clearly defined diagnostic criteria. Even the measurement of existence of cancer is imperfect because pathologists differ in their assessment of pathologic slides. Although measurement error can seldom be eliminated, it is important to reduce it to the extent that is feasible and to understand its effects on study results. Here we will limit the discussion of measurement issues to variables that can take on only two values, such as disease present or absent or exposure present or absent (i.e., binary variables).

In discussing measurement error, several definitions are important (Table 2-3). *Validity* or *accuracy* refers to the closeness with which the measurement approaches the true value, and *reliability* or *reproducibility* refers to the extent to which the same measurement is obtained on the same occasion by the same observer, on multiple occasions by the same observer, or by different observers on the same occasion. *Precision* refers to the amount of variation around the measurement or estimate; a precise measure will have a small amount of variation around it.

Measurement error is said to be *differential* when the magnitude of the error for one variable differs according to the actual value of another variable.

Table 2-3. Important Definitions Pertinent to Measurement

Term	Synonym	Definition
Validity	Accuracy	Closeness of the measure to the true value
Reliability	Reproducibility	Extent to which multiple measurements agree
Precision	—	Amount of variation in the estimate of a measure

For instance, in a case-control study of the association between use of a medication during pregnancy and a congenital malformation in the offspring, mothers of cases might overreport use in their effort to find something to blame, whereas mothers of controls might tend to forget that they had used the medication and underreport its use. In other words, the direction of the error in reporting medication use would depend upon whether a person is a case or a control, and a false association could be observed. Differential measurement error can cause associations to be overestimated or underestimated, depending on the circumstances.

Measurement error is said to be *nondifferential* when the magnitude of the error in one variable does not vary according to the actual value of the other variable of interest. In a 2 × 2 table, nondifferential misclassification always causes the relative risk or odds ratio to be closer to 1.0, provided that errors in measurement of the two variables are independent of each other. Table 2-4 presents a hypothetical case-control study in which misclassification is nondifferential. In this example, the true odds ratio is 2.3. It is assumed that disease is not mismeasured. But exposure, however, is mismeasured by the same amount (100%) in both cases and controls. The odds ratio is observed to be 2.1.

Table 2-5 presents another hypothetical case-control study in which misclassification is nondifferential. In this example, the true odds ratio is 2.3. The disease is assumed to be measured without error, but the exposure is mismeasured. In the first instance, it is mismeasured only in cases. Specifically, 20% more cases are classified as exposed than are exposed in truth. Under these conditions the observed odds ratio is 2.8. The bottom of the table shows what would happen if exposure were mismeasured only in controls. In this instance, it is assumed that 20% more controls are classified as exposed than are exposed in truth. Under these conditions, the odds ratio is odds ratio is 1.8.

Table 2-4. Hypothetical Example of the Effect on the Observed Odds Ratio of Nondifferential Misclassification of Exposure

Exposure	True Status in Case-Control Study[a]			Observed Status in Case-Control Study[b]		
	Cases	Controls	Total	Cases	Controls	Total
+	40	20	60	20	10	30
−	160	180	340	180	190	370
Total	200	200	400	200	200	400

[a] True odds ratio = $(40 \times 180)/(20 \times 160)$ = 2.3.

[b] Assume mismeasurement of exposure but not of disease; 100% more cases and 100% more controls are classified as exposed as are exposed in truth; observed odds ratio = $(20 \times 190)/(10 \times 180)$ = 2.1.

Table 2-5. Hypothetical Examples of the Effect on the Observed Odds Ratio of Differential Misclassification of Exposure

Exposure	True Status[a]		Observed Status[b]		Observed Status[c]	
	Cases	Controls	Cases	Controls	Cases	Controls
+	40	20	48	20	40	24
−	160	180	152	180	160	176
Total	200	200	200	200	200	200

[a] True odds ratio $= (40 \times 180)/(160 \times 20) = 2.3$.

[b] Assume misclassification of exposure but not of disease; assume misclassification of exposure of cases but not controls; 20% more cases are classified as exposed as are exposed in truth; observed odds ratio $= (48 \times 180)/(152 \times 20) = 2.8$.

[c] Assume misclassification of exposure but not of disease; assume misclassification of exposure of controls but not cases; 20% more controls are classified as exposed as are exposed in truth; observed odds ratio $= (40 \times 176)/(160 \times 24) = 1.8$.

When measurement error exists for potentially confounding variables, additional issues arise. If a confounding variable is measured with error, then controlling for it in the analysis will not entirely remove its effect. For instance, if the odds ratio for the association between coffee drinking and delivery of a low-birth weight infant was observed to be 2.0 without controlling for cigarette smoking, and if cigarette smoking was not well measured and was then controlled for in the analysis, the odds ratio might be, say, 1.5. The investigator would not know whether there is some association between coffee drinking and delivery of a low-birth weight infant independent of cigarette smoking, or whether there would be no independent association if cigarette smoking had been accurately measured.

When both the exposure and confounder are measured with error, the effects are less predictable. Also, when estimates are made from tables larger than 2 × 2 tables, there are circumstances under which nondifferential measurement error can make an association appear larger than it really is (Weinberg et al. 1994).

Power and Sample Size

Power

Power can be thought of as the probability that a study will find (or found) a statistically significant difference when, in truth, a difference of a given magnitude exists (or existed). Power is equal to 1 − beta (type II error), where beta is the probability of declaring a difference not to be statistically significant when, in truth, a difference exists. The statistical power of a study to detect an effect of given size is determined by its size. Small studies have lower power than larger studies, all other things being equal.

The danger of conducting a study with low statistical power is that a conclusion that an intervention does not work (or that an exposure is not related to disease) will be drawn when, in truth, the intervention works (or the exposure is related to disease). For example, several small studies of intravenous streptokinase in patients with acute myocardial infarction found no statistically significant difference in postmyocardial infarction outcome between treated and untreated patients. A meta-analysis (Stampfer et al. 1982) and subsequent large study (GISSI 1986) both concluded that streptokinase reduces mortality and reinfarction. The negative findings of initial small studies were a consequence of their small size and low statistical power.

In "negative" studies (i.e., studies that find no effect of the intervention or no association between exposure and disease), the possibility that inadequate statistical power explains the negative result must always be considered. When there are many small studies that are individually statistically insignificant, meta-analysis, described later in this chapter, may sometimes be a useful way to draw conclusions about the body of literature, overcoming the problem of low statistical power in individual studies. Post hoc estimation of power based on observed results and presentation of 95% confidence limits can put negative findings into perspective. The careful planning of studies based on a formal sample size calculation is the best way to prevent erroneous conclusions resulting from inadequate statistical power.

Estimating Sample Size

Although it is important to assure that a study has adequate statistical power in order to avoid erroneous conclusions resulting from inadequate sample size, it is inefficient to include more study subjects than are needed. Furthermore, a study that is too large may declare as statistically significant an effect that is so small in size that it is biologically and clinically meaningless. Determining the optimal sample size for a study is one of the most important aspects of study planning. Determining optimal sample size *a priori* guards against conduct of studies with inadequate power. Many statistical and epidemiologic textbooks provide formulas for estimating sample size for studies with various designs (e.g., Schesselman 1982; Fleiss 1986; Kelsey et al. 1996), and software programs—e.g., EpiInfo (Centers for Disease Control and Prevention [CDC] 1994)—are available to carry out sample size calculations. Here, the most important considerations in the estimation of required sample size for studies of various design are described qualitatively.

First, the investigator must specify a value for alpha, the likelihood that the null hypothesis (of no difference) will be rejected when it is in fact true. Although alpha can be chosen as any value between 0 and 1, by convention it usually taken to be 0.05 based on a two-tailed test of statistical significance. Smaller values of alpha will require larger sample sizes. Specifying a one-tailed test will result in a smaller required sample size, but should be rarely done because it requires that the direction of an association be known with complete certainty.

Second, the investigator must specify a value for beta, the likelihood that the null hypothesis is not rejected (i.e., an observed difference is declared to be "not significant") when the null hypothesis, in fact, is not true. Beta is usually set at 0.10 or 0.20. The power of a statistical test is $1 - $ beta. Thus, with beta equal to 0.10, the power to reject the null hypothesis when it is not true is $1 - 0.10$ or 0.90. The smaller the value of beta, the greater the power, and the larger the sample size that is needed.

Third, the investigator much specify the size of the effect the study is desired to detect. For cohort or experimental studies with outcome measures defined as yes/no, the effect could be either a difference in relative risk or a difference in outcome rates. The effect measure is usually an odds ratio for case-control studies. The smaller the effect size to be detected, the larger the sample size that will be needed.

Finally, the investigator must provide an estimate of the variance in measures of exposure and/or outcome. For cohort and experimental studies, if the outcome of interest is a yes/no variable, the investigator must specify the proportion of the unexposed population expected to develop the condition of interest because the variance depends on this proportion. Rare outcomes require larger sample size. In case-control studies, the investigator must specify the expected proportion of exposed controls. Rare exposures require larger samples sizes in case-control studies. In studies with continuously distributed variables either as exposures or as outcomes (e.g., blood pressure), the required sample size is dependent on the variance of the measure, which must be specified by the investigator. The greater the variance, the larger the sample size that is needed to detect an association of a given size.

Sample-size estimation for more complex study designs may require the investigator to specify other quantities. For example, to estimate the appropriate sample size for a study that involves randomization of units (e.g., communities, physician practices), it necessary to specify the expected correlation of measures within individuals in the randomized unit (see Chapter 6). Estimation of sample size for survival differences in a follow-up study requires specification of the expected rate of loss-to-follow-up and the expected change over time in the rate of disease.

Assessing the Burden of Disease and Contributors to Ill-Health

In applied settings, one of the most important uses of epidemiologic data is to assess the burden of disease and the contributors to ill-health in order to set priorities for interventions and for resource allocation. Measures used to estimate the burden of disease and disability in the population include incidence (the number of new cases in a given time period); prevalence (the number of persons with the disease at a single time period); disability days due to an illness; lives, life-years, or healthy years lost to a condition; the cost of care for persons with the condition; and the contribution of the condition to lost productivity. Special descriptive studies as well as ongoing surveillance are important sources of information on these measures of the burden of illness.

Information from etiologic studies of risk factors for disease or disability is used to help decide which of several risk factors for disease or disability are the most important contributors to the disease. This information, like the descriptive information discussed above, aids in decisions about priorities for intervention and resource allocation.

A number of different measures—measures of attributable risk or attributable fraction—estimate the proportion of disease that can be attributed to a specific exposure. If the association between the exposure and the disease is, in fact, causal, attributable fraction indicates the proportion of the disease that might be eliminated if exposure is eliminated (Last 1995).

Some attributable fraction measures (often referred to as measures of etiologic fraction) apply to the individual. Others (usually called measures of population attributable fraction) apply to the population. Measures of the attributable fraction for the population are most useful. For example, knowing that 80% of cases of lung cancer might be eliminated by elimination of smoking is generally more useful information in a public health setting than knowing that 95% of lung cancer occurrence among smokers can be attributed to their smoking.

The formula for calculating the population attributable fraction using the relative risk or the odds ratio for disease in the exposed is:

$$\text{Population attributable fraction} = P\ (RR - 1.0)/P\ (RR - 1.0) + 1.0$$

where P is the proportion of the population who are exposed and RR is the estimated relative risk of the disease in the exposed.

The population attributable fraction depends on the magnitude of the relative risk and the prevalence of exposure in the population. Exposures of low prevalence cannot account for a large proportion of disease in the population, while common exposures may account for a high proportion of disease even when the relative risk is not very high. For example, in a study done among women in a large urban county (Petitti and Coleman 1990), the relative risk of low birth weight in women who used cocaine during pregnancy was very high (estimated relative risk 10.1), but only 1% of women used cocaine during pregnancy, and it accounted for only about 8% of all low birth weight births in the county (Kooperberg and Petitti 1991).Cigarette smoking was associated with a much more modest increase in the risk of low birth weight (Petitti and Coleman 1990; estimated relative risk 3.8), but 25% of women smoked cigarettes, and smoking accounted for 32% of low birth weight births in the county (Kooperberg and Petitti 1991).

Methods for Combining Studies: Meta-analysis

Basis of Meta-analysis

Because the results of any one study of an issue are seldom definitive, it is often useful to combine results from many studies. Meta-analysis, described in detail by Petitti (1994), Dickersin and Berlin (1992), and Greenland (1987), is one approach to combining results. Specifically, meta-analysis is a quantitative approach for systematically combining the results of previous research in order to arrive at conclusions about the body of research as a whole (Petitti 1994). Petitti describes four steps in undertaking a meta-analysis.

1. *Identify Relevant Studies.* The first step in a meta-analysis is to identify the relevant studies. Systematic, explicit criteria must be established for including studies in a meta-analysis. The establishment of explicit criteria distinguishes meta-analysis from a qualitative literature review. Identifying relevant studies usually involves searching personal reference lists, computerized sources such as Medline, lists of references in other relevant original articles and review articles, the contents of journals in which relevant articles are likely to be published, and doctoral dissertations on the topic. Experts in the area are usually consulted to determine if they know of articles that have been missed through the other sources. In addition, it is important to try to identify unpublished studies, because of "publication bias"—the greater tendency of research with statistically significant results to be submitted and published than results that are not statistically significant and/or null. In other words, published studies are generally not representative of all studies that have been undertaken of an issue. When identifying studies from these various sources, one usually starts with a very broad list of potential studies for inclusion and then narrows it down to studies that are indeed relevant. It should be apparent that identification of relevant studies is usually a time-consuming process.

2. *Inclusion/Exclusion Criteria.* The second step in a meta-analysis is deciding upon inclusion and exclusion criteria for the studies under consideration as relevant. Establishing and applying such criteria increases the likelihood that

the meta-analysis will be reproducible and unbiased. The criteria should be established before data abstraction begins. Criteria for inclusion usually specify the study designs to be included, the years of publication or of data collection, the languages in which the articles are written (e.g., English only or English plus other specified languages), which publication will be selected when more than one publication based on the same or overlapping data is available, the minimum sample size and the extent of follow-up, the treatments and/or exposures, the manner in which the exposures, treatment, and outcomes were measured, and the completeness of information. Finally, study quality needs to be considered. As a minimum, studies whose quality is so poor (by some prespecified criteria) that the results are likely to be invalid should not be included in the meta-analysis. Rating scales may be developed to assess the quality of the included studies. On this basis, studies may be stratified into two or more groups according to their quality. Although in theory studies could be weighted by their score on the rating scale, this has not been done in practice.

3. *Data Abstraction.* The third step in a meta-analysis is data abstraction. The first component of data abstraction is documenting whether or not each identified study is eligible for inclusion. Then, data on the results of the study and characteristics of the study such as its design, number of participants, and other important features are abstracted. The abstraction should produce data that are reliable, valid, and free of bias. Blinding the abstractor to aspects of the study that might influence the data abstraction is the best way to minimize bias in data abstraction.

4. *Statistical Analysis and Exploration of Heterogeneity.* The final step in conducting a meta-analysis is statistical analysis and exploration of heterogeneity if it is present. The analysis generally involves combining the data to obtain a summary estimate of the measure of association, together with its variance and 95% confidence limits. In some situations, dose–response relationships may be presented. The reader is referred to Petitti (1994), Dickersin and Berlin (1992), and Greenland (1987) for further discussion of statistical analysis.

Whether the effect is homogenous across studies should be specifically examined and tested; if not homogenous, reasons for heterogeneity should be sought. An increasingly important use of meta-analysis is to identify reasons for discrepancies in study results.

Application of Meta-analysis

Although meta-analysis is a quite popular way of summarizing data from several studies, its use has generated a fair amount of controversy, particularly when used to combine results of observational studies (Shapiro 1994a,b; Petitti 1994; Greenland 1994). The quality of the meta-analysis depends upon rigorous adherence to the methodology described above, and especially upon delineation of the criteria for selection of the specific studies eligible for inclusion in the meta-analysis. Articles based on meta-analysis need to be read in the same critical manner as original articles. When studies arrive at different conclusions or there are large differences among studies in their estimates of effect size, meta-analysis is most appropriately used to try to identify the reasons for heterogeneity and to suggest further areas for research—not to calculate a single summary estimate of effect (Greenland 1994; Petitti 1994). When properly done, meta-analysis provides a way of summarizing literature that is less subjective than the usual qualitative review.

Notwithstanding concerns about meta-analysis, it has become an extremely important tool in the formulation of public health and clinical policy, and especially in the development of guidelines. A recent example can be seen in the American College of Physicians Guidelines on the Use of Hormone Replacement Therapy, which conducted separate meta-analyses of studies of hormone replacement therapy and coronary artery disease, hip fracture, and breast and endometrial cancer to derive estimates of the relative risk of these conditions. It used this information as input to a decision model estimating life-expectancy in users and nonusers of hormone replacement therapy (Grady et al. 1992). It is likely that the use of meta-analysis for these purposes will increase, not diminish.

Guidance on Interpreting Epidemiologic Evidence

Epidemiologic studies have contributed a great deal to the practice of public health. They provide information that is used on a day-to-day basis to select interventions and to counsel patients about risk. They are important input to clinical guidelines and a variety of policy decisions in the applied setting. Since studies that use epidemiologic methods will continue to provide data that is essential in applied settings, it is important that practitioners have a good understanding of the limitations of these methods and that they be able to evaluate the quality of studies upon which they rely for information. Here we summarize some of the major questions that a person should pose when evaluating studies that use epidemiologic methods.

1. *Was the study design appropriate?* If a case-control or cross-sectional study was used, is it clear what is cause and what is effect? In a case-control study, were the cases and controls appropriately selected, and was the information on exposure to the putative risk factor and to the potential confounding variables obtained in an unbiased manner? If a cohort study was undertaken, was it methodologically sound? Is an experimental study needed to be entirely convincing?

2. *Was the sample size large enough?* Many studies have such small numbers of participants that they have limited ability to detect associations that really do exist. Thus, failure to find a statistically significant association may mean that the association does not exist, or it may mean that the sample size was not large enough to detect a true association.

3. *Was measurement good enough?* One issue is whether the measurements, although of comparable quality in exposed and unexposed cohort members, or in cases and controls in a case-control study, could have been so poor that it was not possible to detect an association that really does exist. In other words, the "noise to signal" ratio is so high that it is impossible to detect the signal. A second possibility to keep in mind is that measurement is not of comparable quality in exposed and unexposed cohort members or in cases and controls. In this instance, one may observe an association that really does not exist, may fail to find one that does exist, or may even find one in the opposite direction to the true association. Results from such a study would be difficult to interpret.

4. *Is confounding present?* Can an association between a putative exposure and a disease be explained by another factor that is associated with both the exposure and disease? If such a confounding variable has been well measured and taken into account either in the study design or the statistical analysis, then valid conclusions may be reached, but if the confounding variable has been poorly measured or not measured at all, then any association may again be difficult to interpret. In addition, what is considered to be a causal association at one point in time may be found to be attributable to a confounding variable not recognized until a later time.

5. *Is effect modification present?* An exposure may not have the same effect in all settings or subgroups of the population. Has this possibility been considered in the existing studies, and, if not, is there reason to believe that such heterogeneity might exist? If so, then one must be cautious in applying information in settings or subgroups where they may not be useful.

6. *Are other biases present?* It has been indicated throughout this chapter that there are many potential sources of bias that can invalidate the results of studies that use epidemiologic methods. The most common sources of bias were described above, and they should be considered when evaluating the quality of these studies.

7. *Can a causal association be inferred?* Criteria commonly used to test causal hypotheses are discussed in detail by others (Hill 1965; Susser 1973; US Dept of Health, Education, and Welfare [USDHEW] 1964). These criteria are useful in reaching judgments about the likelihood of causality. In the end, however, belief in causality is based on an individual's judgment, and different individuals may in good faith reach different conclusions from the same available information.

8. *Should public health action be taken on the basis of available evidence?* Very strong evidence from epidemiologic (and other) studies may mandate that control measures be taken, while, on the other hand, evidence may be so weak that taking action would be premature. Often the strength of evidence is suggestive, but not conclusive, yet one has to make a decision about the desirability of taking action. Here, other factors come into play. How serious are the consequences of taking action or no action, and what other impact will the course of action have? If taking action might reduce the frequency of a lethal disease, would have no adverse effects, and would cost little, then the decision to take action would be clear. If all of these conditions do not exist, then decisions may be more difficult.

9. *Is further study needed? If so, of what kind?* Seldom will any one study provide definitive evidence for or against a hypothesis. Studies are often contradic-

tory, and even results from several consistent studies may not be convincing. What are the weaknesses in studies undertaken to date? Can they be improved upon in subsequent studies, or is it practically or ethnically impossible to reach a conclusion on the basis of even the best epidemiologic studies? Does a study need to be replicated in other subgroups of the population? If more information is needed before reaching a conclusion, and if time and resources are available to conduct such a study, then the wisest course of action will be to wait for the results of more definitive study. On the other hand, if reasonable conclusions can be reached on the basis of currently available, even if slightly flawed data, then it is not prudent to demand that further studies be undertaken before action is taken.

Summary

Methods in epidemiology have grown increasingly sophisticated over the past several decades. Epidemiologic methods are being applied more widely outside the arena of etiologic research. This chapter has briefly described methodologic concepts and issues most pertinent to the application of epidemiology in public health setting and health care organizations. While it is impossible to provide detailed coverage in a single chapter, key concepts and issues are highlighted.

CASE STUDIES

Bicycle Helmet Use and Head Injuries

Background
Bicycling is a popular recreational activity in the United States, where there are approximately 100 million cyclists (National Safety Council 1993). However, bicycling is not without its hazards. Each year in the United States, nearly 1,000 bicyclists die in bicycle crashes. Also, bicycle accidents account for about 550,000 emergency room visits. The most common cause of death and serious disability attributed to bicycle accidents, head injury, is the contributing cause of death in 70–80% of all bicycle fatalities.

To determine the effectiveness of bicycle helmets in reducing the risk of head and brain injury in bicycle accidents, researchers in Seattle, Washington, conducted a case-control study (Thompson et al. 1989). Cases were bicyclists who sought medical care for a bicycle-related head injury in the emergency room of one of five hospitals during the study period ($n = 235$). Two control groups were used. The first consisted of other bicyclists who sought care in the same five emergency rooms for injuries other than head injuries ("emergency room controls"; $n = 433$). A second, population-based, control group consisted of cyclists who had had accidents, regardless of whether or not they were injured or had sought medical care ("population controls"; $n = 558$). This group was identified through the automated files of the Group Health Cooperative using coded data that classify accidents according to cause.

A detailed questionnaire was sent to eligible cases and controls, with telephone follow-up. The questionnaire ascertained household income, education level, the amount of cycling experience, the circumstances surrounding the accident (e.g., the cause, surface, speed), and the ownership and use of helmets. Medical information on the accident was obtained from medical records for cases and emergency room controls and directly from subjects for population controls.

Bicycle riders who wore helmets had a statistically significant reduction in their risk of head injury and brain injury. Results were consistent whether based on emergency room controls or population controls. Based on population controls, riders with helmets had an 85% reduction in their risk of head injury (OR = 0.15; 95% CI = 0.07–0.29) and an 88% reduction in their risk of brain injury (OR = 0.12; 95% CI = 0.04–0.40).

Key Questions

1. What are the major potential sources of bias in this study?

A case-control study such as this one is prone to a number of sources of bias, as noted earlier in this chapter. Among the most important considerations is recall bias. In this instance, it is possible that recall and reporting of helmet usage might not be equally accurate in cases and controls. Based on earlier reports of the recall of discrete events (Harlow and Linet 1989) and a medical record audit, the authors concluded that recall bias was not a major limitation.

It is also important to examine response rates in cases and controls. Differences in rates of response between cases and controls are always a concern.

2. Are the findings from the study generalizable to other populations?

This study was conducted in a single region (i.e., the Seattle metropolitan area), which is relatively affluent and has a low percentage of persons who are ethnic minorities. The effect of helmet use on head injury might differ in areas with populations with a different demographic makeup.

3. Would it be feasible to conduct a randomized trial examining the effects of bicycle helmet use on head injury among cyclists?

Although head injury is the most common cause of death and disability in cyclists, it is still a relatively rare event. A study randomizing individuals would require a very large sample size and would be expensive. There is no easy way to identify bicyclists, and it is hard to envision how large numbers of bicyclists would be recruited to a trial. Convincing bicyclists accustomed to using a helmet that they should stop using it for a study would be difficult.

4. Would it be ethical to conduct a study that randomized bicyclists to use and not use a helmet?

There is strong evidence linking use of motorcycle helmets with reduced risk of head injury and serious disability. There are other nonexperimental data on helmet use and head injury in bicyclists besides the study of Thompson et al. (1989) that show reductions in the risk of head injury in bicyclists. Randomizing individuals to use or not use helmets might be deemed unethical for these reasons.

Implications for Practice

The epidemiologic evidence from this study and others (Zavoski et al. 1995; Thompson et al. 1996) has led to strong advocacy efforts for greater use of bicycle helmets. For example, the CDC has issued a comprehensive set of recommendations that are designed to help increase use of bicycle helmets (CDC 1995). In addition, the

American Academy of Pediatrics recommends the inclusion of counseling for helmet use in pediatric preventive care visits (American Academy of Pediatrics 1990). In some areas of the world, use of bicycle helmets has been mandated (CDC 1993) based on observational studies. It is possible to use data originating solely from observational studies to make public health recommendations.

Measurement and Promotion of Physical Activity Among Sedentary Groups

Background

Physical inactivity is an established risk factor for a range of prevalent chronic diseases and conditions, including cardiovascular disease, non-insulin-dependent diabetes, and some cancers (Bouchard et al. 1994). In addition, regular physical activity has been associated with increases in psychological functioning and well-being and decreases in functional limitations that strongly influence daily functioning and quality of life (Buchner et al. 1992). Despite the clear health benefits that can be accrued through adopting a more active lifestyle, less than one-quarter of US adults are active at the level recommended to achieve such benefits, and approximately 25% of adult Americans report no physical activity at all in their leisure time (US Dept of Health and Human Services [USDHHS] 1996). Low physical activity participation has been noted to be particularly prevalent among specific population subgroups, including persons of low socioeconomic status (SES). Although walking has been identified as one form of exercise that appears to be equally prevalent among persons of differing socioeconomic status, it is unclear whether the apparent preference for walking among low SES persons is independent of other demographic variables, including sex, age, or race.

To better understand the association between walking and SES controlling for other demographic variables, 1990 data from a cross-sectional population survey (the Behavioral Risk Factor Surveillance System [BRFSS]) were analyzed (Siegel et al. 1995). The BRFSS was developed in 1981 by the Centers for Disease Control and provides a flexible, state health-agency-based surveillance system to assist in planning, implementing, and evaluating health promotion and disease prevention programs (Remington et al. 1988). Data are typically collected on modifiable risk factors such as physical inactivity, smoking, diet, alcohol use, and cancer screening practices. Each year, telephone surveys are conducted with a random sample of the adult noninstitutionalized population from each participating state. Data from 81,557 respondents in 45 states and the District of Columbia were analyzed.

Key Questions

1. What were the rates of participation in all forms of physical activity among low versus higher SES persons?

Persons at higher income levels were more likely to participate in some form of physical activity relative to those at lower levels. Unemployed persons and obese persons were less likely to participate in physical activity than the rest of the sample.

2. Were the rates of participation in walking comparable for low versus higher SES persons?

There was relatively little variation in the percentages of those reporting walking for exercise across the population subgroups being compared within income, employment, or body mass strata.

3. Could differences or similarities among group-specific participation rates be accounted for by age, race, or sex?

Adjustment for age, race, and sex did not affect the results.

4. Are there biases in the BRFSS that could account for the differences noted?

The BRFSS is a telephone survey. Therefore, it is subject to a number of biases, most importantly underrepresentation of persons lacking telephones who are typically of lower SES. However, the differences note in this study were relatively large and consistent and are unlikely to be explained by this bias.

Implications for Practice

The researchers concluded that in light of the population preference for walking for exercise, especially among those population subgroups (such as low SES populations) having the lowest prevalence of participation in leisure-time physical activity, increased walking for exercise could have a marked impact on those subgroups who engage in no leisure-time physical activity currently. Walking for exercise appears to be an underutilized tool for promoting regular physical activity that could have a potentially important impact on physical activity levels across the population. The systematic exploration of public health strategies, including those at the public policy level (King et al. 1995), for promoting increased walking are thus indicated. Other similar analysis and dissemination of BRFSS data can bring attention to a variety of important public health issues.

SUGGESTED READINGS

Armenian HK, ed. Applications of the case-control method. Epidemiol Rev 1994;16 [entire issue].

Fleiss JL. Statistical Methods for Rates and Proportions. New York: John Wiley; 1981:218–220.

Hill AB. The environment and disease: association or causation? Proc R Soc Med 1965;58:295–300.

Kelsey JL, Whittemore AS, Evans AS, Thompson WD. Methods in Observational Epidemiology. Second Editon. New York: Oxford University Press; 1996.

Last JM, ed. A Dictionary of Epidemiology. Third Edition. New York: Oxford University Press; 1995.

Meinert CL. Clinical Trials: Design, Conduct, and Analysis. New York: Oxford University Press; 1986.

Petitti DB. Meta-analysis, Decision Analysis, and Cost-Effectiveness Analysis. Methods for Quantitative Synthesis in Medicine. New York: Oxford University Press; 1994.

Schlesselman JJ. Case-Control Studies. Design, Conduct, Analysis. New York: Oxford University Press; 1982.

REFERENCES

American Academy of Pediatrics. Committee on Accident and Poison Prevention. Statement on bicycle helmets. Pediatrics 1990;85:229–230.

Austin H, Hill HA, Flanders WD, Greenberg RS. Limitations in the application of case-control methodology. Epidemiol Rev 1994;16:65–76.

Bouchard C, Shephard RJ, Stephens T, eds. Physical Activity, Fitness, and Health: International Proceedings and Consensus Statement. Champaign, IL: Human Kinetics Publishers; 1994.

Buchner DM, Beresford SA, Larson EB, et al. Effects of physical activity on health status in older adults II: Intervention studies. Annu Rev Pub Health 1992; 13:469–488.

Bullman TA, Kang HK. The risk of suicide among wounded Vietnam veterans. Am J Public Health 1996;86:662–667.

Buring JE, Hennekens CH. The Women's Health Study: summary of the study design. J Myocardial Ischemia 1992;4:27–29.

Centers for Disease Control and Prevention. Mandatory bicycle helmet use in Victoria, Australia. Morb Mortal Wkly Rep 1993;42:359–363.

Centers for Disease Control and Prevention. EpiInfo 6. Version 6.01. Atlanta, GA: Centers for Disease Control and Prevention; August 1994.

Centers for Disease Control and Prevention. Injury-control recommendations: bicycle helmets. Morb Mortal Wkly Rep 1995;44(RR-1):1–18.

Comstock GW. Evaluating vaccination effectiveness and vaccine efficacy by means of case-control studies. Epidemiol Rev 1994;16:77–89.

Dickersin K, Berlin JA. Meta-analysis: State-of-the-science. Epidemiol Rev 1992; 14:154–176.

Fleiss JF. The Design and Analysis of Clinical Experiments. New York: J. Wiley & Sons; 1986.

Forrester HL, Jahnigen DW, LaForce FM. Inefficacy of pneumococcal vaccine in a high-risk population. Am J Med 1987;83:425–430.

Friedman GD. Primer of Epidemiology. Fourth Edition. New York: McGraw-Hill; 1994.

GISSI (Gruppo Italiano per lo Studio Della Streptochiasi Nell'infarcto Miocardico): Effectiveness of intravenous thrombolytic treatment in acute myocardial infarction. Lancet 1986;1:397–402.

Grady D, Rubin SM, Petitti DB, Fox CS, Black D, Ettinger B, et al. Hormone therapy to prevent disease and prolong life in postmenopausal women. Ann Intern Med 1992;117:1016–1037.

Greenland S. Can meta-analysis be salvaged? Am J Epidemiol 1994;140:783–787.

Greenland S. Quantitative methods in the review of epidemiologic literature. Epidemiol Rev 1987;9:1–30.

Greenwald P, Barlow JJ, Nasca PC, Burnett WS. Vaginal cancer after maternal treatment with synthetic hormones. N Engl J Med 1974;285:390–392.

Hannan EL, Kilburn H Jr, Bernard H, O'Donnell JE, Lukccik G, Shields EP. Coronary artery bypass surgery: the relationship between inhospital mortality rate and surgical volume after controlling for clinical risk factors. Med Care 1991;29:1094–1107.

Hennekens CH, Buring JE. Epidemiology in Medicine. Boston: Little, Brown; 1987.

Hennekens CH, Speizer FE, Rosner B, Bain CJ, Belanger C, Peto R. Use of permanent hair dyes and cancer among registered nurses. Lancet 1979;1:1390–1393.

Herbst AL, Ulfelder H, Poskanzer DC. Adenocarcinoma of the vagina: association of maternal stilbestrol therapy with tumor appearance in young women. N Engl J Med 1971;284:878–881.

Hill AB. The environment and disease: association or causation? Proc R Soc Med 1965;58:295–300.

Kelsey JL, Whittemore AS, Evans AS, Thompson WD. Methods in Observational Epidemiology. Second Edition. New York: Oxford University Press; 1996.

King AC, Blair SN, Bild DE, Dishman RK, Dubbert PM, Marcus BH, et al. Determinants of physical activity and interventions in adults. Medicine & Science in Sports and Exercise 1992; S221–236.

King AC, Jeffery RW, Fidinger F, Dusenbury L, Provence S, Hedlund SA, Spangler K. Environmental and policy approaches to cardiovascular disease prevention through physical activity: issues and opportunities. Health Educ Q 1995;22:499–511.

Kjerulff KH, Erickson BA, Langenberg PW. Chronic gynecological conditions reported by U.S. women: findings from the National Health Interview Survey, 1984 to 1992. Am J Public Health 1996;86:195–199.

Kooperberg C, Petitti DB. Using logistic regression to estimate the adjusted attributable risk of low birthweight in an unmatched case-control study. Epidemiology 1991;2:363–366.

Last JM, ed. A Dictionary of Epidemiology. Third Edition. New York: Oxford University Press; 1995.

Levy PS, Lemeshow S. Sampling of Populations: Methods and Applications. New York: Wiley; 1991.

Lipid Research Clinics Program. The Lipid Research Clinics coronary primary prevention trial results. I. Reduction in incidence of coronary heart disease. JAMA 1984;251:351–364.

Looker AC, Harris TB, Madans JH, Sempos CT. Dietary calcium and hip fracture risk: the NHAMES I epidemiologic follow-up study. Osteoporosis Int 1993; 3:177–184.

Los Angeles Department of Health Services. Advanced HIV Disease (AIDS) Surveillance Summary. Los Angeles, CA: Los Angeles Department of Health Services, HIV Epidemiology Program; April 15, 1996.

Luft HS, Garnick DW, Mark DH, et al. Hospital volume, physician volume, and patient outcomes: assessing the evidence. Ann Arbor, MI: Health Administration Press; 1990.

Mason TJ, McKay FW, Hoover R, Blot WJ, Fraumeni JF Jr. Atlas of cancer mortality for U.S. counties: 1950–69. DHEW Publication No. (NIH)75-780. Washington, DC: U.S. Department of Health, Education, and Welfare, 1975.

Mills OF, Rhoads GG. The contribution of the case-control approach to vaccine evaluation: pneumococcal and Haemophilus influenzae type B PRP vaccines. J Clin Epidemiol 1996;49:631–636.

Morrison H, Savitz D, Semenciw R, Hulka B, Mao Y, Morison D, Wigle D. Farming and prostate cancer mortality. Am J Epidemiol 1993;137:270–280.

Petitti DB. Of babies and bathwater. Am J Epidemiol 1994;140:779–782.

Petitti DB, Coleman C. Cocaine and the risk of low birth weight. Am J Public Health 1990;80:25–28.

Remington PL, Smith MY, Williamson DF, Anda RF, Gentry EM, Hogelin GC. Design, characteristics, and usefulness of state-based behavioral risk factor surveillance: 1981–1987. Public Health Rep 1988;103:366–375.

Sackett DL. Bias in analytic research. J Chron Dis 1979;32:51–63.

Schlesselman JJ. Case-Control Studies. Design, Conduct, Analysis. New York: Oxford University Press; 1982.

Selby JV, Friedman GD, Quesenberry CP Jr, Weiss NS. A case-control study of screening sigmoidoscopy and mortality from colorectal cancer. N Engl J Med 1992;326:653–657.

Selby JV. Case-control evaluations of treatment and program efficiency. Epidemiol Rev 1994;16:90–101.

Shapiro ED, Clemens JD. A controlled evaluation of the protective efficacy of pneumococcal vaccine for patients at high risk of serious pneumococcal infections. Ann Intern Med 1984;101:325–330.

Shapiro ED, Berg AT, Austrian R, et al. The protective efficacy of polyvalent pneumococcal polysaccharide vaccine. N Engl J Med 1991;325:1453–1460.

Shapiro S. Is there is or is there ain't no baby?: Dr. Shapiro replies to Drs. Petitti and Greenland. Am J Epidemiol 1994a;140:788–791.

Shapiro S. Point/counterpoint: Meta-analysis of observational studies. Meta-analysis/shmeta-analysis. Am J Epidemiol 1994b;140:771–778.

Showstack JA. Rosenfeld KE. Garnick DW. et al. The association of volume with outcome of coronary bypass surgery: scheduled vs. unscheduled operations. JAMA 1987:257:785–789.

Siegel PZ, Brackbill RM, Heath GW. The epidemiology of walking for exercise: implications for promoting activity among sedentary groups. Am J Public Health 1995;85:706–710.

Sims RV, Steinmann WC, McConville JH, King LR, Zwick WC, Schwartz JA. The clinical effectiveness of pneumococcal vaccine in the elderly. Ann Intern Med 1988;108:653–657.

Stampfer MJ, Goldhaber SZ, Yusuf S, Peto R, Hennekens CH. Effect of intrvenous streptokinase on acute myocardial infarction: pooled results from randomized trials. N Engl J Med 1982;307:1180–1182.

Steenland K, Brown D. Silicosis among gold miners: exposure-response analyses and risk assessment. Am J Public Health 1995;85:1372–1377.

SUDAAN User's Manual. Professional software for survey data analysis. Research Triangle Park, NC: Research Triangle Institute; 1991.

Susser M. Causal Thinking in the Health Sciences: Concepts and Strategies in Epidemiology. New York: Oxford University Press; 1973.

Thaul S, Hotra D, eds. An assessment of the NIH Women's Health Initiative. Institute of Medicine Committee to review the NIH Women's Health Initiative. Washington, DC: National Academy Press; 1993.

Thompson RS, Rivara FP, Thompson DC. A case-control study of the effectiveness of bicycle safety helmets. N Engl J Med 1989;320:1361–1367.

Thompson DC, Rivara FP, Thompson RS. Effectiveness of bicycle safety helments in preventing head injuries. A case-control study. JAMA 1996;276:1968–1973.

US Dept of Health, Education, and Welfare. US Public Health Service. Smoking and Health. Report of the Advisory Committee to the Surgeon General of the Public Health Service. Washington, DC: Center for Disease Control. Publication (PHS) 1103; 1964.

US Dept of Health and Human Services. Physical Activity and Health: A Report of the Surgeon General. Atlanta, GA: US Dept of Health and Human Services; Centers for Disease Control and Prevention; 1996.

Weinberg CR, Umbach DM, Greenland S. When will nondifferential misclassification of an exposure preserve the direction of a trend? Am J Epidemiol 1994;140:565–571.

Weiss NS. Application of the case-control method in the evaluation of screening. Epidemiol Rev 1994;16:102–108.

Wennberg JE, Gittlesohn A. Health care delivery in Maine. I. Patterns of use of common medical procedures. J Maine Med Assoc 1975:66:123–130.

Zavoski R, Lapidus G, Lerer T, Banco L. Bicycle injury in Connecticut. Connecticut Med 1995;59:3–9.

3

Outbreak and Cluster Investigations

ROSS C. BROWNSON

When disease incidence departs from expected patterns, applied epidemiology mounts outbreak and cluster investigations. Outbreaks and clusters are studied for several reasons: to determine etiology quickly so that control measures can be taken to alleviate an immediate health concern; to identify initial etiologic clues, leading to further insights and more methodologically sound studies; and to provide a timely and coherent response to the public when there is outcry over a perceived or real disease outbreak or cluster. These investigations are iterative in nature—ongoing analysis of descriptive epidemiologic data often serves as a basis for more comprehensive studies.

Outbreak and cluster investigations often call for the application of sound epidemiologic methods to resolve an unexpected problem in a limited time. These studies are considered a "core function" of public health (Public Health Foundation 1995). Based on 1993 estimates of core functions and expenditures of state public health agencies (Public Health Foundation 1995), the US expenditures for the "investigation and control of diseases, injuries, and response to natural disasters" was $1.1 billion, about 10% of total state public health expenditures.

Scope and Definitions

An *outbreak* is an "epidemic limited to a localized increase in the incidence of a disease" (Last 1995) and often involves infectious disease. Outbreak epidemiology is conducted under these conditions: The problem is unexpected; an immediate response may be demanded; public health epidemiologists must travel to and work in the field to solve the problem; and the extent of the investigation is likely to be limited because of the need for timely intervention (Goodman and Buechler 1996). In this chapter, the term "outbreak investigation" is used synonymously with terms used by other researchers such as "field investigation" (Goodman et al. 1990a,b) and "epidemic investigation" (Kelsey et al. 1996).

The discipline of outbreak investigation has been refined and formalized in large part due to the work of the Centers for Disease Control and Prevention's (CDC) Epidemic Intelligence Service (EIS). Since 1951, the EIS program has provided 2-year, on-the-job training in applied epidemiology for physicians and other doctorally prepared professionals (Langmuir 1980; Thacker et al. 1990).

A *cluster* is an "aggregation of relatively uncommon events or diseases in space and/or time in amounts that are believed or perceived to be greater than could be expected by chance" (Last 1995). A cluster usually refers to uncommon diseases of noninfectious origin (e.g., leukemia, spontaneous abortions, suicides), which are often perceived to be due to environmental exposures (California Dept of Health Services 1989; Stroup 1994).

Cluster studies are also sometimes called "small area analyses" because they are typically carried out at a subregional level. At this level, routine reporting of disease rates is unlikely (Elliott 1995). As a rough guide, a "small area" has been defined as one containing fewer than 20 cases of the disease of interest (Cuzick and Elliott 1992). Since small area analyses tend to deal with low-incidence events, special considerations and statistical tests may be necessary to deal with small numbers (Diehr et al. 1990).

An *aberration* is a statistical term used to describe departures from a usual distribution (Stroup 1994). An aberration can be distinguished from an outbreak because it denotes changes in the occurrence of health events that are statistically significant compared with usual history—an outbreak or epidemic may be present in the absence of a statistical increase (Stroup 1994). A method for detecting aberrations in time is that used by the CDC in its *Morbidity and Mortality Weekly Report* (Figure 3-1), which compares the number of reported cases of a given health event in the current 4-week period for a given health event with historical data from the previous 5 years (Stroup et al. 1993; Centers for Disease Contol [CDC] 1989).

Many of the studies of outbreaks and clusters at the state and local level are conducted with the assistance of the CDC. Between 1946 and 1987, the CDC participated in 2,900 outbreak and cluster investigations (Goodman et al. 1990b). Of these investigations, 65% were purported to be of infectious origin, 8% were noninfectious, 5% were related to environmental health threats, and 22% were of unknown or "other" origin. A more detailed examination of a random subsample of 370 investigations showed that most investigations were conducted in residential or community settings (50%), followed by hospitals (15%), schools or universities (11%), agricultural or rural settings (10%), workplaces (8%), military bases (4%), and recreational settings (2%). Among designs, cross-sectional studies were conducted in 90% of investiga-

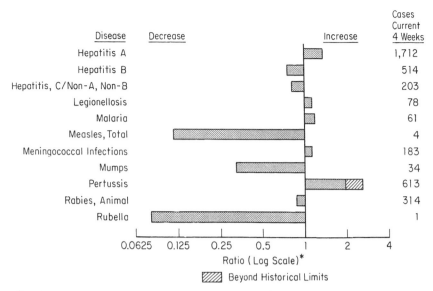

*Ratio of current 4-week total to mean of 15 4-week totals (from previous, comparable, and subsequent 4-week periods for the past 5 years). The point where the hatched area begins is based on the mean and two standard deviations of these 4-week totals.

Figure 3-1. Deviation bar chart of notifiable disease reports, comparision of 4-week totals ending June 1, 1996, with historical data—United States; *Source:* CDC (1997)

tions, followed by case-control studies (15%) and cohort studies (5%). (Percentages for study types do not add to 100% due to multiple study designs in some investigations.) It is important to note that the 2,900 investigations reported are those formally classified by the CDC; the actual number of outbreak investigations at the state and local levels over this period is in the many thousands.

This chapter discusses the significance and basic methods of outbreak and cluster investigations, some of the epidemiologic challenges in these studies, and summary recommendations for public health practice. Although there are many similarities between outbreak and cluster investigations, there are also important differences (Table 3-1); therefore, outbreak and cluster investigations are discussed separately in this chapter, with areas of overlap noted.

Outbreak Investigations

Outbreaks are commonly identified by reports from affected persons, members of a facility (e.g., a hospital, nursing home, school, or child care center), or a health care provider, or by review of existing surveillance data. There may be enormous financial and legal consequences (Dwyer et al. 1994). Costs to businesses and individuals may result from closing of restaurants, destruc-

Table 3-1. Comparison of Outbreak and Cluster Investigations

Characteristics	Outbreak Investigation	Cluster Investigation
Disease/condition	Infectious (e.g., *Salmonella* poisoning, hepatitis A)	Noninfectious (e.g., cancer, birth defects)
Etiologic agent	Transmissible microorganism (e.g., bacterium, virus)	Often unknown or combined agents (e.g., environmental exposures, personal risk factors such as smoking)
Time frame for investigation	Short (days or weeks)	Longer (weeks or months)
Effect estimates	Generally moderate to large	Generally weak to moderate
Exposure level	Moderate to high	Low
Exposure period	Acute (hours or days)	Chronic (years or decades)
Laboratory confirmation of cases and/or exposures	Common	Less common
Possibility of establishing cause and effect	Moderate to high	Low
Most common analytic study design	Retrospective cohort study	Case-control study

tion of contaminated livestock, removal of a contaminated product from the market, or product liability. This discussion of outbreak investigations focuses on the public sector practice of outbreak epidemiology; such investigations would frequently be carried out by state and local health departments with assistance from other experts (e.g., the CDC, academic researchers).

Outbreak investigations are distinct from many other types of epidemiologic studies in several important ways. First, outbreak investigations are usually retrospective, often relying on recall of affected persons to identify causal linkages (Palmer 1995). Second, because they begin without clear hypotheses, outbreak investigations require descriptive studies to generate hypotheses before analytic studies can be conducted (Goodman et al. 1990a). Third, since outbreak investigations are driven by an immediate health concern in the community, the need for responsiveness to community needs and effective risk communication is heightened. And finally, outbreaks require public health officials to weigh the evidence, often in the absence of a clear etiologic connection, and determine when the data are sufficient to take controversial and sometimes unwelcome action (e.g., close a restaurant) (Palmer 1995; Goodman and Buechler 1996).

In addition, outbreak investigations often attain national or international prominence. A few examples are highlighted. In the case of an infectious agent transmitted by a fomite (i.e., an inanimate object that may harbor a pathogen), the illness known as toxic-shock syndrome was reported to the CDC by five state health departments and individual physicians beginning in October 1979 (CDC 1980). Toxic-shock syndrome began with high fever, vomiting, and profuse, watery diarrhea and progressed to hypotensive shock. Among the first 55 cases, the case-fatality ratio was 13%. The bacterium *Staphylococcus aureus* was found to be responsible for the syndrome. Through a nationwide case-control study of 52 cases and 52 matched controls, the mode of transmission was determined to be the use of high-absorbency (fluid capacity) tampons in women (Shands et al. 1980). Public health recommendations were made to women regarding safe use of tampons. The Rely brand was voluntarily removed from the market. Subsequently, the absorbency of all brands of tampons was lowered (Schuchat and Broome 1991). Substantial reductions in the incidence of toxic shock syndrome resulted.

Due to a multistate foodborne outbreak, excess cases of hemolytic uremic syndrome (bloody diarrhea) were identified. From November 1992 through February 1993, over 500 laboratory-confirmed cases of *E. coli* 0157:H7 infection occurred, including four associated deaths (CDC 1993). Case-control studies in the affected geographic areas revealed that consumption of hamburgers from a specific fast food chain was strongly associated with confirmed illness (relative risk estimates ranging from 6 to 13). The findings from this outbreak investigation led to new recommendations for cooking ground beef to lessen the likelihood of a future similar outbreak.

Types of Outbreaks

Epidemics (outbreaks) can be classified according to the method of spread or propagation, nature and length of exposure to the infectious agent, and duration (Goodman and Peavy 1996; Kelsey et al. 1996). There are a few main categories.

Common Source Epidemic. Disease occurs as a result of exposure of a group of susceptible persons to a common source of a pathogen, often at the same time or within a brief time period. When the exposure is simultaneous, the resulting cases develop within one incubation period (a point source epidemic) (Last 1995). The epidemic curve in a common source outbreak will commonly show tight temporal clustering (Figure 3-2). The data shown from

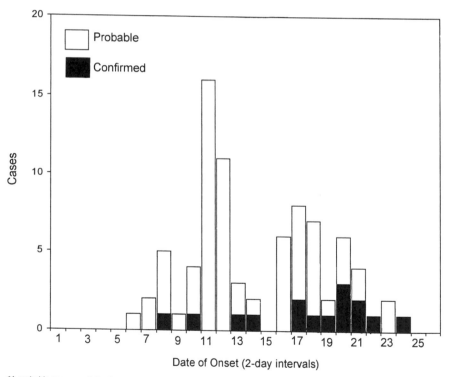

*A probable case was defined as onset of diarrhea (two or more loose stools during a 24-hour period) with either fever or bloody stools while at the resort or within 11 days of leaving the resort. A confirmed case additionally required *Shigella sonnei* isolated from stool. A total of 82 cases were identified, including 67 probable and 15 confirmed.

Figure 3-2. Epidemic curve showing the number of cases of confirmed and probable cases of *Shigella sonnei*,* by date of onset—Idaho, August 6–24, 1995; *Source:* CDC (1996)

the outbreak of *Shigella sonnei* also show the effect of a case definition based on laboratory confirmation versus that based on signs and symptoms. When a common source is present, a sharp upslope and a more gentle downslope are common (Figure 3-3). A waterborne outbreak that is spread through a contaminated community water supply is an example of a common source epidemic.

Propagative Epidemics. The infectious agent is transferred from one host to another. Generally, this involves multiplication and excretion of an infectious agent in the host and sometimes intermediate animal–human or arthropod–human multiplication cycles (Kelsey et al. 1996). Propagative spread usually results in an epidemic curve with a relatively gently upslope and somewhat steeper tail, sometimes including a second but less prominent group of cases later in time (Goodman and Peavy). An example of a propagative epidemic is an outbreak of hepatitis B virus due to intravenous drug use.

Mixed Epidemics. In this category, the epidemic begins with a single, common source of an infectious agent with subsequent propagative spread. Many foodborne pathogens result in mixed epidemics.

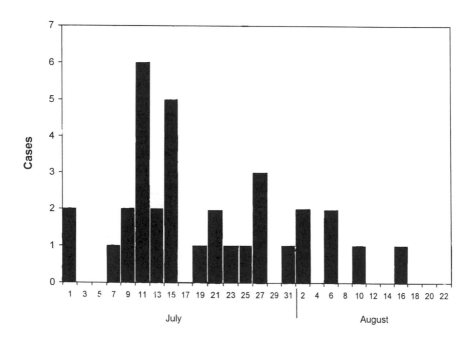

Date of Symptom Onset

Figure 3-3. Epidemic curve showing the number of cases of *Shigella dysenteriae* type 1 detected at Suan Phung Hospital, Thailand, July–August, 1992; *Source:* Hoge et al. (1995)

Steps in the Outbreak Investigation Process in the Community Setting

Several public health epidemiologists (Goodman et al. 1990a; Tyler and Last 1992; Gregg 1996a) have described a series of steps that should be considered when conducting an outbreak investigation (Table 3-2). While there is considerable overlap between steps and certain aspects may assume more importance depending on the nature of the individual outbreak, the following framework provides a useful guide. A comprehensive discussion of outbreak investigation methods is provided in Gregg et al. (1996).

Determine the Existence of an Epidemic. Ongoing disease surveillance conducted by state and local health agencies can be used to determine whether an excess of disease is occurring (Thacker 1996). Observed numbers can be compared with expected frequencies based on past trends by week, month, or year. This initial determination is often made on the basis of preliminary data, lacking laboratory confirmation of cases.

Confirm the Diagnosis. Clinical diagnosis can be obtained through standard laboratory techniques such as serology and/or isolation and characterization of the agent (Gregg 1996a). Information on the signs and symptoms among cases must be obtained early in an outbreak investigation (Tyler and Last 1992). It is frequently impractical to confirm every case with laboratory evidence; if every reported case has signs and symptoms consistent with laboratory-confirmed cases it is necessary to obtain laboratory verification on approximately 15–20% of cases.

Define a Case and Estimate the Number of Cases. Usually on the basis of preliminary information, the epidemiologist must develop a case definition.

Table 3-2. Ten Key Steps in an Outbreak Investigation

1.	Determine the existence of an epidemic
2.	Confirm the diagnosis
3.	Define a case and estimate the number of cases
4.	Orient the data in terms of time, place, and person
5.	Determine who is at risk of having the health problem
6.	Develop an explanatory hypothesis
7.	Compare the hypothesis with the established facts
8.	Plan and execute a more systematic study
9.	Prepare a written report
10.	Execute control and prevention measures

Sources: Goodman et al. (1990a); Tyler and Last (1992); Goodman and Buechler (1996).

In general, the simplest and most objective criteria for case definition are the best (e.g., fever, blood in the stool, elevated white blood cell count) (Gregg 1996a). Often, a preliminary case definition is adequate as an outbreak is unfolding and this definition can later be refined. After a usable case definition has been established, the field epidemiologist should count the cases, collect data on the cases, and determine common features (Tyler and Last 1992). The case definition must be applied without bias to all persons under investigation.

Orient the Data in Terms of Time, Place, and Person. Each case must be defined according to standard epidemiologic parameters: the date of onset of the illness, the place where the person lives or became ill, and the socio-demographic characteristics (e.g., age, sex, education level, occupation). Graphic depiction of cases will aid in showing the relationship between case frequency and their time of occurrence (known as the "epidemic curve") (Figure 3-2). Graphical representation typically shows the number of cases (y axis) over the appropriate time interval of the date of onset (x axis). In addition, a spot map can be useful in determining the spatial relation of cases (Figure 3-4). Although initial description of cases may superficially seem simple, it can lead to complex and difficult issues. For example, if one is investigating an outbreak in a multiracial population, public health surveillance information may be ambiguous in the classification of race and ethnicity due to lack of consensus in measuring these variables (Hahn and Stroup 1994).

Determine Who is at Risk of Having the Health Problem. Preliminary analysis of the data to this point often provides enough information to determine with reasonable certainty how and why the outbreak started (Gregg 1996a). However, in outbreaks that cover large geographic areas, it may be extremely difficult to determine who is at risk. A preliminary survey may be necessary to obtain more specific information about the group of ill persons.

Develop an Explanatory Hypothesis. This step, the first real foray into analytic epidemiology, involves the assessment of the data collected to date and the generation of hypotheses that may explain the outbreak. The goal is to explain the specific exposure(s) that caused the outbreak. This step is often the most difficult to perform. In nearly every outbreak investigation, a priori hypotheses are voiced by public health professionals, affected persons, the media, employers, or others (Palmer 1989). Careful examination of descriptive epidemiologic data can exclude many possible hypotheses and will often stimulate alternative hypotheses.

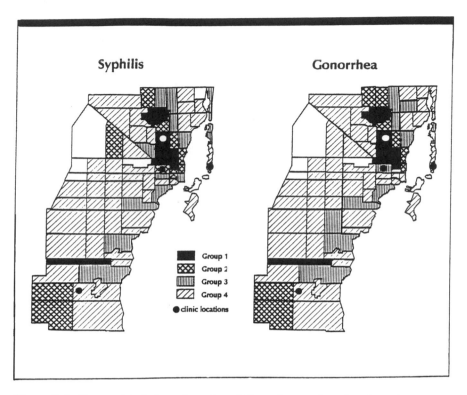

Figure 3-4. Geographical clustering of syphilis and gonorrhea, by zip code group, Dade County, Florida, 1986–1990; *Source:* Hamers et al. (1995)

Compare the Hypothesis with the Established Facts. At this point, the goal is to compare the hypothesis with the clinical, laboratory, and other epidemiologic data. The key issue is whether the data collected thus far fit with what is known about the disease (i.e., its method of spread, incubation period, duration of illness, population affected).

Plan and Execute a More Systematic Study. After completion of the initial outbreak investigation, a more systematic study may be necessary, depending on whether there is a need to find more cases, better define the extent of the outbreak, or evaluate a new laboratory or case-finding method. The epidemiologic approaches most commonly used in this phase are case-control and retrospective cohort studies. Both of these designs are discussed in the later section on "Analytic Study Designs" and in Chapter 2. In planning a detailed epidemiologic study of an outbreak it is important to carefully address ethical issues related to informed consent, protections of confidentiality, and reporting of results (see Chapter 1 and Coughlin and Beauchamp 1996).

Prepare a Written Report. The development of a written summary of an outbreak is an essential part of the investigation, just as a hospital discharge summary is key for patient care (Tyler and Last 1992). Of utmost importance, the written report serves as a basis for public health action—namely, implementing prevention and control measures outlined in the next section. The process of writing the report and the report itself can provide (1) information to the public about the outbreak, (2) new insights into the characteristics of the outbreak including the agent and its spread, (3) a record of performance of the outbreak investigation team, (4) documentation of potential legal issues, and (5) a means for teaching epidemiology (Gregg 1996a).

Execute Control and Prevention Measures. The underlying purpose of most outbreak investigations is to develop and implement appropriate measures of prevention and control. Methods to eliminate the current outbreak and to prevent future similar outbreaks may involve one or more of the following: (1) eliminate the source of the pathogen or the exposure of susceptibles to it; (2) interrupt the spread from the source to the susceptibles, and (3) protect the susceptibles from the consequences of exposure even when the source or method of transmission cannot be controlled (Kelsey et al. 1996) (Table 3-3). After a control measure has been implemented, ongoing evaluation is necessary to determine effectiveness.

Several examples illustrate the interplay between etiology, mode of transmission, and disease control measures (Figure 3-5) (Goodman et al. 1990a). A single case of hepatitis A in a daycare setting can lead to prophylactic administration of immune globulin to an entire group of children and staff (CDC 1985). A multistate outbreak of *Salmonella muenchen* required extensive outbreak investigation, including a case-control study. This investigation found

Table 3-3. Elements of Outbreak Control

Action	*Example*
Control the source of the pathogen	Remove the source of contamination
	Remove persons from exposure
	Inactivate or neutralize the pathogen
	Isolate and/or treat the infected person(s)
Interrupt the transmission	Sterilize or interrupt environmental sources of spread (e.g., water, milk, air)
	Control mosquito or insect transmission
	Improve personal sanitation (e.g., hand washing)
Control or modify the host response to exposure	Immunize the susceptibles
	Use prophylactic chemotherapy

Source: Kelsey et al. (1996).

Source/Transmission Mode

	known	unknown
known	Investigation: + Control: +++ Example: Hepatitis A in day care (CDC 1985)	Investigation: +++ Control: + Example: Salmonellosis and marijuana (Taylor et al. 1982)
unknown	Investigation: +++ Control: +++ Example: Parathion poisoning (Etzel et al. 1987)	Investigation: +++ Control: + Example: Legionnaires' disease (Fraser et al. 1977)

Etiology (row axis label)

Figure 3-5. Relative emphasis of investigative and control efforts (response options) in disease outbreaks as influenced by levels of certainty about etiology and source/ mode of transmission. "Investigation" means extent of the investigation; "control" means the basis for rapid implementation of control measures. Pluses show the level of response indicated: +, low; + +, intermediate; + + +, high. *Source:* Goodman et al. (1990a)

the mode of transmission to be personal use of or household exposure to marijuana (Taylor et al. 1982). In an outbreak of acute organophosphate poisoning, contaminated bread was shown as the source of exposure, allowing public health officials to make preventive recommendations before the etiologic agent (i.e., parathion) was isolated in the laboratory (Etzel et al. 1987). In the Legionnaires' disease outbreak of 1976, extensive field investigation failed to identify either the etiology or source of the outbreak in sufficient time to control the acute problem (Fraser et al. 1977).

Analytic Study Designs

The case-control study and the retrospective cohort study are the two most common designs used in outbreak investigations (Dwyer et al. 1994; Buehler and Dicker 1996). Each of these designs has advantages and disadvantages. Rather than a detailed review of each study design, this chapter will present a brief discussion of the use of each study design in outbreak investigations. Detailed descriptions are available elsewhere (Schlesselman 1982; Hennekens and Buring 1987; Lilienfeld and Stolley 1994; Kelsey et al. 1996).

Case-Control Studies. Over the past few decades, the case-control method has grown in prominence as an important tool for outbreak investigation. A comparison of the use of case-control studies within 6-year periods of the 1960s, 1970s, and 1980s showed a clear increase in frequency of use (Fonseca and Armenian 1991). The proportion of published outbreak investigations that used case-control methods increased from 0.2% in the 1960 period to 5.7% in the 1970 period to 17.0% in the 1980 period. Methodologic improvements were increasingly noted over time including more frequent reporting of control selection, exposures, possible biases, and control of confounders.

Three specific circumstances have been cited where case-control studies are the most appropriate method of formally testing hypotheses in outbreak investigations (Dwyer et al. 1994). These situations take into account the advantages and disadvantages of each study design. First, in a large outbreak where it would be necessary to enumerate (i.e., obtain a complete list of individuals) an entire cohort to conduct a retrospective cohort study, a case-control sample is much faster and less costly because full enumeration is not necessary. Second, the complete cohort at risk cannot be adequately defined or a discrete cohort cannot be fully enumerated. Third, case-control studies can be conducted within cohort studies ("nested case-control studies") to test specific hypotheses that would be too expensive or infeasible to study in an entire cohort.

Retrospective Cohort Studies. The retrospective cohort study is a commonly used design in outbreak investigations. In a retrospective cohort study, the outcomes (i.e., a disease or health condition) have all occurred prior to the start of the investigation and the experience of cohorts is reconstructed through existing records. The general characteristics of a retrospective cohort design are discussed in Chapter 2. They often measure the association between exposure and disease by means of the risk ratio or relative risk (i.e., the attack rate in the exposed divided by the attack rate in the unexposed).

Advantages and Disadvantages. The advantages of the case-control method tend to highlight the disadvantages of the cohort method. The main advantages of the case-control method (and disadvantages of the cohort design) are that results can be obtained relatively quickly, at relatively low costs; multiple exposures can be studied; and enumeration of the whole cohort is not required when a representative sample of cases can be obtained. The major disadvantages of case-control studies (and advantages of the cohort design) include the inability to directly measure the attack rate, higher potential for bias in retrospectively measuring risk factors, the inability to evaluate multiple disease outcomes, and the potential for bias in control group selection.

Epidemiologic Challenges in Outbreak Investigations

In this section, we highlight a few biases and unique challenges in outbreak investigations that are likely to be encountered and particularly problematic. Some of these issues are common to any epidemiologic study and are discussed further in Chapter 2.

Sampling Bias. Sampling is a method of gathering information that otherwise would not be available (Peavy 1996). Sampling bias is a "systematic error due to study of a nonrandom sample of a population" (Last 1995). Outbreak investigations may be particularly prone to sampling bias because persons involved in an outbreak may have a particular interest in not cooperating in the study (e.g., employees of a restaurant concerned about job loss). As noted earlier, appropriate selection of controls is a key issue in conducting a sound case-control study. In other situations, affected persons in an outbreak may be dispersed (e.g., illness among airline passengers), making full enumeration of cases difficult.

Measurement Bias. Measurement bias is a systematic error resulting from inaccurate classification of study subjects (i.e., misclassification bias). Such a bias can result in misclassification of exposure and/or disease status. For example, in an outbreak investigation, laboratory confirmation may not be possible and cases may be classified based on signs and symptoms. If cases are misclassified and have disparate etiologies, erroneous conclusions may be drawn. Information in an outbreak investigation is frequently collected by questionnaire. The sensitivity and specificity of outbreak questionnaires have not been frequently evaluated (Palmer 1989). Techniques to minimize differential misclassification in assessment of risk factors include using standardized questionnaire designs when possible, checking data against other sources (e.g., menus, discussion with relatives), and providing background details of events to enhance recall (Palmer 1989).

Small Sample Sizes. Unlike analytic epidemiologic studies that are designed and implemented over a period of years, outbreak investigations are "natural experiments" and the researcher has relatively little control over the number of affected subjects available for study (Goodman et al. 1990a). This can impose a serious restriction on the statistical power of the study, making detection of moderate or weak risk factors extremely difficult.

Publicity. Frequently, outbreak investigations are conducted in the midst of considerable publicity. Such public attention may occur at local, regional, national, and occasionally international levels (CDC 1995a). Publicity can be both beneficial and detrimental to the investigation process. On the positive side, public attention may encourage full participation of study subjects in the investigation, and the early involvement of the media and the public may be beneficial if and when control measures are implemented. Conversely, widespread publicity may lead to study subjects having a preconception about the cause(s) of an outbreak, potentially resulting in biased study conclusions (Goodman et al. 1990a).

Lack of Public Health Infrastructure. Although nearly all public health departments commonly have some level of resources dedicated to outbreak investigation, a shortage of trained epidemiologists in the public health setting may result in less than optimal outbreak investigation.

Cluster Investigations

Clustering of disease has intrigued public health professionals for many years and some cluster investigations have led to important scientific discoveries. For example, the investigation of spatial clustering of enamel discoloration early in the twentieth century led to discovery of the relation between flouride levels in drinking water and dental caries (Rothman 1987). Another notable cluster investigation led to the epidemiologic discovery that clustering of vaginal cancer was linked with diethylstibesterol use during pregnancy (Herbst et al. 1971).

Most cluster investigations focus on cancer etiology. The role of cluster investigations in the discovery of 35 carcinogens has been summarized (International Agency for Research on Cancer 1987; Neutra 1990). Many of these carcinogens were discovered through occupational (46%) or medical (29%) cluster investigations. Only one, the mineral erionite, was discovered from the investigation of a neighborhood cluster (Neutra 1990). Even this single case was not a classic space–time cluster but was only a space cluster (Neutra 1990). Investigations of potential cancer clusters began at the CDC in 1961, largely to determine if there was a single infectious, causative agent for some types of cancer, most likely a virus (Caldwell 1990). Over a period of 22 years, 108 reported cancer clusters were investigated. Among these, the majority involved leukemia only (38%) or leukemia and lymphoma (30%). In the summary of these investigations, no clear-cut etiologic relationships were established.

A real or perceived cluster can have a significant impact on the psychosocial and economic well-being of a community. Such an impact was illustrated in a case study from two suburbs of Edmonton, Alberta (Guidotti and Jacobs 1993). Initial analysis of epidemiologic data suggested a cancer excess for most major sites and types of cancer in men and women although many individual sites were not statistically significantly elevated. However, reanalysis of these data several months later revealed an error in the population figures used in the original calculations that had artificially elevated incidence rates. After correction of the error, the sole elevation occurred for bladder cancer in women (Guidotti and Jacobs 1993). Due to the incident and considerable media coverage, public opinions and property values were assessed in the affected communities and a nearby comparison community. Despite the lack of a true cluster, survey data showed a significant increase in perception of personal, family, and community risk in the affected communities. Property values in one affected community temporarily lost 5% of total value, compared with a similar adjacent housing market.

Types of Clusters

A spatial cluster occurs when the disease in question has a higher incidence rate in some places than in others (Rothman 1990). Virtually every disease shows some degree of spatial clustering. A temporal cluster occurs when a disease has a higher rate at some times than at others. Temporal clustering also includes cyclic variation, in which the change in incidence rates occurs at regular intervals (Rothman 1990). In a space–time cluster, more than the expected number of cases of a given disease occurs in a defined locality during some period of time (e.g., an excess of childhood leukemia in a neighborhood over a given time period). A time–cohort cluster is more than the expected number of cases of a given disease in a group of people who have some other characteristic in common besides their place of residence (e.g., an occupational cancer cluster).

Guidelines for Cluster Investigations in the Community Setting

Public health agencies will frequently receive requests to investigate potential clusters of noninfectious diseases from health professionals, policy-makers, community activists, and the general public. Knowing that the scientific value of cluster investigations may be limited, should a public health agency provide an investigation of potential disease clusters? If the goal is to determine the cause(s) of a particular disease cluster, the answer is probably "No." However, if the goal is to provide a service to the public that will not be available elsewhere, there is a definite need to investigate potential disease clusters.

If one accepts the premise that clusters should be investigated, the question becomes, "should a more active or passive approach be taken?" The active approach involves continually examining disease registries and systems to search out clusters. In a passive approach, public health agencies evaluate potential clusters that are brought to their attention. After about a decade of relying mainly on the passive approach in cluster investigations, the California Department of Health Services has determined that most clusters should be followed up after they are brought to attention (Smith and Neutra 1993). Active surveillance is reserved for new or emerging environmental issues and may have the most utility in the occupational setting where exposures are generally more limited and defined. In practical terms, most state health agencies lack the resources to actively seek out and investigate noninfectious disease clusters.

Most practitioners and researchers (Schulte et al. 1987; California Dept of Health Services 1989; Bender et al. 1990; Devier et al. 1990) agree that the most useful method for responding to potential clusters is a staged or stepwise approach, with a strong emphasis on public health education. A public health agency framework for cluster investigation is shown in Table 3-4. Although not explicitly stated, an advisory committee, with diverse membership, can provide valuable review and assistance in determining closure or continuation of a particular investigation at various stages (CDC 1990; Devier et al. 1990). Although this may appear as a linear process, several steps may be occurring simultaneously and the staged approach allows opportunities for closure of a particular cluster investigation at numerous points. In most states, linkage of the cluster investigation process with other programs and registries (e.g., cancer registries, birth defects registries) is possible and will enhance the investigation. The framework for cancer cluster investigations outlined by the CDC (CDC 1990) also has been successfully applied to other noninfectious diseases such as spontaneous abortions (McDiarmid et al. 1994).

Experience in cancer cluster investigations from California has shown the utility of this staged, systematic approach (Smith and Neutra 1993). During 1991, from a total of 41 reports of potential cancer clusters, 56% were resolved with a phone call or visit. Of the remaining 44% that required additional follow-up (e.g., index case verification, case finding, statistical calculations), three investigations (7% of the total) became an epidemiologic or exposure assessment study.

Similarly, the value of a systematic protocol was illustrated in a descriptive study of 141 noninfectious disease cluster investigations from Wisconsin (Fiore et al. 1990). Most of these investigations (77%) focused on potential cancer clusters, followed by reproductive outcomes (10%) and other chronic diseases (13%). Forty-four percent of reports were adequately addressed through the initial contact and investigation, 43% required descriptive analyses but no site visit, and 13% (n = 18) required a site visit including

Table 3-4. Framework for a Cluster Investigation in a State or Local Health Agency

Major Stage	Question/Procedure
1. Initial contact and response	What are the characteristics of the reporting party and the potential cluster? • gather identifying information on the caller • gather initial data on the potential cluster • discuss initial impressions with the caller • request further information, schedule follow-up contact • provide assurance that a written response will be issued • maintain a log of each contact • notify health agency public information office
2. Assessment: preliminary evaluation ("in-house" evaluation)	What are the descriptive epidemiologic characteristics of the potential cluster? • determine the appropriate geographic area and the period in which to study the cluster • determine which cases will be included in the analysis • determine an appropriate reference population • if case size is sufficient, calculate rates and ratios • if case size is not sufficient for rates, determine the appropriate use of alternative statistical tests
Case evaluation	• verify the diagnosis by reviewing health registry data and/or contacting physicians • obtain pathology and/or medical examiner's reports • if relevant, obtain histologic evaluation
Occurrence evaluation (requires field evaluation)	• determine the appropriate geographic area and temporal boundaries • ascertain all potential cases

(continued)

simple exposure assessment (e.g., well water testing). None of the reports resulted in a full analytic investigation.

When using a staged approach, others have estimated that the majority (50–60%) of investigations can be closed after the initial contact and response (Aldrich et al. 1993). An additional 20–30% of investigations can be closed during some phase of the assessment. Only about 5% of investigations should be considered for a full etiologic investigation. A full investigation should be carefully considered as it can be extremely resource intensive with relatively little chance of producing scientifically meaningful results.

Cluster Investigations in the Occupational Setting

Although the study of disease clusters in the workplace has received relatively little systematic attention (Fleming et al. 1992), studies of clustering in the occupational setting have identified important exposure–disease relationships

Table 3-4. (continued)

Major Stage	Question/Procedure
	• identify the appropriate data bases for numerators and denominators
	• identify statistical and epidemiologic procedures to be used
	• perform an in-depth review of the literature
	• assess the likelihood that an exposure–event relationship may be established
	• complete the proposed descriptive epidemiologic study
3. Major Feasibility Study	What is the feasibility and utility of conducting an epidemiologic study linking the putative exposure to the health event?
	• review the detailed literature with particular attention to the exposure–health outcome of interest
	• consider the appropriate study design and alternatives
	• determine the data that would need to be collected
	• delineate the logistics of data collection and processing
	• determine the appropriate plan of analysis, including hypotheses to be tested and study power
	• assess the current social and political climate and the potential impact of study findings
	• assess the resource requirements and implications
4. Etiologic investigation	What are the etiologic factors responsible for the disease cluster?
	• conduct a full investigation of the cluster using established methods in epidemiology[a]

Source: CDC (1990); California Dept of Health Services (1989); Devier et al. (1990).

[a] See Chapter 2 and other epidemiology texts (Schlesselman 1982; Hennekens and Buring 1987; Kelsey et al. 1996) for full coverage of methods.

(e.g., vinyl chloride exposure and angiosarcoma of the liver, dibromochloropropane and male infertility). Occupational clusters may be investigated by public health agencies or in larger worksites, by epidemiologic or medical personnel of the company.

In contrast to several of the disadvantages encountered when investigating clusters in the general community, a number of advantages can be cited for studying the relationships between various occupational exposures and potential clusters, including: the clear definition of a population at risk, allowing identification of a denominator; shared, measurable exposures that are often higher than those in the general populations; useful intermediate hypotheses that may identify a job classification (e.g., a painter or a printer) associated with a disease outcome prior to establishment of the specific exposure; and availability of comparable populations to test etiologic hypotheses in retrospective cohort studies (Fleming et al. 1991, 1992).

Even with these advantages for cluster studies in the occupational setting, epidemiologic challenges are substantial. Several of the scientific and pragmatic issues encountered in occupational cluster investigation are illustrated by the experience of the National Institute for Occupational Safety and Health (NIOSH) in investigating 61 potential clusters of cancer in the workplace (Schulte et al. 1987). Investigation of a potential cancer cluster by NIOSH was prompted by one of the following: (1) more than one relatively young person in a workforce developed cancer; (2) workers or employers noticed more than one case of apparently the same type of cancer in a workforce or there was a general feeling among workers or employers that there was too much cancer in a workforce; or (3) there was a realization that workers were potentially exposed to a carcinogen (Schulte et al. 1987). Of the 61 reported clusters, only 16 had an observed versus expected excess of cancer. Among these 16, only five were plausible in terms of an occupational etiology. For most situations, there was no identified environmental exposure, and in some instances, there was an insufficient induction period. The researchers noted scientific issues that add to the difficulty of clearly identifying occupational cancer clusters that are biologically plausible: (1) numerous large cancer risks due to occupational carcinogens have been previously identified and in many cases controlled, making evaluation of current potential clusters more subtle; (2) most of the cases studied involved exposures within the past 5 years, yet induction periods for many occupational cancers are considerably longer (most often between 10 and 20 years); and (3) many of the cancer types identified (e.g., breast cancer, Hodgkin's disease) are not generally considered to have occupational etiologies. Despite the scientific difficulties, the researchers acknowledged the obligation and importance of occupational cluster investigations. Many investigations of perceived cancer clusters involve less epidemiologic methodology and more epidemiologic interpretation and explanation.

Epidemiologic Challenges in Cluster Investigations

Several of the difficulties encountered in cluster investigations parallel those discussed earlier for investigations of outbreaks and occupational clusters; others are more applicable to cluster studies due to their noninfectious nature. Limitations have been summarized by several researchers (CDC 1990; Rothman 1990; Neutra 1990). Rothman (1990) has suggested that there is "little scientific or public health purpose to investigate individual disease clusters at all." While it is likely that scientific potential is limited, cluster investigations can serve important public health functions. The following section outlines a few of the most important challenges one may encounter in a cluster investigation. The difficulties stem in part from the constraints of available information in a typical cluster investigation (Reynolds et al. 1996).

Rare Health Events. Cluster investigations tend to focus on relatively rare health events (e.g., those with incidence rates less than 10 per 100,000 persons). Due to these relatively small numbers, standard statistical methods that rely on normal or near-normal distributions cannot be used in most cluster investigations. Therefore, alternative statistical tests are needed (see the next section, "Statistical Methods for Cluster Investigations").

Vague Definition and/or Heterogeneity of Cases. Accurate definition and enumeration of cases are essential elements of cluster investigations. Frequently, reported clusters have vague case definitions, or cases that may appear to represent one disease may actually represent many diseases. For example, a citizen may be concerned that "we have an excess of cancer." After investigation, it may be revealed that many types of cancer are present, each with a distinct etiology.

Lack of a Population Base for Rate Calculation. A population at risk must be determined in order to calculate rates. In a cluster investigation, the geographic distribution of the reported cases commonly does not coincide with boundaries for population (denominator) data such as counties, zip codes, or census tracts. This makes accurate calculation of rates difficult and sometimes impossible.

Weak Associations and Multiple Risk Factors. The difficulties in measuring weak associations are discussed elsewhere in this book (Chapters 1 and 2). Many noninfectious disease clusters are purported to be environmentally related, and if an association exists, relative risk estimates are likely to be less than three. Statistical power calculations for many chronic disease clusters have suggested that relative risk estimates must be 8 or larger to achieve statistical significance (Neutra 1990). Such a large risk estimate in most cluster investigations is unlikely.

In addition, noninfectious diseases, in particular chronic diseases, have multifactoral etiologies (Brownson et al. 1993). As noted in Chapters 1 and 2, these risk factors can be especially subject to methodologic biases. In practice, this combination of weak, multiple risk factors means that an analytic study to assess causation may require hundreds or thousands of cases to detect a statistically significant relative risk estimate.

Long Induction Periods. The induction period is the interval from the time from the exposure and causal action of a risk factor to the initiation of the disease (Last 1995). With infectious diseases and chemical outbreaks, the relevant exposures occurred only hours or days earlier. Yet for many chronic diseases with long induction periods (years or decades), assessment of relevant exposure is extremely difficult.

Multiple Comparisons. An epidemiologic study has a higher probability of producing a statistically significant result when a large number of comparisons or associations are examined. Therefore, it may be relatively easy to detect statistical clusters because of the vast number of comparisons by geographic area, number of conditions (e.g., types of cancer), and temporal options. Therefore, active public health surveillance for clusters may lead to false positives.

Low-Level, Long-Term, Heterogeneous Exposures. As noted earlier, relevant exposures in noninfectious disease clusters may have occurred years or decades prior to disease initiation. In addition, cluster investigations with a suspected environmental etiology commonly involve exposures that are much too low to produce measurable effects. For example, it is estimated that one would need about 70% of a maximum tolerate dose of a carcinogen for a full year to produce a sevenfold increase in a moderately rare cancer (Neutra et al. 1989; Neutra 1990). Advances in molecular epidemiology cited in Chapter 1 may assist in determining appropriate biomarkers to measure exposure.

Intense Publicity. As noted earlier for outbreak investigations, media publicity and public controversy can make the unbiased investigation of clusters difficult.

Resource Intensiveness of Full Investigations. Conducting an analytic epidemiologic study of a disease cluster requires considerable resources and takes months or years to complete. These investigations can seriously impact the resources of state and local health departments and are not always the best use of public resources. In addition, the time needed to complete a sound investigation may be perceived as "foot-dragging" by members of the public who desire a more immediate answer. It has been proposed that full investigations should be limited to clusters that have potentially large relative risk estimates, at least five confirmed cases, and good estimates of personal exposure (Neutra 1990).

Statistical Methods for Cluster Investigations

Traditional statistical methods used in descriptive epidemiology (e.g., calculations of rates and ratios) were primarily developed to reflect large sample sizes and a definable population at risk. Because cluster investigations commonly involve small numbers of cases that may have developed over several years, alternative statistical techniques have been developed to determine whether a disease cluster can be attributed to chance alone (Lilienfeld and Stolley 1994). The uses and limitations of these techniques constitute a controversial area in epidemiology in part due to the diverse and complicated nature of clusters (CDC 1990; Rothenberg et al. 1990). It is important to note that these statistical methods for cluster evaluation are exploratory methods— their greatest value may be in attempting to prove or disprove a report of a cluster, yet do not infer etiology (Aldrich et al. 1993).

Most statistical tests for clusters have been developed through cancer cluster investigations and fall into two categories: cell occupancy tests and interval approaches. To illustrate the use of statistical methods in cluster investigations, these two common methods are discussed.

Many of the statistical tests developed to test the statistical significance of clusters use the Poisson distribution, which is a distribution function designed to test the occurrence of rare events in a continuum of time or space (Last 1995). The number of events has a Poisson distribution with parameter λ (lambda) if the probability of observing k events ($k = 0, 1, \ldots$) is equal to:

$$p(x = k) = \frac{e^{-\lambda} \lambda^k}{k!}$$

where e is the base of natural logarithm (2.7183) and the mean and variance of the distribution are both equal to λ. This distribution is used in modeling person-time incidence rates (Last 1995).

The cell occupancy method begins by defining discrete units of time or space (Ederer et al. 1964). The study area is divided into "subareas" (e.g., census tracts, townships). The study period over which the events are identified is divided into a number of k intervals of constant length (e.g., months, 1-year intervals). From a total of r cases, events are classified according to the time interval and the largest number of cases (m_I) in any single time interval is noted. The sum of these frequencies across all subareas results in the chi-square statistic (χ^2) that is used to test for space–time clustering. The null distribution of m_I is multinomial $(1/k + \ldots + 1/k)^r$. A limitation of this method is that it assumes that no important population changes have occurred over time in the study area over time (Mantel 1967; Stroup 1994).

To address the limitation of equal population density across all cells, the interval approach attempts to measure actual observed time and space intervals between cases (Knox 1964a). All possible pairs of cases are examined and each of the $n(n - 1)/2$ pairs is scrutinized as being close or far apart in space to form a 2×2 contingency table.

Using the data from Table 3-5, Knox's method can be illustrated. Based

Table 3-5. Illustration of the Interval Approach to Detection of Space–Time Clustering: 96 Cases of Leukemia in Children Under 6 Years of Age in Northumberland and Durham, 1951–1961

Time Apart (days)	Distance Apart (km)		Total
	0–1	>1	
0–59	5	147	152
60–3,651	20	4,388	4,408
Total	25	4,535	4,560

Source: Knox (1964b); the table shows the space–time distances between all possible pairs (n = 4,560) of cases.

on leukemia occurrence in 96 children, there is a possibility of 4,560 pairs (96 × 95/2). A pair of cases is classified as close in space if the members resided within 1 km of each other and close in time if the cases occurred within 59 or fewer days of each other. Of the 4,560 pairs, 25 were close in space and 152 were close in time. The expected number is calculated for the 2 × 2 table (i.e., 25 × 152/4,560 = 0.83). Under the Poisson distribution, the five close pairs are in excess of the expected 0.83 ($p < 0.01$).

Although this method is useful, in part due to its conceptual simplicity, there are limitations. The choice of space and time distances can arbitrarily determine the extent of clustering (Smith 1982). It also does not allow for "edge effects" that may arise from natural geographic boundaries or lack of inclusion of unrecorded cases outside the specified study region (Stroup 1994).

This brief discussion on statistical methods illustrates a few common approaches to assessment of clustering. There are dozens of other statistical tests for detection of clusters and a software program called *CLUSTER* designed to perform many of these tests (Mantel 1967; Aldrich and Drane 1990).

Legal Considerations

Legal issues pertaining to outbreak and cluster investigations fall into three general areas: the legal basis for epidemiologic investigations, implications for field research, and legal considerations when epidemiologists and epidemiologic data become involved in litigation.

Both federal and state governments have inherent powers to protect the health of the public (Neslund 1996). The federal government has broad oversight for health-related activities such as licensure and regulation of drugs, biological substances, and medical devices (Neslund 1996). States have more extensive legal powers rooted in the mandate to protect the peace, safety, health, and general welfare of their citizens. Under this rubric is the public health authority to conduct epidemiologic investigations of outbreaks and clusters.

Given this authority, outbreak and cluster researchers should consider several key issues when embarking on a field investigation. Investigators must be aware of legal protections for records and information that will be examined in conjunction with outbreak and cluster investigations. Most states have specific laws to protect the confidentiality of medical and public health records. In many cases, only authorized individuals are afforded access to such records and these must be retained in a secure manner (Neslund 1996). Investigations may identify "reportable diseases" (see Chapter 4) and researchers may have an obligation to report these to the proper public health authorities. Because investigations involve human subjects, attention must be paid to federal and state regulations that require the informed consent of individuals who are interviewed or studied.

Epidemiologic evidence is increasingly being used in court cases (Lilienfeld and Black 1986); data from both outbreak and cluster investigations are likely to be used as testimony in civil or criminal trials (Black 1990; Goodman et al. 1990a). Governing this type of litigation is the law of torts, which applies when a person seeks legal redress for personal injuries (Black 1990). In most tort cases, a plaintiff must show that the evidence presented shows the alleged facts are more likely than not true (Cleary et al. 1984). These cases often put epidemiologists in unfamiliar territory—scientific training seldom prepares one to examine such issues in a legal setting. The epidemiologic concept of attributable risk coincides nicely with certain legal cases, particularly so-called toxic tort cases. If more than 50% of the cases in an exposed population can be attributed to an exposure and if the basic causal criteria of epidemiology are satisfied, it can be legally deemed that more likely than not his or her illness was caused by the exposure (Black and Lilienfeld 1984; Black 1990). This contrasts sharply with the epidemiologic level of proof commonly applied in which demonstration of 95% or greater probability suggests that the results of a given study were not due to chance (Hoffman 1984). Since an epidemiologist involved in any outbreak or cluster investigation may become part of a legal action, it is imperative to maintain meticulous study records and if necessary, consult with an expert in health law. In some instances, affected persons in an outbreak or cluster investigation may become clients of a toxic tort attorney and due to legal considerations may be counseled not to cooperate in an investigation.

Summary

This review of the current state of the art in outbreak and cluster investigations gives rise to several summary conclusions and recommendations.

Scientific Opportunities and Public Health Roles

In general, outbreak investigations have been more fruitful in leading to scientific discoveries in epidemiology than have studies of clusters. Because outbreak investigations are "natural experiments" and their methods are relatively well established, they provide unique opportunities in applied epidemiology (Goodman et al. 1990a; Gregg et al. 1996). A properly conducted outbreak investigation can lead to rapid implementation of control measures, to new discoveries about risk factors, and to important field training opportunities through programs such as the EIS (Langmuir 1980).

In spite of the relatively low scientific value of cluster investigations, there is an obligation for the public health system to quickly and systematically respond to reports of potential disease clusters (Neutra 1990). The lack of a response can foster an atmosphere of skepticism and may lead the community or the media to perceive a cover-up.

During a cluster investigation, the appropriate role of the public health agency is to maintain objectivity, develop effective communication strategies, provide leadership on controversial issues, and conduct sound science in the investigation (Bender et al. 1990). State public health agencies and larger city and county public health agencies should have official policies that describe how they will respond to reports of perceived disease clusters. The work of selected state health agencies (e.g., California, Minnesota, Missouri, Wisconsin) and the CDC has been useful in providing an initial framework for such guidelines. Public health professionals should view cluster investigations as an important opportunity for public education.

In most states, the state health officer or designee (typically the "state epidemiologist") has statutory authority for outbreak investigations (Dwyer et al. 1994). It seems appropriate and useful to designate a similar authority for investigation of potential clusters of noninfectious diseases. There is now a "state chronic disease epidemiologist" designated in every state and this person is likely to be qualified to oversee cluster investigations.

In addition, outbreak and cluster investigations in the public health setting provide an ideal opportunity for collaborations between public health officials at the local, state, and federal levels, academic researchers, and medical professionals.

Methodological Issues

Methodology in outbreak and cluster investigation has become increasingly refined. Case-control studies are becoming more frequently used in outbreak investigations and this may become the single most frequently used application of the case-control method (Fonseca and Armenian 1991). Statistical methods to detect clusters are fairly well established, yet major limitations remain when analytic epidemiology is invoked to determine etiology. As biomarker research evolves, it may prove a useful adjunct to cluster investigations by allowing detection of intermediate markers of exposure and disease. Studies of outbreaks and clusters are subject to many sources of methodologic bias, most notably sampling and measurement biases.

Communication and Media Considerations

Perhaps more important than many of the scientific issues concerning outbreak and cluster investigations, effective communication is a key component of the investigation process. Data are not useful to the public and to other scientists unless findings are convincingly communicated (King 1991). Essential ingredients of successful communication of information to a scientific audience have been outlined by others (Gregg 1996b) and are summarized in Chapter 11.

Communication is often necessary with the general public, affected workers, the media, and policy-makers. The best advice to an epidemiologist involved in communication of health risk information about an outbreak or cluster investigation is probably to seek out the help of an expert in health communication (e.g., a health psychologist). In some circumstances, qualitative methods such as focus groups may serve an important purpose in assessing risk perceptions among population subgroups.

In the media setting, several recommendations have been proposed on how epidemiologists can improve news coverage of disease outbreaks and clusters (Greenberg and Wartenberg 1990a,b; Dan 1996). Several important points:

- Epidemiologists should summarize the two or three most important pieces of health risk information for any given story; these key points should be repeated early and often during the interview.
- For television and radio, 15–30-second-long quotable statements should be prepared on each key point.
- Avoid jargon; language should be understandable and interesting to the general public.
- Quotable statements should address what the citizens can and should do to protect their health.

In summary, this chapter has highlighted the important public health role in outbreak and cluster investigations. Methodologic advances (e.g., more refined case-control methods) have improved over the past decade, yet substantial challenges remain. A combination of scientific and communication skills are needed to effectively deal with reports of outbreaks and clusters.

CASE STUDIES

Outbreak Investigation of Ebola Viral Hemorrhagic Fever

Background

Ebola virus and Marburg virus are the two known members of the filovirus family (CDC 1995a). The Ebola virus is responsible for viral hemorrhagic fever (VHF), which is initially characterized by fever, headache, chills, myalgia, and malaise. Subsequent manifestations include severe abdominal pain, vomiting, and diarrhea. In reported outbreaks of VHF, case-fatality rates have ranged between 50% and 90% (CDC 1995a). Ebola viruses were first isolated from humans during concurrent outbreaks of VHF in northern Zaire and southern Sudan in 1976. Four additional outbreaks of VHF in humans have been reported. In 1989, an outbreak of Ebola virus infection occurred among monkeys imported into the United States but was not associated with human disease.

Most recently, an outbreak of VHF occurred in Kikwit, Zaire, between January and June 1995 (CDC 1995a). This outbreak received international attention due to the high fatality rate and unknown reservoir and mode of spread. During this period, 315 persons developed VHF and 244 died of the disease, a case fatality rate of 77% (Stoekle and Douglas 1996). The World Health Organization and the CDC investigated the 1995 outbreak, based on the request of the government of Zaire.

Key Questions

1. How can modern laboratory technologies be used to determine objective case definitions for VHF?

In the 1995 outbreak investigation of VHF, two laboratory tests were used to verify cases: an enzyme-linked immunosorbent assay and reverse transcription-polymerase chain reaction (CDC 1995a).

2. Which high-risk groups were identified during the course of outbreak investigation of VHF?

Among ill persons, the median age was 37 years; cases were evenly distributed between men and women (CDC 1995b). One third of cases involved health care workers.

3. What is the mode of transmission for Ebola virus infection?

Transmission of VHF is suspected to occur from direct contact with ill persons or their body or body fluids (CDC 1996). The natural reservoir remains a mystery and effective prevention and control of VHF depends on identification of this reservoir (Stoekle and Douglas 1996).

4. What prevention measures can be implemented to control Ebola virus infection?

During the course of the outbreak in 1995, educational and quarantine measures were implemented to avoid further spread of VHF (CDC 1995a). Aggressive measures were needed due to the lack of a proven specific treatment or vaccine.

Implications for Practice
Active surveillance for VHF has been implemented in 13 clinics in Kikwit and 15 remote sites within a 150-mile radius of Kikwit (CDC 1995a). To minimize the potential of spread of Ebola virus to the United States, precautionary measures have been implemented: (1) issuance of a travel advisory to state and local health departments, federal agencies, airlines, travel agents, and travel clinics; (2) distribution of the routine Health Alert Notice to all passengers arriving in the United States from Europe and Africa; and (3) distribution of an Ebola Virus Hemorrhagic Fever Alert Notice to any travelers who have recently been in Zaire (CDC 1995b).

Suicide Clustering Among Teenagers

Background
Suicide is the third leading cause of death among adolescents and young adults, accounting for more than 5,000 deaths annually (National Center for Health Statistics 1996). From 1952 to 1992, the incidence of suicide among adolescents and young adults nearly tripled (CDC 1995c). An alarming aspect of youth suicides has been the contention that suicides tend to cluster.

Between February 1983 and October 1984, two clusters of teenage suicides were reported in Texas (Davidson et al. 1989). Descriptive data were collected on the eight reported suicides in site I and the six in site II; cases were verified by reviewing the official death investigations, autopsies, and toxicologic studies.

To better understand the factors responsible for these two clusters, a case-control study was conducted (Davidson et al. 1989). Three control teenagers were matched to each case on the basis of school district, grade, race, and sex. Researchers examined whether study subjects actually knew the person who committed suicide ("direct" exposure) or whether cases and controls knew the person who committed suicide only through news accounts or word of mouth ("indirect" exposure). Other study variables included exposure to personal violence, demographic data, physical and emotional health, behavioral patterns, and life events. Information on cases and controls was obtained from interviews with one or both parents.

Key Questions
1. What risk factors for teenage suicide can be identified from this analytic study of a cluster?

Cases were more likely to have attempted or threatened suicide previously (odds ratio [OR] = 79.5]), to have damaged themselves physically (OR = 85), to have known someone closely who died violently (OR = 12.6), and to have broken up with their girlfriends or boyfriends lately (OR = 42.8). Cases were not more likely than controls to have direct exposure to suicide as measured by their acquaintance with a person who committed suicide.

2. Are any of these risk factors modifiable?

Many of the risk factors identified could be modified; however, they are generally complex social and interpersonal risk factors that are not easily modified.

3. Are there sources of bias in the study that can explain these findings?

Use of surrogate respondents in studies of suicide may lead to recall bias. In addition, the small number of cases and controls makes effect estimates unstable, with large standard errors.

4. Could other unmeasured factors explain the clusters?

Given the complex nature of a behavior like suicide, there is likely an array of risk factors involved in etiology. However, given the large effect estimates identified by Davidson et al., it is likely that the risk factors noted are important determinants.

Implications for Practice

Researchers concluded that an analytic study of a suicide cluster can help identify high-risk youth and help direct preventive services. For example, identifying and treating youths with certain behaviors (e.g., violence, antisocial behavior) may collaterally reduce their risk of suicide. In addition, the CDC (1992) has suggested seven general strategies for preventing suicide among youth: (1) training school and community leaders to identify youth at highest risk; (2) educating young people about suicide, risk factors, and interventions; (3) implementing screening and referral programs; (4) developing peer-support programs; (5) establishing and operating suicide crisis centers and hotlines; (6) restricting access to highly lethal methods of suicide; and (7) intervening after a suicide crisis to prevent other young persons from attempting suicide.

SUGGESTED READINGS

Centers for Disease Control. Guidelines for investigating clusters of health events. Morb Mortal Wkly Rep 1990;39(RR-11):1–16.

Goodman RA, Buehler JW, Koplan JP. The epidemiologic field investigation: science and judgment in public health practice. Am J Epidemiol 1990;132:9–16.

Gregg MB, Dicker RC, Goodman RA. Field Epidemiology. New York: Oxford University Press; 1996.

National Conference on Clustering of Health Events. Am J Epidemiol 1990;132 (Suppl):S1–S202 [entire issue].

REFERENCES

Aldrich TE, Drane W. CLUSTER: User's Manual for Software to Assist with Investigations of Rare Health Events. Atlanta, GA: Agency for Toxic Substances and Disease Registries, Centers for Disease Control; 1990.

Aldrich TE, Drane W, Griffith J. Disease clusters. In: Aldrich TE, Griffith J, eds. Environmental Epidemiology and Risk Assessment. New York: Van Nostrand Reinhold; 1993:61–82.

Bender AP, Williams AN, Johnson RA, Jagger HG. Appropriate public health responses to clusters: the art of being responsibly responsive. Am J Epidemiol 1990;132:S48–S52.

Black B, Lilienfeld DE. Epidemiologic proof in toxic tort litigation. Fordham Law Rev 1984;52:732–785.

Black B. Matching evidence about clustered health events with tort law requirements. Am J Epidemiol 1990;132:S79–S86.

Brownson RC, Remington PL, Davis JR, eds. Chronic Disease Epidemiology and Control. Washington, DC: American Public Health Association; 1993.

Buehler JW, Dicker RC. Designing studies in the field. In: Gregg MB, Dicker RC, Goodman RA, eds. Field Epidemiology. New York: Oxford University Press; 1996:81–91.

Caldwell GG. Twenty-two years of cancer cluster investigations at the Centers for Disease Control. Am J Epidemiol 1990;132:S43–S47.

California Dept of Health Services. Investigating Possible Non-Infectious Disease Clusters. Berkeley, CA: Environmental Epidemiology and Toxicology Branch, California Department of Health Services; 1989.

Centers for Disease Control and Prevention. Toxic-shock syndrome—United States. Morb Mortal Wkly Rep 1980;29:229–230.

Centers for Disease Control and Prevention. Recommendations for protection against viral hepatitis. Morb Mortal Wkly Rep 1985;34:313–316.

Centers for Disease Control and Prevention. Proposed changes in format for presentation of notifiable disease report data. Morb Mortal Wkly Rep 1989;38:805–809.

Centers for Disease Control and Prevention. Guidelines for investigating clusters of health events. Morb Mortal Wkly Rep 1990;39(RR-11):1–16.

Centers for Disease Control and Prevention. Youth Suicide Prevention Programs: A Resource Guide. Atlanta, GA: US Dept Health and Human Services, CDC; 1992.

Centers for Disease Control and Prevention. Update: multistate outbreak of Escherichia coli O157:H7 infections from hamburgers—Western United States, 1992–1993. Morb Mortal Wkly Rep 1993;42:258–263.

Centers for Disease Control and Prevention. Outbreak of Ebola viral hemorrhagic fever—Zaire, 1995. Morb Mortal Wkly Rep 1995a;44:381–382.

Centers for Disease Control and Prevention. Update: outbreak of Ebola viral hemorrhagic fever—Zaire, 1995. Morb Mortal Wkly Rep 1995b;44:399.

Centers for Disease Control and Prevention. Suicide among children, adolescents, and young adults—United States, 1980–1992. Morb Mortal Wkly Rep 1995c;44:289–291.

Centers for Disease Control and Prevention. Shigella sonnei outbreak associated with contaminated drinking water—Island Park, Idaho, August 1995. Morb Mortal Wkly Rep 1996;45:229–231.

Centers for Disease Control and Prevention. Summary of Notifiable Diseases. Morb Mortal Wkly Rep 1997;46:13.

Cleary EW, Broun KS, Dix GE, et al. McCormick on Evidence. Third Edition. St. Paul, MN: West; 1984.

Coughlin SS, Beauchamp TL, eds. Ethics and Epidemiology. New York: Oxford University Press; 1996.

Cuzick J, Elliott P. Small area studies: purpose and methods. In: Elliott P, Cuzick J, English D, Stern R, eds. Geographical and Environmental Epidemiology: Methods for Small Area Studies. Oxford: Oxford University Press; 1992:14–21.

Dan BB. Dealing with the public and the media. In: Gregg MB, Dicker RC, Goodman RA, eds. Field Epidemiology. New York: Oxford University Press; 1996:181–193.

Davidson LE, Rosenberg ML, Mercy JA, Franklin J, Simmons JT. An epidemiologic study of risk factors in two teenage suicide clusters. JAMA 1989;262:2687–2692.

Devier JR, Brownson RC, Bagby JR Jr, Carlson GM, Crellin JR. A public health response to cancer clusters in Missouri. Am J Epidemiol 1990:132:S23–S31.

Diehr P, Cain K, Connell F, Volinn E. What is too much variation? The null hypothesis in small-area analysis. Health Services Res 1990;24:741–771.

Dwyer DM, Strickler H, Goodman RA, Armenian HK. Use of case-control studies in outbreak investigations. Epidemiol Rev 1994;16:109–123.

Ederer F, Myers MH, Mantel N. A statistical problem in space and time: do leukemia cases come in clusters? Biometrics 1964;20:626–638.

Elliott P. Investigation of disease risks in small areas. Occup Environ Med 1995; 52:785–789.

Etzel RA, Forthal DN, Hill RH Jr, et al. Fatal parathion poisoning in Sierra Leone. Bull WHO 1987;65:645–649.

Fiore BJ, Hanrahan LP, Anderson HA. State health department response to disease cluster reports: a protocol for investigation. Am J Epidemiol 1990;132:S14–S22.

Fleming LE, Ducatman AM, Shalat SL. Disease clusters: a central and ongoing role in occupational medicine. J Occup Med 1991;33:818–825.

Fleming LE, Ducatman AM, Shalat SL. Disease clusters in occupational medicine: a protocol for their investigation in the workplace. Am J Ind Med 1992;22:33–47.

Fonseca MGP, Armenian HK. Use of the case-control method in outbreak investigations. Am J Epidemiol 1991;133:748–752.

Fraser DW, Tsai TR, Orenstein W, et al. Legionnaires' disease: description of an epidemic of pneumonia. N Engl J Med 1977;297:1189–1197.

Goodman RA, Buehler JW, Koplan JP. The epidemiologic field investigation: science and judgment in public health practice. Am J Epidemiol 1990a;132:9–16.

Goodman RA, Bauman CF, Gregg MB, Videtto JF, Stroup DF, Chalmers NP. Epidemiologic field investigations by the Centers for Disease Control and Epidemic Intelligence Service, 1946–87. Public Health Rep 1990b;105:604–610.

Goodman RA, Buechler JW. Field epidemiology defined. In: Gregg MB, Dicker RC, Goodman RA, eds. Field Epidemiology. New York: Oxford University Press; 1996:3–8.

Goodman RA, Peavy JV. Describing epidemiologic data. In: Gregg MB, Dicker RC, Goodman RA, eds. Field Epidemiology. New York: Oxford University Press; 1996:60–80.

Greenberg M, Wartenberg D. Understanding mass media coverage of disease clusters. Am J Epidemiol 1990a;132:S192–S195.

Greenberg M, Wartenberg D. How epidemiologists can improve television network news coverage of disease cluster reports. Epidemiol 1990b;1:167–170.

Gregg MB. Conducting a field investigation. In: Gregg MB, Dicker RC, Goodman RA, eds. Field Epidemiology. New York: Oxford University Press; 1996a:44–59.

Gregg MB. Communicating epidemiologic findings. In: Gregg MB, Dicker RC, Goodman RA, eds. Field Epidemiology. New York: Oxford University Press; 1996b: 139–151.

Gregg MB, Dicker RC, Goodman RA, eds. Field Epidemiology. New York: Oxford University Press; 1996.

Guidotti TL, Jacobs P. The implications of an epidemiological mistake: a community's response to a perceived excess cancer risk. Am J Public Health 1993;83: 233–239.

Hahn RA, Stroup DF. Race and ethnicity in public health surveillance: criteria for the scientific use of social categories. Public Health Rep 1994;109:7–15.

Hamers FF, Peterman TA, Zaidi AA, Ransom RL, Wroten JE, Witte JJ. Syphilis and gonorrhea in Miami: similar clustering, different trends. Am J Public Health 1995;85:1104–1108.

Hennekens CH, Buring JE. Epidemiology in Medicine. Boston, MA: Little, Brown; 1987.

Herbst AL, Ulfelder H, Poskanzer DC. Adenocarcinoma of the vagina: association of maternal stilbestrol therapy with tumor appearance in young women. N Engl J Med 1971;284:878–881.

Hoffman RE. The use of epidemiologic data in the courts. Am J Epidemiol 1984;120:190–202.

Hoge CW, Bodhidatta L, Tungtaem C, Echeverria P. Emergence of nalidixic acid resistant Shigella dysenteriae type 1 in Thailand: an outbreak associated with consumption of coconut milk desert. Int J Epidemiol 1995;24:1228–1232.

International Agency for Research on Cancer. Monographs on the Evaluation of Carcinogenic Risk to Humans. Supplement 7. Overall Evaluations of Carcinogenicity: An Updating of IARC Monographs Volumes 1–42. Lyon, France: International Agency for Research on Cancer; 1987.

Kelsey JL, Whittemore AS, Evans AS, Thompson WD. Methods in Observational Epidemiology. Second Edition. New York: Oxford University Press; 1996.

King LS. Why Not Say It Clearly: A Guide to Expository Writing. Second Edition. Boston: Little, Brown; 1991.

Knox EG. The detection of space-time interactions. Appl Stat 1964a;13:25–29.

Knox EG. Epidemiology of childhood leukaemia in Northumberland and Durham. Br J Prev Soc Med 1964b;18:17–24.

Langmuir AD. The Epidemic Intelligence Service of the Centers for Disease Control. Public Health Rep 1980;95:470–477.

Last JM, ed. A Dictionary of Epidemiology. Third Edition. New York: Oxford University Press; 1995.

Lilienfeld DE, Black B. The epidemiologist in court: some comments. Am J Epidemiol 1986;123:961–964.

Lilienfeld DE, Stolley PD. Foundations of Epidemiology. Third Edition. New York: Oxford University Press; 1994.

Mantel N. The detection of disease clustering and a generalized regression approach. Cancer Res 1967;27:209–220.

McDiarmid MA, Breysse P, Lees PSJ, Curbow B, Kolodner K. Investigation of a spontaneous abortion cluster: lessons learned. Am J Ind Med 1994;25:463–475.

National Center for Health Statistics. Health, United States, 1995. Hyattsville, MD: Public Health Service; DHHS publication no. (PHS) 96–1232; 1996.

Neslund VJ. Legal considerations in a field investigation. In: Gregg MB, Dicker RC, Goodman RA, eds. Field Epidemiology. New York: Oxford University Press; 1996:197–207.

Neutra RR, Swan SH, Freedman, et al. Clusters Galore. (Abstract). Brookhaven, NY: First International Meeting of the International Society for Environmental Epidemiology; September 1989.

Neutra RR. Counterpoint from a cluster buster. Am J Epidemiol 1990;132:1–8.

Palmer SR. Epidemiology in search of infectious diseases: methods in outbreak investigation. J Epidemiol Commun Health 1989;43:311–314.

Palmer SR. Outbreak investigation: the need for 'quick and clean' epidemiology. Int J Epidemiol 1995;24(Suppl 1):S34–S38.

Peavy JV. Surveys and sampling. In: Gregg MB, Dicker RC, Goodman RA, eds. Field Epidemiology. New York: Oxford University Press; 1996:152–163.

Public Health Foundation. Measuring state expenditures for core public health functions. Am J Prev Med 1995;11(Suppl 2):58–73.

Reynolds P, Smith DF, Satariano E, Nelson DO, Goldman LR, Neutra RR. The four county study of childhood cancer: clusters in context. Stat Med 1996;15:683–697.

Rothenberg RB, Steinberg KK, Thacker SB. The public health importance of clusters: a note from the Centers for Disease Control. Am J Epidemiol 1990;132:S3–S5.

Rothman KJ. Clustering of disease. Am J Public Health 1987;77:13–15.

Rothman KJ. A sobering start to the cluster busters' conference. Am J Epidemiol 1990;132:S6–S13.

Schlesselman JJ. Case-Control Studies. Design, Conduct, Analysis. New York: Oxford University Press; 1982.

Schuchat A, Broome CV. Toxic shock syndrome and tampons. Epidemiol Rev 1991;13:99–112.

Schulte PA, Ehrenberg RL, Singal M. Investigation of occupational cancer clusters: theory and practice. Am J Public Health 1987;77:52–56.

Shands KN, Schmid GP, Dan BB, et al. Toxic-shock syndrome in menstruating women: association with tampon use and Staphylococcus aureus and clinical features in 52 cases. New Engl J Med 1980;303:1436–1442.

Smith PG. Spatial and temporal clustering. In: Schottenfeld D, Fraumeni JF Jr, eds. Cancer Epidemiology and Prevention. Philadelphia, PA: W.B. Saunders; 1982.

Smith D, Neutra R. Approaches to disease cluster investigations in a state health department. Stat Med 1993;12:1757–1762.

Stoekle MY, Douglas RG. Infectious diseases. JAMA 1996;275:1816–1817.

Stroup DF, Wharton M, Kafadar K, Dean AG. An evaluation of a method for detecting aberrations in public health surveillance data. Am J Epidemiol 1993;137:373–380.

Stroup DF. Special analytic issues. In: Teutsch SM, Churchill RE, eds. Principles and Practices of Public Health Surveillance. New York, NY: Oxford University Press; 1994:136–149.

Taylor DN, Wachsmuth K, Yung-Hui S, et al. Salmonellosis associated with marijuana: a multistate outbreak traced by plasmid fingerprinting. N Engl J Med 1982;306:1249–1253.

Thacker SB, Goodman RA, Dicker RC. Training and service in public health practice, 1951–90—CDC's Epidemic Intelligence Service. Public Health Rep 1990;105:599–604.

Thacker SB. Surveillance. In: Gregg MB, Dicker RC, Goodman RA, eds. Field Epidemiology. New York: Oxford University Press; 1996:16–32.

Tyler CW Jr, Last JM. Epidemiology. In: Last JM, Wallace RB, eds. Maxcy-Rosenau-Last Public Health & Preventive Medicine. Norwalk, CT: Appleton & Lange; 1992:11–39.

4

Public Health Surveillance

STEPHEN B. THACKER
DONNA F. STROUP

Public health and health care practitioners are concerned with a wide spectrum of health issues including infectious diseases, chronic conditions, reproductive outcomes, environmental health, and health events related to occupation, injuries, and behaviors. This array of problems requires a variety of intervention strategies for populations in addition to the need to provide clinical preventive services for individuals. Some critical examples are the provision of prophylactic measures (e.g., vaccination or postexposure rabies prophylaxis), educational services (e.g., public health messages to diverse populations or counseling and prophylaxis for contacts of persons with certain infectious diseases), inspection of food establishments, and control of infectious and noninfectious conditions.

For these activities, the rational development of health policy depends on public health information. For example, information on the age of children with vaccine-preventable diseases has been used to establish policy on appropriate ages for delivering vaccinations (Centers for Disease Control and Prevention [CDC] 1994a). Documentation of the prevalence of elevated levels of lead (a known toxicant) in blood in the US population has been used as the justification for eliminating lead from gasoline and for documenting the effects of this intervention (Annest et al. 1983), and information on the rate at which breast cancer is detected has led to new policies regarding the ages at which to recommend mammograms (Day 1991).

Public health information is understood most basically in terms of time, place, and person. Descriptive analysis of surveillance data over *time* shows patterns which generate hypotheses or merely reflect patterns in reporting behavior rather than underlying disease incidence (Figure 4-1). Furthermore, the approach to the prevention and control of disease and injury is often determined by circumstances unique to the *place* or geographic distribution of the disease or of its causative exposures or risk-associated behavior. For example, elevated blood-lead levels in children may represent exposure to

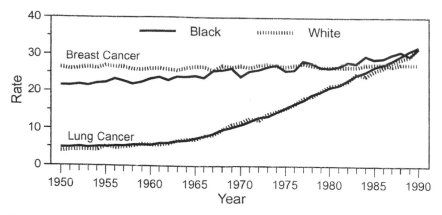

Figure 4-1. Age-adjusted lung and breast cancer death rates per 100,000 women, standardized to the 1970 age distribution of the U.S. population, for women, by race—United States, 1950–1990

lead hazards in their environment and may require both medical and environmental interventions. Distributions of some forms of cancer (e.g., melanoma of the skin) show a definite spatial distribution (Pickle et al. 1987).

Finally, the characteristics of the *person* or groups who develop specific diseases or who sustain specific injuries are important in understanding the disease or injury, identifying those at high risk, and targeting intervention efforts. For example, disparities in health (incidence or severity of disease) among members of different population groups highlight the need to identify cultural, economic, or social factors associated with these health problems (CDC 1993a).

Definition and Brief History

Public health surveillance (in some literature called epidemiological surveillance) is the ongoing systematic collection, analysis, and interpretation of outcome-specific health data, closely integrated with the timely dissemination of these data to those responsible for preventing and controlling disease or injury (Thacker and Berkelman 1992). Public health surveillance systems should have the capacity to collect and analyze data (Cates and Williamson 1994), disseminate data to public health programs (Langmuir 1963), and regularly evaluate the effectiveness of the use of the disseminated data (Klaucke et al. 1988). Public health information systems, on the other hand, have been defined to include a variety of data sources essential to public health and are often used for surveillance; however, historically, they lack some critical elements of surveillance systems (Thacker 1992). For example, they may not focus on specific outcomes (e.g., vital statistics), are not ongoing (e.g., a one-time or occasional survey), or are not linked directly to public health practices (e.g., insurance claims data).

The history of public health surveillance can be traced back to efforts to control the bubonic plague in the 14th century and includes such key figures as von Leibnitz, Graunt, Shattuck, and Farr (Thacker 1992). Following the discoveries of infectious disease agents in the late 1800s, the first use of scientifically based surveillance concepts in public health practice was the monitoring of contacts of persons with serious communicable diseases such as plague, smallpox, typhus, and yellow fever to detect the first signs and symptoms of disease and to begin prompt isolation. For many decades, this was the function of foreign quarantine stations throughout the world.

In the late 1940s, Alexander D. Langmuir, then the chief epidemiologist of the Communicable Disease Center (now the Centers for Disease Control and Prevention [CDC]), began to broaden the concept of surveillance. Although surveillance of persons at risk for specific disease continued at quarantine stations, Langmuir and his colleagues changed the focus of attention from individuals to diseases such as malaria and smallpox. They emphasized rapid collection and analysis of data on a particular disease with quick dissemination of the findings to those who needed to know (Langmuir 1963). As later stated by Foege et al. (1976): "The reason for collecting, analyzing, and disseminating information on a disease is to control that disease. Collection and analysis should not be allowed to consume resources if action does not follow." Although surveillance was originally concerned with protection of the population against infectious disease (Langmuir 1963), more recently a wide variety of health events, such as childhood lead poisoning, birth defects, injuries, and behavioral risk factors, have been included in surveillance activities (Thacker and Stroup 1994).

Unless those who set policy and implement programs have ready access to data, the use is limited to archives and academic pursuits, and the material is therefore appropriately considered health information rather than surveillance data (Terris 1992). Thus, the boundary of surveillance practice meets with—but does not extend to—actual research and implementation of intervention programs (Ballard and Duncan 1994). For example, although patient identifiers are not collected for most surveillance activities, state and local health departments may need this information for effective prevention of the spread of sexually transmitted diseases (i.e., contacting the partners of infected persons to deliver treatment and prevention information). A central difference between public health work and other biomedical research is that the boundary in public health between research and nonresearch activities is ill-defined (Last 1996). Specifically, state and local health departments use surveillance information for control and prevention of disease, and most surveillance activities are mandated (or permitted) by state statute (CDC 1990b). If persons with contagious diseases were allowed to refuse appropriate intervention, this would have an adverse effect on the health of communities (Chorba et al. 1989). At the same time, surveillance is *more than* the collection of reports of health events, and data collected for other purposes may enhance surveillance activities. This extension of activities can be seen in the 1957 national weekly influenza surveillance system established by CDC which used morbidity and laboratory data from state health departments, school and industrial absenteeism, mortality data from 108 US cities, and acute respiratory illness rates from the National Health Interview Survey (Langmuir 1987).

Uses

The uses of surveillance information can be organized on the basis of three categories of timeliness: *immediate, annual,* and *archival* (Thacker and Stroup 1994) (Figure 4-2).

- Immediate detection of:
  - epidemics
  - newly emerging health problems
  - changes in health practices
  - changes in antibiotic resistance

- Annual dissemination for:
  - estimating the magnitude of the health problem, including cost
  - assessing control activities
  - setting research priorities
  - testing hypotheses
  - facilitating planning
  - monitoring risk factors
  - monitoring changes in health practices
  - documenting distribution and spread

- Archival information for:
  - describing natural history of diseases
  - facilitating epidemiologic and laboratory research
  - validating use of preliminary data
  - setting research priorities
  - documenting distribution and spread

Figure 4-2. Uses of surveillance data

Immediate

For detecting epidemics, a surveillance system should allow public health officials immediate access to new information (Kilbourne 1992). For example, detection of a disease related to contaminated food or biological products should immediately trigger intervention and control efforts. As soon as, say, unusual clusters of specific birth defects or geographic clusters or pedestrian injuries are detected (by use of automated triggers defined by sentinel health events [Kilbourne 1992]), public health officials should respond (CDC 1990a).

In hospital and health department laboratories, various infectious agents are monitored for changes in bacterial resistance to antibiotics or antigenic composition. The detection of penicillinase-producing *Neisseria gonorrhea* in the United States through surveillance activities has provided critical information for the proper treatment of gonorrhea (CDC 1976). The National Nosocomial Infection Surveillance System monitors the occurrence of hospital-acquired infections, including changes in antibiotic resistance. Surveillance of influenza monitors the continual change in the influenza virus structure, information vital to vaccine formulation (Emori et al. 1991).

Annual

Timely annual data summaries would provide immediate estimates of the magnitude of a health problem, thus assisting policy-makers to modify priorities and plan intervention programs. These same data would be useful to those assessing control activities and would help researchers establish research priorities in applied epidemiology and laboratory research.

Surveillance data are used to assess control activities programs. For example, they have demonstrated the decrease in poliomyelitis rates following the introduction of both the inactivated and oral polio vaccines (Figure 4-3) and the effect on motor vehicle-associated injury of broad-based community interventions such as increased legal age of driving and seat-belt laws (Loeb 1993).

The traditional use of surveillance was to quarantine persons infected with or exposed to a particular disease and to monitor isolation activities. While this measure is rarely used today, isolation and surveillance of individuals is done for patients with multidrug-resistant tuberculosis and patients suspected of having serious, imported diseases such as the hemorrhagic fevers.

Surveillance has been used to monitor health practices such as hysterectomy, cesarean delivery, mammography, and tubal sterilization (Thacker et al. 1995). In the United States, a sociological trend is shifting in the health care industry from one dominated by a large number of small offices to one characterized by a small number of large managed-care organizations with

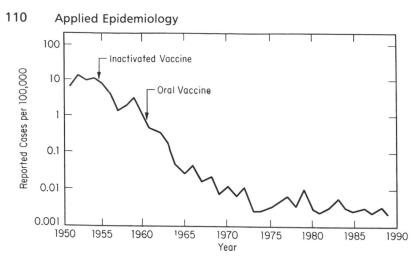

Figure 4-3. Semilogarithmic-scale line graph of reported cases of paralytic poliomyelitis—United States, 1951–1989

computerized patient records. For example, as of June 1995, 32% of Medicaid beneficiaries were enrolled in managed-care organizations, compared with 14% in 1994 (CDC 1995a). Data systems developed for managed-care activities will have tremendous potential for public health surveillance.

Surveillance data serve as the cornerstone of epidemiologic and public health practice. Representative and relevant health surveillance data give the necessary framework to facilitate planning and management of public programs. For example, Missouri health officials used existing chronic disease surveillance data to develop a cardiovascular disease health plan (Thacker et al. 1995). Data used were from existing sources, including mortality, data on behavioral risk factors, and data on population distribution. The resulting plan included a task force to establish priorities and monitor progress, a plan for chronic disease control, a resource directory, and training in cardiovascular disease control strategies. As discussed later in the case study section of this chapter, officials cite the appropriate use of surveillance data as the integral component in local coalition development (Brownson et al. 1992).

The health of populations may be adversely affected by time required to do special studies. Although surveillance information has limitations, it can often be used to test hypotheses. For example, the reported occurrence of lung cancer in the United States over the past 50 years has shown the impact of changes in the prevalence of smoking behaviors in women (Figure 4-1). For example, the passage of smoking legislation in the United States was shown to increase the age of initiation of smoking (United States Department of Health and Human Services 1994) (Figure 4-4). Surveillance data on cancer from the Surveillance, Epidemiology, and End Results (SEER) Program of the Na-

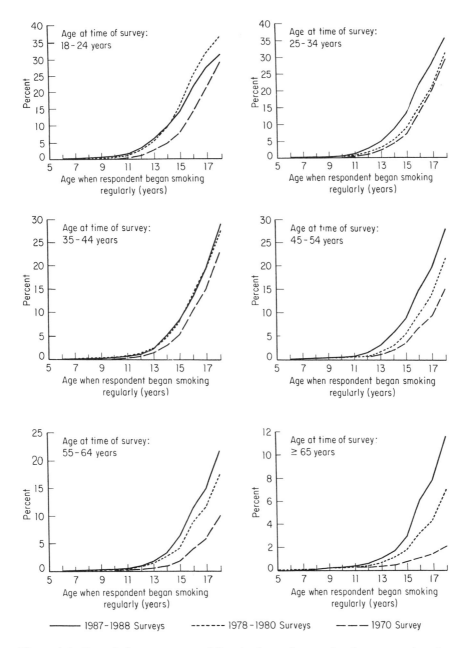

Figure 4-4. Cumulative percentage of females becoming regular cigarette smokers by age 18, by age at time of survey, United States, 1970, 1978–1980, and 1987–1988

tional Cancer Institute (Gloeckler-Ries et al. 1990) has been used as the basis of etiologic studies (Tejeda et al. 1996).

Archival

Surveillance data should be retained in readily accessible archival form, not only to document the evolving health status of a population but also to help us understand the predictors of disease and injury. For example, as we better understand spatial spread of infectious diseases such as influenza or measles, more effective prevention strategies may be possible (Longini et al. 1986; Cliff et al. 1992a). Carefully maintained archival data can provide the most accurate portrayal of the natural history of a disease in a population (Thacker and Berkelman 1992), effective measurements of the long-term effects of public policies or social changes (CDC 1991), and validation of interim data (CDC 1992; Thacker 1996).

Archival surveillance data can be used at the local, and to a lesser degree national, level to develop prevention and control activities. Missouri investigators used surveillance data to provide quantitative estimates of the magnitude of heart disease and to demonstrate an epidemic in that population. As a result, policy-makers adopted a cardiovascular health plan, enhancing its disease control program (Thacker et al. 1995). Conversely, surveillance data suggested that diabetic patients using continuous subcutaneous insulin infusion pumps suffered excess mortality; an investigation triggered by these data showed that this important technology was not associated with mortality (Teutsch et al. 1984).

Sources of Public Health Surveillance Data

Langmuir's credo of rapid reporting, analysis, and action now applies to over 100 infectious diseases and health events of noninfectious etiology nationally (Osterholm et al. 1996). Some ongoing systems of reporting have resulted from national emergencies such as contaminated lots of polio vaccine (Langmuir 1987), the Asian influenza epidemic of 1957, shellfish-associated hepatitis type A in 1961, and toxic-shock syndrome in 1980. Following the investigation of L-tryptophan-associated eosinophilia-myalgia syndrome (EMS) in 1990, within days a national surveillance system was put into place (Philen et al. 1993).

For such activities, public health agencies need several categories of information: (1) reports of health events affecting individuals; (2) vital statistics on the entire population; (3) information on the health status, risk behaviors, and experiences of populations; (4) information on potential exposure to environmental agents; (5) information on existing public health programs; (6) information useful to public health but obtained by organizations not directly involved in public health practice; and (7) information on the health care system and the impact of the health care system on health.

Reports of Health Events

Reports of cases of specific diseases of public health importance serve as the basis of many national surveillance programs in the United States (e.g., the National Notifiable Disease Surveillance System [NNDSS]; CDC 1991; Koo and Wetterhall 1996). Public health information needs may dictate the level of detail needed in data collection. For example, on a weekly basis, the NNDSS seeks reports on all cases of more than 40 conditions in the United States but collects only a small amount of information for each case, in order to minimize the burden placed on those who report. NNDSS data are used to monitor trends in disease, to evaluate public health programs, and to identify unusual occurrences of conditions that may require further epidemiologic investigation at the local level.

For some public health purposes, however, effective action requires additional detail on each case. For this reason, supplemental data collection systems have been developed for some of the diseases involved in the NNDSS. Such supplemental systems are sometimes less comprehensive in terms of the population represented but provide more detailed information on characteristics of the occurrence of disease (CDC 1991). For example, cases of hepatitis are reported weekly to NNDSS for publication in the *Morbidity and Mortality Weekly Report* (*MMWR*). In addition, the Viral Hepatitis Surveillance Project collects data on specific risk factors for different types of viral hepatitis in selected geographic areas. These data have been used to evaluate the importance of behavior associated with sexual activity and drug use as risk factors for transmitting hepatitis type B and to target educational and vaccination programs. Other uses of data may require the ability to identify the patient whose case is reported and sometimes persons who have contact with the patient, as in the identification and treatment of persons in contact with cases of sexually transmitted disease or tuberculosis.

Intervention and control of some conditions require more detailed information than can be obtained from a large group of clinicians or institutions. As a result, networks of selected health care providers have been organized to meet these targeted information needs. For example, CDC's Sentinel Event Notification System for Occupational Risks (SENSOR) targets select groups of health care providers as a component of a comprehensive approach that uses multiple data sources to provide information used in directing efforts to prevent workplace-related morbidity (Maizlish et al. 1995). Data from this system were used by states to institute intervention programs for occupational asthma. As a result, investigations of workplaces where occupational asthma cases have occurred have identified substantial numbers of symptomatic co-workers and inadequacies in engineering controls and work practices. These findings have led to preventive measures by the Office for Safety and Health Administration, health departments, and employers (Reilly et al. 1994). The National Nosocomial Infections Surveillance System receives reports from a selected group of hospitals on the incidence and characteristics of hospital-acquired infections; data from this system have been instrumental in alerting health authorities to the emergence of antibiotic-resistant strains of bacteria, which in turn has led to the development of specific recommendations regarding use of antibiotics (CDC 1996d).

Sometimes it is easier, more practical, or more useful to count epidemics rather than single cases of disease. This is particularly true of common diseases that have epidemic potential, may be poorly reported, or have a wide clinical spectrum. For example, surveillance of influenza includes a report of level of illness incidence assessed by each state. During early phases of the smallpox eradication program of West Africa in the early 1970s, the field teams stopped counting cases, and counted only epidemics, defined as one or more cases (Foege et al. 1975). This saved much time and effort, focusing most of the effort on control.

Reporting From Laboratories and Other Health Facilities

For diseases diagnosed through laboratory tests, data obtained from laboratories provide useful information about specific characteristics of a pathogen or toxic substance. State public health laboratories currently analyze 41 million specimens annually (Bean et al. 1991). Some of the data from these analyses immediately enter the electronic public health laboratory information system (PHLIS) and are used in monitoring both short- and long-range trends in the incidence of disease. In addition, private laboratories report several times as many data as the state public health laboratories; most of this information is available in electronic form.

For example, serotypes of *Salmonella* reported by laboratories can complement the use of data reported through NNDSS; such information is commonly used in identifying outbreaks that might otherwise not be detected. Increases in microbial isolates, recognition of rare or unusual sero- or biotypes, or even simply an increase in demands for laboratory facilities provides essential data in the detection and investigation of epidemics caused by such agents as salmonella, shigella, *Escherichia coli* O157:H7, and staphylococcus. Pivotal information used for control and prevention efforts has also come from ongoing surveillance of influenza and poliomyelitis isolates as well as laboratory studies of lead and other environmental hazards (Brody et al. 1994). With the rapid sophistication of laboratory tools in environmental health, the laboratory is playing an increasingly important role in surveillance of exposure to such toxicants as lead, mercury, pesticides, and volatile organic compounds.

Data from health facilities are increasingly important, particularly for the surveillance of chronic conditions. For example, the National Hospital Discharge Survey, a continuing nationwide sample survey of short-stay hospitals in the United States conducted since 1965 (National Center for Health Statistics 1977), has been used for ectopic pregnancy surveillance (CDC 1988) and to ascertain morbidity for surveillance of certain chronic conditions (Higgins and Thom 1989).

Registries

Registries provide detailed and periodically updated information on individuals. For example, ATSDR's National Exposure Registry is a system for collecting and maintaining information on persons with documented environmental exposure(s). The stated purpose of the registry is to aid in assessing long-term health consequences to the general population from exposure(s) to Superfund-related hazardous substances. This is accomplished through facilitating epidemiologic or health studies by (1) verifying what are thought to be known adverse health outcomes (hypothesis testing) and (2) identifying previously unknown, undetermined adverse health outcomes should they exist (hypothesis generating). This information assists ATSDR in providing advice on appropriate actions to be taken for a specific community (Markowitz 1992).

The SEER Registry (Miller et al. 1991) can be used to show differences between trends in morbidity and mortality due to cancer. Specifically, the annual incidence of breast cancer among women increased approximately 52% during 1950–1990, while the death rate increased 4% during the same period (CDC 1994b). In addition, the data can be used to show that survival rates vary substantially by race. Immunization registries enable public health practitioners to target children in need of services and direct resources effectively (Gostin and Lazzarini 1995).

Vital Statistics

The registration of all births and deaths has been legally mandated in the United States since 1903 (Grebenik 1978). Because the systems established to collect these data also contain other health-related information (e.g., birth weight and cause of death), they can be used in monitoring the public's health. For example, the mortality information system provides data (from death certificates) on virtually all deaths and is extremely useful for assessing the impact of different causes of death and for establishing priorities. Mortality data are regularly available at the local and state level, and because of burial laws, mortality statistics can be used at the local level within a matter of days. Mortality data are available on a weekly basis from 121 large United States cities as part of a national influenza surveillance system (Baron et al. 1988). Maintained and published weekly by CDC in collaboration with local health jurisdictions, these mortality statistics come from cities that represent about 27% of the nation's population and give a useful timely index of the extent and impact of influenza at local, state, and national levels (Simonsen et al. 1997).

Medical examiners and coroners are excellent sources of data on sudden or unexpected deaths. Data are available at the state or county level and include detailed information about the cause and the nature of death that is unavailable on the death certificate. These data are especially valuable for surveillance of intentional and unintentional injuries, as well as for sudden deaths of unknown cause. Data from the national system have been used to investigate the magnitude of the problem of use of methamphetamine, the most widely illegally manufactured, distributed, and abused type of stimulant drug (Greenblatt et al. 1995).

Information on Health Status, Risk Factors, and Experiences of Populations

Since the determinants of many important public health problems are behavioral, health agencies need information that is not readily available from medical records on the prevalence of various types of behavior and on access to care. Thus, regularly conducted *surveys* of the general population are needed for public health surveillance. These surveys may range from large-scale assessments of the general population to assessments targeted at high-risk (i.e., particularly vulnerable) populations. This need is particularly acute at the state and local level. For example, the National Health and Nutrition Examination Survey (NHANES) (CDC 1994c) provides data to monitor changes in the dietary, nutritional, and health status of the US population. The National Health Interview Survey (NHIS) (Massey et al. 1989) is an annual cross-sectional household interview survey of the civilian, noninstitutionalized US population, which can be used to estimate a variety of health status measures such as smoking prevalence (CDC 1994d) and vaccine coverage. The National Ambulatory Medical Care Survey (NAMCS) (Schappert 1992) can be used to quantify utilization of medical services. For example, the data show a lower rate of mammography use by women aged over 50 years (who are at greatest risk for breast cancer), perhaps due to the finding that these women are less likely to visit gynecologists, and of all physician specialists, gynecologists are most likely to recommend mammograms (CDC 1995b).

The surveillance of risk factors is useful, especially for chronic conditions. Prevalence of specific behavioral risk factors can be measured by the Behavioral Risk Factor Surveillance System (Siegel et al. 1993), by the Youth Risk Factor Behavioral Surveillance System (Serdula et al. 1993), by medical risk factors (e.g., NHANES and Pregnancy Risk Assessment and Monitoring System), by use of health care services and identification of underserved populations (e.g., NHIS), and by potential for exposure to toxic agents (e.g., the National Occupational Exposure Survey [Lyles and Kupper 1996]).

One example of an internal performance measurement and quality improvement system associated with managed care is the "report card" known as the Health Plan Employer Data and Information Set (HEDIS) (Corrigan and Nielsen 1993; Campion and Rosenblatt 1996). Several of the indicators are preventive: incidence of low birth weight infants, utilization of vaccinations, mammography, cervical cancer screening, screening for cholesterol, prenatal care, and retinal examinations for persons with diabetes (Cooper 1995) (see Chapter 10).

Information on Potential Exposure to Environmental Agents

Information on exposures to environmental agents can be used in evaluating the risk to health represented by noninfectious diseases, injuries, and certain infectious diseases. For example, measurement of airborne particulates is useful in assessing risks related to certain pulmonary disorders (e.g., asthma and lung cancer). Information on vectors that may carry agents of infectious disease (e.g., ticks as vectors for Lyme disease and Rocky Mountain spotted fever, mosquitoes as vectors for viral encephalitides, and raccoons as vectors for rabies) is important in evaluating the risk of infection. Information on exposures to known risks supports the development and implementation of rational public health interventions (e.g., ATSDR's Hazardous Substances Emergency Events Surveillance System provides information on the public health consequences associated with the release of hazardous substances) (CDC 1994e). In addition, information on exposures provides the basis for issuing alerts to the public and bulletins for clinicians on how to recognize and treat persons for health problems acquired through specific exposures. For example, concerns about heat-related morbidity during the 1996 Centennial Games in Atlanta prompted public health officials to design and implement a surveillance system that collected information daily to monitor infectious diseases, injuries, and heat-related illnesses that required medical attention (CDC 1996a).

Information From Other Organizations

Data useful for public health are currently or potentially available from organizations whose functions may not be related directly to those of public health agencies. Data from the Bureau of the Census, for example, are necessary both for the reliable computation of rates and for the proper adjustment of rates for comparisons over time or in different geographic areas. The Environmental Protection Agency (EPA) compiles environmental air-monitoring data to assess compliance with standards for air pollutants established by the Clean Air Act. Data collected through this system are also used by public health officials for hazard alerts when pollutants exceed federal standards and in studies of the effects of air pollutants on morbidity associated with respiratory diseases (McClellan 1994). The Occupational Safety and Health Administration (OSHA) and the Bureau of Labor Statistics compile data on the occurrence of work-related injuries and illnesses and exposure to hazards in the workplace which can be used for surveillance and research purposes (Smith 1995; CDC 1996b). Similarly, many states compile workers' compensation claims data in administering their worker's compensation programs; these same data can be used for surveillance purposes. The Department of Transportation operates the Fatal Accident Reporting System (FARS), which is used in public health to assess risk factors for motor-vehicle-related injuries and deaths (CDC 1995c). The Federal Bureau of Investigation (FBI) crime statistics assist in evaluating the public health impact of intentional injuries (CDC 1996c), and the Consumer Product Safety Commission (CPSC) collects data on injuries related to consumer products (Mattison and Sandler 1994).

Establishing a Surveillance System

The usefulness of surveillance activities can be increased by early attention to the components of establishing a public health surveillance system (Figure 4-5).

Establish Goals

At the beginning, it is important to understand clearly the purpose of establishing or maintaining a surveillance program. This includes a determination of priority health events for surveillance, which surveillance data elements are necessary, and how and when they are to be used. A particular surveillance program may have more than one goal, including monitoring the occurrence of fatal and nonfatal disease, evaluating the effect of a public health program, or detecting epidemics for control and prevention activities. These needs, then, may require data from multiple surveillance systems to monitor a single

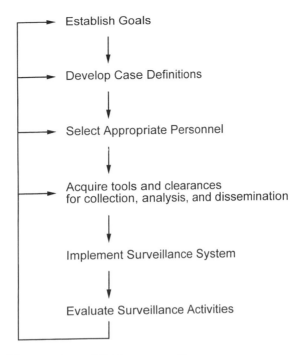

Figure 4-5. Elements in establishing a surveillance system

condition such as data to track morbidity, mortality, laboratory tests, exposures, or risk factors.

Develop Case Definitions

Clear and simple case definitions that are practical and quantifiable are essential to the utility of surveillance data. Minimal criteria (clinical and laboratory) for definition of a case must be made explicit (Wharton et al. 1990). For a newly emergent disease, the case definition is often broad, sometimes depending on clinical and epidemiological criteria in the absence of laboratory data. As a grasp of the disease process increases, a more refined definition may be used. Surveillance case definitions should distinguish confirmed cases from probable or possible cases, for with the proper analysis, this often enhances an understanding of the causes of an outbreak while not losing sight of its scope and impact.

Select Appropriate Personnel

It is essential to know not only who is responsible for overseeing the surveillance activities but also who will be providing the data, collecting and tabulating the data, analyzing and preparing the data for display, and, finally, who will be interpreting these data and disseminating them to those who need to know. For example, information for technically oriented public health workers may not take the same form as information for policy-makers (CDC 1993b). The entire surveillance system in a small area may have only one person doing essentially all these tasks. At the state, regional, and national levels, several persons will likely be involved in the surveillance of specific health events. In an acute outbreak setting, a large number of people at various professional levels may be involved in starting and conducting the necessary surveillance. As time progresses and the epidemic becomes better understood, the participants will likely assume a more well-defined and permanent role.

Acquire Tools and Clearances for Collection, Analysis, and Dissemination

Before establishing any surveillance system, whether an emergency assessment during a field investigation or a process of continued monitoring for months or years to come, the public health practitioner should first be very clear about the legal aspects of such a plan. In most instances, surveillance is conducted under the aegis of state health laws or regulations, rather than federal legislation. In epidemic investigations, the field team is usually given oral approval for setting up emergency surveillance systems, but when long-term programs of surveillance evolve into a longer-term study with generalizable results, suitable review for informed consent and human subjects issues may be required.

Confidentiality of data and the public's right to know information influencing health can be in conflict with each other, and these must be carefully considered at all steps in the surveillance process (Gostin et al. 1996). Usually, many persons are involved at each level of surveillance, including individuals in the community; patients (both within and outside of institutions); practitioners, including physicians, nurses, and others involved in the health care delivery system; members of the local health department; and, of course, members of one's immediate staff. Failure to recognize potential conflicts of interest or unacceptability of reporting to any of these persons could derail the surveillance process.

The capability of computers and technology creates great opportunity for surveillance activities (Lasker et al. 1995; Baker and Ross 1996). High-capacity storage devices, networks, new programming tools, video capacity, and enhanced transmission capabilities all offer tremendous benefit to surveillance. However, the utility of such tools will likely require education, as well as changes in societal expectation and mandatory statute (Dean et al. 1994).

Implement the Surveillance System

During the floods in the midwestern United States in 1993, it became clear that a surveillance system was essential to assess the magnitude of the health problem created, as well as the nature and distribution of flood-related illness and injury (O'Carroll et al. 1995). Previous examples include the emergence of AIDS (Buehler et al. 1996), toxic-shock syndrome (Schucat and Broome 1991), and eosinophilia-myalgia syndrome (Swygert et al. 1990). In establishing an ongoing system, a natural tendency at the start will be to make the case definition both as specific and sensitive as possible. Logical and defensible though this may be, it should not stand in the way of getting the system off the ground. Many a system has languished for months, even years, because of needless worry over missing or misclassifying a case or two—thus losing interest, cooperation, and potential impact. Since surveillance is a fluid process, as populations or health problems change, the surveillance system must adapt (Spitalny 1996).

Evaluate Surveillance Activities

The evaluation of the usefulness of public health surveillance systems is necessary for making rational decisions in the allocation of limited resources. The first step in evaluating a public health surveillance system is to describe the preventability and public health importance of the event under surveillance (Klaucke et al. 1988; Thacker et al. 1995). This can be done using the total number of incident and prevalent cases, mortality, and case-fatality ratio of the outcome under surveillance. In the health services research context, an evaluation also should consider intermediate outcomes (e.g., control of hypertension) which are incontrovertibly linked to long-term outcomes (e.g., stroke). The description of the surveillance system should include objectives, case definitions, and the specific components of data collection, analysis, and dissemination. Most important, the actions that will be taken and the results expected based on the data from the surveillance system should be included.

Subsequently, an evaluation of a surveillance system should include assessment of system attributes: simplicity, flexibility (i.e., can it adapt to changing disease characteristics and population structure), and acceptability to both data collectors and users. More quantitative attributes to be evaluated include sensitivity, positive predictive value, representativeness, and timeliness (Simpson 1996; Meek et al. 1996). For example, while a sensitive system is very important in detecting acute events for intervention, high sensitivity comes at a cost (e.g., increased false positives). On the other hand, the positive predictive value of a system is important in efficient uses of resources. As a condition becomes rarer (such as during eradication), the case definition often becomes more sensitive, as each probable case may be investigated.

Another aspect of surveillance evaluation is the timeliness of reporting. For all health conditions, a measurable delay occurs between the exposure and the report of a problem to health authorities. In the case of disease (as opposed to most injuries), an interval exists between exposure and expression of symptoms, in addition to the interval between (1) onset of symptoms and diagnosis of the problem, (2) eventual reporting of the illness to public health authorities, and (3) dissemination of that information for public health action. For an infectious disease, these intervals may represent days or weeks, whereas for a chronic disease, they may be measured in years. For example, a cluster of meningoccal meningitis cases among schoolchildren represents a public health emergency that requires immediate intervention. Other public health actions may require detailed data but in a less urgent time frame.

The system should represent the population under consideration not only as to demographics and geography, but also with regard to the appropriate time frame under investigation. Historical data may not be helpful in addressing current health problems affected by shifting demographic patterns or changes in case definitions. Rapid dissemination of data is needed to address acute outbreaks of communicable diseases; on the other hand, monitoring long-term patterns of illness may permit less timely data. Finally, a cost analysis of the system should delineate the resources used to operate the entire system, including costs incurred by providers, insurers, and other elements of the health services activity (Osterholm et al. 1996).

Several states have made noteworthy efforts in evaluation of surveillance activities (Baker et al. 1995). These evaluations have identified priority activities in data linkage and standardization, computerization, allocation of resources, and policies on data sharing. For example, in 1993, Iowa identified five areas of strategic importance to public health: health care reform, primary care, prevention, integrated services, and assessment. To address these areas, approximately 100 separate databases were identified, including surveillance data. Priority was given to integrating, combining, or linking data in the allocation of resources within the state. Other components included electronic transmission, attention to the cost of data collection, system documentation, staff resources, standardization of variables, and data sharing (Blood 1995).

Analysis and Dissemination of Surveillance Data

As with all descriptive epidemiologic data, surveillance information can be analyzed in terms of time, place, and person. Simple tabular and graphic techniques can be applied for display and analysis (Cates et al. 1994). More sophisticated methods such as cluster and time-series analyses and computer mapping techniques may be appropriate after initial descriptive presentations (Stroup and Thacker 1993; Stroup 1994).

The timely dissemination of surveillance data to those who need to know is critical to the usefulness of surveillance systems (see Chapter 11). Whatever format is chosen, the nature of the audience will affect data collection and interpretation as well as the dissemination process. The data should be distributed in a predictable and timely manner so that control and prevention measures can be implemented. Some of "those who need to know" include policy-makers and administrators, people whose needs are different from those of epidemiologists; thus, the data presentation should take this viewpoint into account (CDC 1993b). Finally, recognizing people who have contributed to the surveillance process not only gives them credit, but it gives them a degree of responsibility as well.

CDC and other federal agencies give information to those who need to know through the *MMWR*, the *MMWR Surveillance Summaries, Recommendations and Reports*, the *Annual Summary of Notifiable Diseases*, and special, condition-specific reports. State and local health departments, as well as other countries, often have their own reports, analogous to the *MMWR*, that are disseminated to health care providers and other interested persons in the relevant states or communities. In addition, surveillance data for some conditions are disseminated in more detail (Hoy 1996; Cantoni et al. 1995). Also, surveillance data are analyzed and published in the medical literature, typically presenting cumulative data for several years (Cliff et al. 1992b). One major trend that will affect public health surveillance dissemination is the explosive growth in hardware, software, and spatial aspects of the transfer of electronic data, currently characterized by the explosive growth of the Internet. Appropriate use of these developments should lead to more timely, complete, and accessible surveillance data.

Public Health Informatics

The term *public health informatics* is used to describe the rapidly evolving fields of information science, engineering, and technology applied to public health (Kilbourne 1992). The goal of professionals working in this field is to facilitate effective and efficient collection and presentation of relevant data and information to both public health and health care practitioners, as well as the general public. Objectives of these activities are to permit rapid, comprehensive assessments of community health, early identification of outbreaks and hazards, and provision of timely, accurate information and guidelines for clinical and public health practice.

Three elements are essential to the evolution of integrated public health information systems in this context: data standards, a communications infrastructure, and policy-level agreements on data access, sharing, and reduction of burden on data providers (Stratton 1996). Each element is necessary, but not sufficient. Although technical systems may be compatible, data will not be shared unless there are policy-level agreements to do so. Likewise, agreements on a policy level cannot be implemented unless adequate technical systems are in place (Morris et al. 1996).

Standards

Integrated information systems require that users and providers agree on standards for factors common to many public health systems. This list includes common definitions of data elements and terms, common classification systems, compatible telecommunication protocols, and other technical specifications that allow different systems to be compared, linked, and otherwise integrated. Public health practitioners should stimulate and facilitate the development of standards in the areas of (1) core variables and other data elements, (2) software applications, (3) data transmission, (4) data access, and (5) confidentiality and security (Madans and Hunter 1996).

Communications Infrastructure

An integrated public health surveillance system is dependent upon an information network infrastructure (Lasker et al. 1995). Public health data tend to be distributed, i.e., they are created in numerous locations, for numerous reasons, and often remain as local databases. Today, many of these data are stored in electronic format. In its most general terms, an electronic communications infrastructure includes the equipment, protocols, and software that allow users to connect and exchange data with other users via local- and wide-area networks. The means of communication are typically dial-up telephone connections for data communications but are moving toward local-area networks (LANs) that link the components of a group (such as a local health department) together. Wide-area networks (WANs) link these smaller components together with others involved in the same enterprise (e.g., linking local health departments with state and federal public health agencies). Thus, sources of information become available to members of networks through their personal computers or other electronic equipment.

Policies, Legislative Mandates, Regulations, and Organizational Practices

An integrated public health surveillance system is the result of agreements that exist between those who provide data and those who use these data.

These agreements provide for the efficient flow of data to appropriate users by avoiding duplication, minimizing burden, protecting confidentiality, and maximizing analytic utility. In this chapter, we have noted that health information exists in a variety of settings: Individuals have knowledge about their own situations, lifestyles, attitudes, etc.; health providers maintain patients' records about diagnosis and care delivered; laboratories report information on test results; government agencies routinely conduct surveys and generate information about their services. Users (e.g., public health officials, policy makers, and researchers) describe a wide variety of needs for information (e.g., disease surveillance, epidemiologic and prevention research, trend statistics, and policy research) and, to some extent, bear the burden of demonstrating that these needs are legitimate enough to justify the burden imposed on those who provide data (Ehling 1996).

In many cases, organizations serve multiple roles—as initial sources of data, as intermediaries that add value before passing data on to other users, and as end users of data from a variety of sources. Currently, however, a variety of barriers exist that tend to divide and isolate users and sources and have led to the creation of multiple, independent information systems to meet the needs of diverse users. Such barriers include policies, legislation, and organizational practices that unnecessarily impede access to data; end users that specify system requirements that exceed real needs, necessitating unique systems; categorical funding for surveillance and data systems; and a "turf and control" culture that encourages independence rather than cooperation. Finally, concerns about confidentiality and a conflict between the individual's right to privacy and the public's need to know have not been resolved (Neslund 1996).

Summary

Public health surveillance is a cornerstone of public health practice, providing the scientific and factual database essential to informed decision-making and action. Surveillance data have many uses but, in general, are needed for the assessment of the health status of a population in order to set public health priorities and determine appropriate actions. Surveillance is based on morbidity, mortality, and risk factor data, as well as information from outside of the traditional public health system.

Surveillance systems are established for the identification of specific outcomes, such as a disease or injury, or for risk factors, and must have clearly expressed goals. Explicit case definitions are essential for a useful surveillance system. The initiation and maintenance of any successful surveillance system will reflect recognition of the human element in surveillance practice—in data collection, analysis, and data dissemination. Attention to the people involved in such a system will increase its use.

The science and practice of prevention have advanced greatly in this century, and the technology for diagnosis and treatment of diseases has become highly sophisticated. Likewise, the technology for processing and managing information has greatly altered the way public health conducts business. In 1980, few public health professionals operated personal computers at their desks. Today, such computers, with greatly enhanced capabilities and with appropriate software, are not only common, but they are one of the essential tools of public health practice (Friede and O'Carroll 1996). Public health must now maximize the efficiency of existing information systems while finding new, more innovative ways of conducting public health surveillance.

CASE STUDIES

Surveillance for Eosinophilia-Myalgia Syndrome

Background

In 1989, a state health department and the CDC were notified about a few cases of patients with severe myalgia and peripheral eosinophilia. Upon investigation, it was found that all three had taken an amino acid preparation of L-tryptophan (CDC 1989). Because this preparation was distributed nationally, the CDC, in collaboration with state and territorial health departments, established a national, state-based surveillance system for eosinophilia and severe myalgia within 1 week of the reported outbreak (Swygert et al. 1990).

An early step was the identification of a case definition using descriptive epidemiology from the early reports. Initially, laboratory data were required to rule out trichinosis; however, this part of the definition was dropped after data for 1 week showed that the laboratory testing was not always clinically indicated (CDC 1990c). Probable cases were reported on a voluntary basis by physicians in all 50 states, the District of Columbia, and Puerto Rico. Standardized collection forms were used to collect demographic, clinical, and laboratory information, and aggregate numbers were telephoned weekly to the CDC. Case report forms were then mailed. State and territorial health departments conducted follow-up investigations of all deaths of patients confirmed as having eosinophilia-myalgia syndrome (EMS). Disease latency was calculated using the period from the date of first tryptophan use to date of onset of illness. Frequencies of multiple- versus single-brand use and of reported brand names were also used to assess association with specific products.

Key Questions

1. How does a public health surveillance system lead to accurate detection and control of an emerging health condition such as EMS?

For a public health surveillance system to lead to detection and control, it is essential that the steps outlined earlier in this chapter for establishing a surveillance system be followed closely.

2. What are the epidemiologic characteristics of EMS in the United States?

During the acute phase of the epidemic, more than 1,500 cases of EMS were reported nationwide. Of these, 46 had died and 36 met the case definition for a death related to EMS (Swygert et al. 1993). Of these deaths, the majority were female, non-Hispanic whites, with a median age of 58 years. Those who died were significantly older than other reported patients. Of the 36 deaths related to EMS, 34 had used L-tryptophan before illness onset. Most deaths occurred within 6 months of illness onset. Follow-up of reported deaths revealed that the disease involved at least two organ systems.

3. How can public health surveillance for a condition such as EMS lead to important health policy actions?

Public health action is possible when surveillance systems are already in place, or as in this case, when they can be established quickly. In the cases of EMS, the US Food and Drug Administration recalled the amino acid preparation L-tryptophan.

Implications for Practice
The success of this national surveillance effort depended on physicians' knowledge of the disease and their willingness to report. Since cases were dispersed throughout the country, national surveillance data were necessary to look at patterns in their distribution. The rapid establishment of a previously unrecognized syndrome required an initial case definition specific enough to ensure consistent case reporting. This strict case definition was accurate enough for policy decisions (FDA recall of the product), but the definition was broadened subsequently to allow for early detection of any undue increase in EMS incidence and to document decrease in cases following withdrawal of L-tryptophan.

State-Based Surveillance to Prevent Cardiovascular Disease

Background
Although cardiovascular disease mortality has declined nearly 40% in the last 20 years (CDC 1996e), it remains the leading causes of morbidity and mortality in the United States. The State of Missouri used existing data systems for chronic disease surveillance to develop a cardiovascular health plan (Missouri Cardiovascular Health Task Force 1991).

Data from the Missouri Center for Health Statistics were used to quantify that cardiovascular disease was the cause of death in more than 40% of all deaths attributed to cardiovascular diseases (Thacker et al. 1995). Age-adjusted mortality rates were used to document the distribution and spread of the disease among populations in that state. Data from the Behavioral Risk Factor Surveillance System allowed testing hypotheses of intervention programs (e.g., worksite smoking cessation programs). Hospital discharge data were used to estimate the burden of chronic disease.

Key Questions
1. Which public health surveillance systems are readily available in a state health department for addressing and important health condition such as cardiovascular disease?

A variety of surveillance systems are available, including those noted above and those noted in Table 4-1. These data sets are commonly underutilized in public health practice.

2. What was the descriptive profile of cardiovascular disease in Missouri and the associated risk factors?

Table 4-1. Selected Uses and Illustrative Sources of Public Health Surveillance Data

Use	Selected Data Source	Strengths	Limitations
Portray of trends in disease and health	Vital statistics	Essentially complete Length of history	Inaccuracies for selected causes Variation in reporting across regions Underreporting for chronic conditions (Percy et al. 1981, Percy and Muir 1989)
Evaluate control measures	Immunization registries	Population-based Links immunization surveillance and intervention	Confidentiality concerns New data collection system
Monitor changes in infectious agents	Reporting from laboratories	Provides laboratory confirmation	Incomplete (mostly public laboratories) Lack of epidemiologic information
Estimate magnitude of health problems	Notifiable diseases	National coverage Timely Length of history	Incomplete reporting Low sensitivity for some diseases
Monitor health practice	Hospital discharge data	National estimate	Sample, not enumeration Measures discharges, not people Cannot detect infrequent events
Plan public health practice	Risk factor surveillance	Timely	Sample Limited epidemiologic information Self-reported data
Test hypotheses	Cancer registries	Detailed information	No national coverage No uniform standards for reporting

In 1988, cardiovascular disease was responsible for almost half of all deaths in Missouri, with ischemic heart disease listed as the primary cause of death for over half of these (Brownson et al. 1990). Use of hospital discharge data showed that over half of those people discharged from a hospital with diagnosis of ischemic heart disease were under the age of 65. At the same time, data from the Behavioral Risk Factor Surveillance System showed information on several risk factors for cardiovascular disease: Over half of adult Missourians were physically inactive, about one-fourth were overweight, one-fourth were smokers, and 20% had self-reported hypertension.

3. How can these types of data be used in statewide and community-based efforts to control cardiovascular disease?

In part due to this effort, Missouri established a cardiovascular disease control program. A task force established priorities and monitored progress, a resource directory was compiled, and communities offered training in cardiovascular disease control strategies. Activities of local health coalitions were guided in part by routinely collected surveillance data.

Implications for Practice

Control of chronic diseases such as cardiovascular disease has become an important priority for the United States and state public health agencies (US Dept of Health and Human Services 1990; Schwartz et al. 1993). There are numerous sources of surveillance data that can be essential for priority setting, program development, and evaluation. However, the quality and completeness of surveillance systems may vary considerably so attention to the methodologic issues outlined in this chapter is needed.

SUGGESTED READINGS

Gostin LO, Lazzarini Z. Childhood immunization registries: a national review of public health information systems and the protection of privacy. JAMA 1995; 274:1793–1799.

Klaucke DN, Buehler JW, Thacker SB, et al. Guidelines for evaluating surveillance systems. Morb Mortal Wkly Rep 1988;37(SS-5):1–18.

Langmuir AD. The surveillance of communicable diseases of national importance. N Engl J Med 1963;288:182–192.

Teutsch SM, Churchill RE, eds. Principles and Practices of Public Health Surveillance. New York: Oxford University Press; 1994.

Thacker SB, Choi K, Brachman PS. The surveillance of infectious diseases. JAMA 1983;249:1181–1185.

Thacker SB, Stroup DF. Future directions of comprehensive public health surveillance and health information systems in the United States. Am J Epidemiol 1994;140(5):383–397.

Thacker SB, Stroup DF, Rothenberg RR, Brownson R. Public health surveillance for chronic conditions: a scientific basis for decisions. Stat Med 1995;14:629–642.

Wharton M, Chorba TL, Vogt RL, Morse DL, Buehler JW. Case definitions for public health surveillance. Morb Mortal Wkly Rep 1990;39(RR-13):1–43.

REFERENCES

Annest JL, Pirkle JL, Makuc D, et al. Chronological trend in blood lead levels between 1976 and 1980. N Engl J Med 1983;308:1373–1377.

Baker EL, Friede A, Moulton AD, Ross DA. CDC's Information Network for Public Health Officials (INPHO): a framework for integrated public health information and practice. J Public Health Management Practice 1995;1:43–47.

Baker EL, Ross DA. Information and surveillance systems and community health: buidling the public health information infrastructure. J Public Health Management Practice 1996;2(4):58–60.

Ballard DJ, Duncan PW. Role of population-based epidemiologic surveillance in clinical practice guideline development. In: McCormick KA, Moore SR, Siegel RA, eds. Methodology Perspectives. U.S. Department of Health and Human Services, Public Health Service, Agency for Health Care Policy and Research; AHCPR pub. no. 95-0009; November 1994.

Baron RC, Dicker RC, Bussell KE, Herndon JL. Assessing trends in mortality in 121 U.S. cities, 1970–79, from all causes and from pneumonia and influenza. Public Health Rep 1988;103(2):120–128.

Bean NH, Martin SM, Bradford H. PHLIS: an electronic system for reporting public health data from remote sites. Am J Public Health 1991;89(9):1273–1276.

Blood P. Evaluating public health data systems: a practical approach. Centers for Disease Control and Prevention, National Center for Health Statistics; DHHS pub. no. (PHS) 95-1237; 1995.

Brody DJ, Pirkle JL, Kramer RA, et al. Blood lead levels in the U. S. population from phase 1 of the Third National Health and Nutrition Examination survey. JAMA 1994;272:277–283.

Brownson RC, Van Tuinen M, Smith CA. Cardiovascular disease in Missouri: mortality, hospital discharges and risk factors. MO Med 1990;87(4):225–227.

Brownson RC, Smith CA, Jorge NE, et al. The role of data-driven planning and coalition development in preventing cardiovascular disease. Public Health Rep 1992;10:721–737.

Buehler JW, Petersen LR, Ward JW. Future issues in HIV/AIDS surveillance. J Public Health Management Practice 1996;2(4):52–57.

Campion FX, Rosenblatt MS. Quality assurance and medical outcomes in the era of cost containment. Surg Clin of North Am 1996;76(1):139–159.

Cantoni M, Cozzi Lepri A, Grossi P, Pezzotti P, Rezza G, Verdecchia A. Use of AIDS surveillance data to describe subepidemic dynamics. Int J Epidemiol 1995;24(4):804–812.

Cates W, Williamson GD. Descriptive epidemiology: analyzing and interpreting surveillance data. In: Teutsch SM, Churchill RE, eds. Principles and Practice of Public Health Surveillance. New York: Oxford University Press; 1994:96–135.

Centers for Disease Control and Prevention. Penicillinase-producing *Neisseria gonorrhoeae*. Morb Mortal Wkly Rep 1976;25:261.

Centers for Disease Control and Prevention. Ectopic pregnancy surveillance, United States, 1970–1985. Morb Mortal Wkly Rep CDC Surveill Summ 1988;37 (SS-5):9–18.

Centers for Disease Control and Prevention. Eosinophilia-myalgia syndrome—New Mexico. Morb Mortal Wkly Rep 1989;38:765–767.

Centers for Disease Control and Prevention. Guidelines for the investigation of clusters. Morb Mortal Wkly Rep 1990a;39(RR-11):1–16.

Centers for Disease Control and Prevention. Mandatory reporting of infectious diseases by clinicians. Morb Mortal Wkly Rep 1990b;39(RR-9):1–18.

Centers for Disease Control and Prevention. Update: eosinophilia-myalgia syndrome associated with ingestion of L-tryptophan—United States, January 9, 1990. Morb Mortal Wkly Rep 1990c;39:14–15.

Centers for Disease Control and Prevention. National electronic telecommunication system for surveillance—United States, 1990–1991. Morb Mortal Wkly Rep 1991;40:502–503.

Centers for Disease Control and Prevention. Years of potential life lost before ages 65 and 85—United States, 1989–1990. Morb Mortal Wkly Rep 1992;41(18):313–315.

Centers for Disease Control and Prevention. Use of race and ethnicity in public health surveillance: summary of the CDC/ATSDR Workshop. Morb Mortal Wkly Rep 1993a;42(RR-10).

Centers for Disease Control and Prevention. Surveillance for Cholera—Cochabamba Department, Bolivia, January–June 1992. Morb Mortal Wkly Rep 1993b;32: 636–639.

Centers for Disease Control and Prevention. General recommendations on immunization: recommendations of the Advisory Committee on Immunization Practices (ACIP). Morb Mortal Wkly Rep 1994a;43(RR-1).

Centers for Disease Control and Prevention. Deaths from breast cancer—United States, 1991. Morb Mortal Wkly Rep 1994b;43:273–281.

Centers for Disease Control and Prevention. National Center for Health Statistics. Plan and operation of the Third National Health and Nutrition Examination Survey, 1988–94. Hyattsville, MD. US Department of Health and Human Services, Public Health Service, CDC, 1994c; DHHS publication no. (PHS)94–1308. (Vital and health statistics; series 1, no. 32).

Centers for Disease Control and Prevention. Cigarette smoking among adults—United States, 1993. Morb Mortal Wkly Rep 1994d;43:925–930.

Centers for Disease Control and Prevention. Surveillance for emergency events involving hazardous substances, United States 1990–1992. Morb Mortal Wkly Rep 1994e;43(SS-2):1–6.

Centers for Disease Control and Prevention. Prevention and Managed care: Opportunities for managed care organizations, purchasers of health care, and public health agencies. Morb Mortal Wkly Rep 1995a; 44(no.RR-14).

Centers for Disease Control and Prevention. Trends in cancer screening C United States, 1987 and 1992. Morb Mortal Wkly Rep 1995b;45:57–60.

Centers for Disease Control and Prevention. Update: alcohol-related traffic crashes and fatalities among youth and young adults C United States, 1982–1994. Morb Mortal Wkly Rep 1995c;44:969–975.

Centers for Disease Control and Prevention. Public health surveillance during the XVII Central American and Caribbean Games —Puerto Rico, November 1993. Morb Mortal Wkly Rep 1996a;45:581–584.

Centers for Disease Control and Prevention. Work-related injuries and illnesses associated with child labor—United States, 1993. Morb Mortal Wkly Rep 1996b; 45(22):464–468.

Centers for Disease Control and Prevetion. Trends in rates of homicide—United States, 1985–1994. Morb Mortal Wkly Rep 1996c;45(22):460–464.

Centers for Disease Control and Prevention. Assessment of testing. Morb Mortal Wkly Rep 1996d;45(14):289–291.

Centers for Disease Control and Prevention. National Center for Health Statistics. Health, United States, 1995. Hyattsville, MD: Public Health Service; 1996e.

Chorba TL, Berkelman RL, Safford SK, Gibbs NP, Hull HF. Mandatory reporting of infectious diseases by clinicians. JAMA 1989;262:3018–3026.

Cliff AD, Haggett P, Stroup DF. The geographical structure of measles epidemics in the northeastern United States. Am J Epidemiol 1992a;136:592–602.

Cliff AD, Haggett P, Stroup DF, Cheney E. The changing geographical coherence of measles morbidity in the United States. Stat Med 1992b;11:1409–1424.

Cooper JK. Accountability for clinical preventive services. Mil Med 1995;160(6):297–299.

Corrigan JM, Neilson DM. Toward the development of uniform reporting standards for managed case organizations: The Health Plan Employer Data and Information Set (Version 2.0). J Quality Improvement 1993;19:566–575.

Day NE. Screening for breast cancer. Br Med Bull 1991;47:400–415.

Dean AD, Fagan RF, Panter-Connah BJ. Computerizing public health surveillance systems. In: Teutsch SM, Churchill RE, eds. Principles and Practice of Public Health Surveillance. New York: Oxford University Press; 1994:200-217.

Ehling LR. In practice: forcing the task. J Public Health Management Practice 1996;2(4):77–79.

Emori TG, Culver DH, Horan TC, et al. National Nosocomial Infections Surveillance Systems (NNISS): description of surveillance methods. Am J Infect Control 1991;19:19–35.

Foege WH, Millar JD, Henderson DA. Smallpox eradication in West and Central Africa. Bull WHO 1975;52(2):209–222.

Foege WH, Hogan RC, Newton LH. Surveillance projects for selected diseases. Int J Epidemiol 1976;5:29–37.

Friede A, O'Carroll PW. CDC and ATSDR electronic information resources for health officers. J Public Health Management Practice 1996;2(3):10–24.

Gloeckler-Ries LA, Hankey BF, Edwards BK, eds. Cancer statistics review. 1973–1987. Bethesda, MD: National Cancer Institute; NIH pub. No. 90-2789; 1990.

Gostin LO, Lazzarini Z. Childhood immunization registries: a national review of public health information systems and the protection of privacy. JAMA 1995;274:1793–1799.

Gostin LO, Lazzarini Z, Neslund VS, Osterholm MT. The public health information infrastructure. A national review of the law on health information privacy. JAMA 1996;275(24):1921–1927.

Grebenik E. Vital statistics. In: Kruskal WH, Tanur JM, eds. International Encyclopedia of Statistics. New York: Macmillan; 1978:1225–1227.

Greenblatt JC, Gfroerer JC, Melnick D. Increasing morbidity and mortality associated with abuse of methamphetamine—United States, 1991B1994. Morb Mortal Wkly Rep 1995;44:882–886.

Higgins M, Thom T. Trends in CHD in the United States. Int J Epidemiol 1989;18(Suppl):s58–s66.

Hoy WE. Nonmelanoma skin carcinoma in Albuquerque, New Mexico: experience of a major health care provider. Cancer 1996; 77(12):2489–2495.

Kilbourne EM. Informatics in public health surveillance: current issues and future perspectives. In: Wetterhall SF, ed. Proceedings of the 1992 International Symposium on Public Health Surveillance. Morb Mortal Wkly Rep 1992;41 (Suppl):91–99.

Klaucke DN, Buehler JW, Thacker SB, et al. Guidelines for evaluating surveillance systems. Morb Mortal Wkly Rep 1988;37(SS-5):1–18.

Koo D, Wetterhall SF. History and current status of the National Notifiable Diseases Surveillance System. J Public Health Management Practice 1996;2(4):4–10.

Langmuir AD. The surveillance of communicable diseases of national importance. N Engl J Med 1963;288:182–192.

Langmuir AD. The territory of epidemiology: pentimento. J Infect Dis 1987;155:349.

Lasker RD, Humphreys BL, Braithwaite WR. Making a Powerful Connection: The Health of the Public and the National Information Infrastructure. Washington, DC: Report of the U.S. Public Health Service Public Health Data Policy Coordinating Committee; 1995.

Last J. Professional standard of conduct for epidemiologists. In: Coughlin SS, Beauchamp TL, eds. Ethics and Epidemiology. New York: Oxford University Press; 1996.

Loeb PD. The effectiveness of seat belt legislation in reducing various driver-involved injury rates in California. Accid Anal Prev 1993;25(2):189–197.

Longini IM, Fine PEM, Thacker SB. Predicting the global spread of new infectious agents. Am J Epidemiol 1986;123:383–391.

Lyles RH, Kupper LL. On strategies for comparing occupational exposure data to limits. Am Ind Hyg Assoc J 1996;57(1):6–15.

Madans JH, Hunter EL. Improving and integrating data systems for public health surveillance. J Public Health Management Practice 1996;2(4):42–44.

Maizlish N, Rudolph L, Dervin K, Sankaranarayan M. Surveillance and prevention of work-related carpal tunnel syndrome: an application of the Sentinel Events Notification System for Occupational Risks. Am J Ind Med 1995;27(5):715–729.

Markowitz S. The role of surveillance in occupational health. In: Rom WN, ed. Environmental and Occupational Medicine. Second Edition. Boston: Little, Brown; 1992:19–28.

Massey JT, Moore TF, Parsons VL, Tadros W. Design and estimation for the National Health Interview Survey, 1985B1994. Hyattsville, MD: US Department of Health and Human Services, Public Health Service, CDC; 1989. (Vital and health statistics; series 2, no. 110).

Mattison DR, Sandler JD. Summary of the workshop on issues in risk assessment: quantitative methods for developmental toxicology. Risk Anal 1994;14(4):595–604.

McClellan RO. A commentary on the NRC report "Science and judgment in risk assessment" [published erratum appears in Regul Toxicol Pharmacol 1995 Jun;21(3):439]. Regulatory Toxicol Pharmacol 1994;20(3 Pt 2):S142–168.

Meek JI, Roberts CL, Smith EV, Cartter ML. Underreporting of lyme disease by Connecticut physicians, 1992. J Public Health Management Practice 1996;2 (4)61–65.

Miller BA, Reis LAG, Hankey BF, et al., eds. SEER cancer statistics review, 1973B90. Bethesda, MD: US Department of Health and Human Services, Public Health Service, National Institutes of Health, National Cancer Institute; IV.1BIV.24; DHHS pub. no. (NIH)93-2789; 1991.

Missouri Cardiovascular Health Task Force. The Missouri Cardiovascular Health Plan, 1991.

Morris G, Snider D, Katz M. Integrating public health information and surveillance systems. J Public Health Management Practice 1996;2(4):24–27.

National Center for Health Statistics. Development of the design of the NCHS hospital discharge survey. Washington, DC: US Government Printing Office; 1977. (Vital and health statistics; series 2, no. 39).

Neslund VJ. Legal considerations in a field investigation. In: Gregg MB, Dickey RC, Goodman RA, eds. Field Epidemiology. New York: Oxford University Press; 1996:197–207.

O'Carroll PW, Friede A, Noji EK, et al. The rapid implementation of a state-wide emergency health information system during the 1993 Iowa flood. Am J Public Health 1995;85(4):564–567.

Osterholm MT, Birkhead GS, Meriwether RA. Impediments to public health surveillance in the 1990s: the lack of resources and the need for priorities. J Public Health Management Practice, 1996;2(4):11–15.

Percy C, Stanek E, Gloeckler L. Accuracy of cancer death certificates and its effect on cancer mortality statistics. Am J Public Health 1981;71(3):242–250.

Percy C, Muir C. The international comparability of cancer mortality data. Results of an international death certificate study. Am J Epidemiol 1989;129(5):934–946.

Philen RM, Hill RH Jr, Flanders WD, et al. Tryptophan contaminants associated with eosinophilia-myalgia syndrome. The eosinophilia-myalgia studies of Oregon, New York and New Mexico. Am J Epidemiol 1993;138:154–159.

Pickle LW, Mason JJ, Howard N, Hoover R, Fraumeni JF Jr. Atlas of United States Cancer Mortality Among Whites: 1950–1980. Washington, DC: US Department of Health and Human Services; DHHS Publication No. (NIH) 87-2900; 1987.

Reilly MJ, Rosenman KD, Watt FC, et al. Surveillance for occupational asthma—Michigan and New Jersey, 1988–1992. In: CDC Surveillance Summaries (June 10). Morb Mortal Wkly Rep 1994;43(SS-1):9–17.

Schappert SM. National Ambulatory Medical Care Survey: 1989 summary. Hyattsville, MD: US Department of Health and Human Services, Public Health Service, CDC, NCHS; 1992. (Vital and health statistics; series 13, no. 110).

Schucat A, Broome CV. Toxic shock syndrome and tampons. Epidemiol Rev 1991;13:99–112.

Schwartz R, Smith C, Speers MA, et al. Capacity building and resource needs of state health agencies to implement community-based cardiovascular disease programs. J Public Health Policy. 1993;14:480–494.

Serdula MK, Collins ME, Williamson DF, Anda RF, Pamuk E, Byers TE. Weight control practices of U.S. adolescents and adults. Ann Int Med 1993;119(7 Pt 2):667–671.

Siegel PZ, Frazier EL, Mariolis P, Brackbill RM, et al. Behavioral risk factor surveillance, 1991: monitoring progress toward the nation's Year 2000 Health Objectives. Morb Mortal Wkly Rep 1993;42(SS42).

Simonsen L, Clark M, Stroup DF, et al. The impact of influenza epidemics on mortality: introducing a severity index. Epidemiol 1997;8:390–395.

Simpson DM. Improving the reporting of notifiable diseases in Texas: suggestions from an ad hoc committee of providers. J Public Health Management Practice 1996;2(4):37–39.

Smith RB. Recordkeeping rule aims for accuracy, wiser use of injury and illness data. OSHA hopes better documentation will lead to analysis that is precise. Occup Health Safety 1995;64(1):37, 40–41.

Spitalny KC. Learning to design new systems: communicable disease surveillance. J Public Health Management Practice 1996;2(4):40–41.

Stratton J. Systems development and integration: policy implications. Presented at: Second National Conference, Information Network for Public Health Officials, Atlanta, GA; 1996.

Stroup DF. Special statistical issues. In: Teutsch SM, Churchill RE, eds. Principles and Practice of Public Health Surveillance. New York: Oxford University Press; 1994:136–149.

Stroup DF, Thacker SB. A Bayesian approach to the detection of aberrations in public health surveillance data. Am J Epidemiol 1993;4(5):435–443.

Swygert LA, Maes EF, Sewell LE, et al. Eosinophilia-myalgia syndrome: results of national surveillance. JAMA 1990;264(3):1696–1703.

Swygert LA, Back EE, et al. Eosinophilia-myalgia syndrome: mortality data from the US National Surveillance System. J Rheumatol 1993;20:1711–1717.

Tejeda HA, Green SB, et al. Representation of African-Americans, Hispanics, and whites in National Cancer Institute cancer treatment trials. J Natl Cancer Inst 1996;88(12):812–816.

Terris M. The Society for Epidemiologic Research (SER) and the future of epidemiology. Am J Epidemiol 1992;136:909–915.

Teutsch SM, Herman WH, Dwyer DM, Lane JM. Mortality among diabetic patients using continuous subcutaneous insulin-infusion pumps. N Engl J Med 1984; 310:361–368.

Thacker SB. The principles and practice of public health surveillance: use of data in public health practice. Sante Publique 1992;4:43–49.

Thacker SB. Surveillance. In: Gregg MB, Goodman RA, eds. Field Epidemiology. New York: Oxford University Press; 1996:16–34.

Thacker SB, Berkelman RL. History of public health surveillance. In: Halperin WE, Baker EL, Monson RR, eds. Public Health Surveillance. New York: Van Nostrand Reinhold; 1992: 1–15.

Thacker SB, Stroup DF. Future directions of comprehensive public health surveillance and health information systems in the United States. Am J Epidemiol 1994;140(5):383–397.

Thacker SB, Berkelman RL, Stroup DF. The science of public health surveillance. J Public Health Policy 1989;10:187–203.

Thacker SB, Stroup DF, Rothenberg RR, Brownson R. Public health surveillance for chronic conditions: a scientific basis for decisions. Stat Med 1995;14:629–642.

US Dept of Health and Human Services. Healthy People 2000: National Health Promotion and Disease Prevention. Washington, DC: US Govt Printing Office; pub. no. 017-001-00473-1;1990.

US Dept of Health and Human Services. Preventing Tobacco Use among Young People. A Report of the Surgeon General. Atlanta, GA: US Dept of Health and Human Services, Centers for Disease Control and Prevention; 1994.

Wharton M, Chorba TL, Vogt RL, Morse DL, Buehler JW. Case definitions for public health surveillance. Morb Mortal Wkly Rep 1990;39(RR-13):1–43.

5

Epidemiology and Risk Assessment

JONATHAN M. SAMET
THOMAS A. BURKE

Overview and Definitions

Risk assessment is now a widely used term for a systematic approach to characterizing the risks posed to individuals and populations by environmental pollutants and other potentially adverse exposures. Risk assessment is increasingly applied as a translational tool for moving from research findings to the implementation and evaluation of policies. In the United States, its use is either explicitly or implicitly required by a number of federal statutes (Table 5-1), and its application worldwide is mounting. This chapter provides an introduction to risk assessment, focusing on those aspects of its methodology most pertinent to epidemiologists and addressing the use of epidemiologic data in risk assessment. The topic is assuming ever greater relevance for epidemiologists as the findings of epidemiologic research are incorporated into risk assessments both to determine the existence of a hazard and to gauge its extent of the hazard.

A seminal 1983 National Research Council report, *Risk Assessment in the Federal Government: Managing the Process* (often called the "Red Book" because of its cover), defined risk assessment as "the use of the factual base to define the health effects of exposure of individuals or populations to hazardous materials and situations (National Research Council [NRC] 1983)." This conceptualization of risk assessment is both qualitative and quantitative, although quantitative risk assessment should be considered as a component of risk assessment in its broadest context. The term "risk," as used in the context of risk assessment, conveys the same meaning as in its standard epidemiologic formulation: the probability of an event, e.g., disease occurrence, taking place. Depending on the context, risks sustained by individuals or by populations may be of interest. Some other health-related applications

Table 5-1. Principal US Environmental Health And Safety Laws: Agencies And Mandates Related To Risk

Statute	Responsible Agency	Mandate
Federal Food, Drug, and Cosmetic Act, 21 U.S.C. 301 *et seq.*	Department of Health and Human services Environmental Protection Agency	Prohibit, *inter alia*, distribution of foods, food and color additives, drugs, medical devices, and cosmetics that are "unsafe" or "injurious to health"; set standards for environmental contaminants in food as "necessary for the protection of public health"; set "safe" tolerances "to protect the public health" from pesticide residues on raw agricultural commodities (EPA sets the tolerances)
Federal Insecticide, Fungicide, and Rodenticide Act, 7 U.S.C. 136 *et seq.*	Environmental Protection Agency	Disallow use of pesticides that pose "any unreasonable risk to human health or the environment, taking into account the economic, social, and environment costs and benefits of the use of [the] pesticide"
Clean Air Act, 42 U.S.C. 7401 *et seq.*	Environmental Protection Agency	Issue ambient standards sufficient to "protect the public health" "with an adequate margin of safety"; issue "maximum achievable" standards for sources of hazardous pollutants which are "known or anticipated to cause adverse effects"; and set supplemental emission standards if it is found that the "maximum achievable" standards do not provide an "ample margin of safety" (defined for known or potential carcinogens as a risk level of less than one in one million for the most exposed individual)
Clean Water Act, 33 U.S.C. 1251 *et seq.*	Environmental Protection Agency	Prohibit discharges of pollutants in quantities "which may reasonably be anticipated to pose an unacceptable risk to human health or the environment" or "which present an imminent and substantial danger to the public health or welfare"
Safe Drinking Water Act, 42 U.S.C. 300f *et seq.*	Environmental Protection Agency	Set maximum contaminant level goals (MCLGs) to prevent "known or anticipated adverse [health] effects" with an "adequate margin of safety" and set maximum contaminant levels "as close as feasible" to the MCLGs

Statute	Agency	Description
Resource Conservation and Recovery Act, 42 U.S.C. 6901 *et seq.*	Environmental Protection Agency	Could disposal of solid wastes which "may cause, or significantly contribute to an increase in mortality or . . . serious irreversible, or incapacitating reversible, illness; or . . . pose a substantial present or potential hazard to human health or the environment" or which "endanger health [when present in excess of certain levels]"
Toxic Substances Control Act, 7 U.S.C. 136 *et seq.*	Environmental Protection Agency	Prevent "unreasonable risk of injury to health or the environment" from chemical substances or mixtures (as defined, with specified exceptions such as pesticides, drugs, and food additives)
Comprehensive Environmental Response, Compensation and Liability Act, 42 U.S.C. 9601 *et seq.*	Environmental Protection Agency	Hazardous waste cleanup levels must assure "protection of human health and the environment" against contaminants that "will, or may reasonably be anticipated to cause" certain adverse health effects, and must, under certain circumstances, meet standards set under other Acts, such as the Safe Drinking Water Act
Consumer Product Safety Act, 15 U.S.C. 2051 *et seq.*	Consumer Product Safety Commission	Set standards for, or prohibit distribution of, "consumer products" (with certain exceptions such as pesticides, drugs, and foods covered by other laws) that present an "unreasonable risk" of "death, personal injury, or serious or frequent illness"
Federal Mine Safety and Health Act, 30 U.S.C. 801 *et seq.*	Department of Labor	Set standards for the protection of life and prevention of injuries

Source: Federal Focus Inc. (1996).

of the term *risk*, as in "risk adjustment" for underlying disease severity, are not related to risk assessment.

The 1983 National Research Council report explicitly positioned risk assessment as a tool for translating the findings of research into science-based risk management strategies (Figure 5-1). Risk assessment evaluates and incorporates the findings of all relevant lines of investigation, from the molecular to population levels, through the application of a systematic process with four sequential steps: hazard identification, dose–response assessment, exposure assessment, and risk characterization (Table 5-2). If there is no positive determination of the existence of a hazard, then the subsequent steps are not warranted. Risk assessment also provides a comprehensive framework for bringing together all relevant information on the existence of a hazard to health and on the magnitude of the hazard. Thus, the hazard identification step could involve consideration of structure–activity relationships for a toxin, laboratory findings from in vitro and in vivo experiments, and epidemiologic evidence. dose–response assessment may also draw on multiple types of data. While the figure separates research from risk assessment, there is continued interplay between researchers and risk assessors as key gaps in evidence are identified and research is initiated to address them.

Risk assessments are performed by a variety of institutions. Some are conducted within federal and state agencies because of mandated requirements (Table 5-1). For example, the Occupational Safety and Health Administration uses risk assessment to establish that the agent considered for regulation causes "significant risk of harm," as mandated by the Supreme Court's "Benzene" decision. In this significant Supreme Court decision, the Occupational Safety and Health Administration was required to conduct a risk assessment for exposure of workers to benzene in order to show that benzene caused a significant risk to health. The Environmental Protection Agency, under the 1990 Clean Air Act amendments, has been required to evaluate the risks of 189 hazardous air pollutants to ensure that exposures to populations have "an ample margin of safety." Private sector entities including pollutant-emitting industries may also use risk assessment to determine potential consequences of exposures to workers or to the general population from processes that may lead to environmental contamination. Voluntary health organizations, such as the American Lung Association, or environmental organizations may themselves apply risk assessment methods to gauge the magnitude of hazards posed by environmental toxins and then use the results to promote prevention and influence the public and policy-makers.

Risk management follows and builds from risk assessment. Risk management involves the evaluation of alternative regulatory actions and the selection of the strategy to be applied. Risk communication is the transmission of the findings of risk assessments to the many "stake-holders" who need to

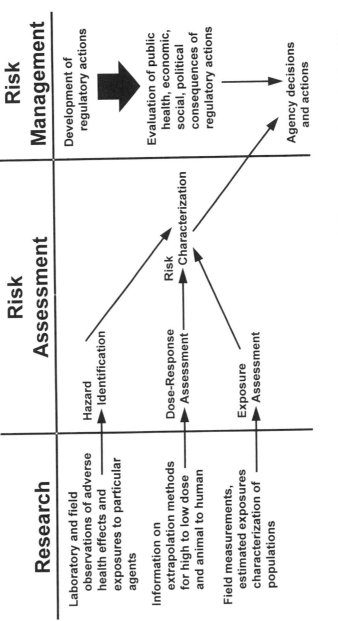

Figure 5-1. Schematic relations among research, risk assessment, and risk management. *Source:* NCR (1983)

Table 5-2. The "Red Book" Paradigm: the Four Steps of Risk Assessment

Hazard identification:	A review of the relevant biological and chemical information bearing on whether or not an agent may pose a carcinogenic hazard and whether toxic effects in one setting will occur in other settings
Dose response:	The process of quantifying a dosage and evaluating its relationship to the incidence of adverse health effects response
Exposure assessment:	The determination or estimation (qualitative or quantitative) of the magnitude, duration, and route of exposure
Risk characterization:	An integration and summary of hazard identification, dose-response assessment, and exposure assessment presented with assumptions and uncertainties. This final step provides an estimate of the risk to public health and a framework to define the significance of the risk

Source: NRC (1983).

know the results to participate in the policy-making process and to the general public. In this formalism, and in practice to some degree, those performing the risk assessment—risk assessors—and those managing the risks—risk managers—are separate groups of professionals and distinct from the researchers who develop the data used in risk assessments. At present, risk assessors come from diverse disciplinary backgrounds and many have moved from scientific- or policy-based positions into conducting risk assessments.

Epidemiologists have diverse potential roles in risk assessment and risk management. First, the findings of epidemiologic studies may be key in the steps of hazard identification and dose–response assessment, and may also contribute to exposure assessment. Consequently, epidemiologists may become partners in the conduct of a risk assessment and assist in assuring that the findings of epidemiologic studies have been interpreted appropriately by risk assessors. This type of engagement by epidemiologists may involve committee service, consultation, peer review, or testimony. Second, epidemiologists may assume the roles of risk assessors or risk managers, leaving behind the primary role of epidemiologic researcher. Finally, epidemiologists may be called on to devise surveillance systems to document the consequences of an implemented risk management strategy.

While epidemiologists and epidemiologic data may have prominent roles in risk assessments, the epidemiologic literature contains surprisingly few discussions of risk assessment. The topic was treated directly in a 1985 conference (Gordis 1988) and again in a 1994 conference (Graham 1995). Hertz-Picciotto (1995) provided a cogent summary in a recent review, emphasizing the use of epidemiologic data to characterize dose–response relationships. Risk assessment in general is covered in a series of landmark reports on the topic by committees of the US National Research Council: the 1983 report, *Risk Assessment in the Federal Government: Managing the Process* (NRC 1983); a 1989 report on risk communication, *Improving Risk Communication* (NRC 1989); a 1994 report that comprehensively evaluated risk assessment methods, *Science and Judgment in Risk Assessment* (known as the "Blue Book") (NRC 1994a); and a 1996 report on risk characterization, *Understanding Risk. Informing Decisions in a Democratic Society* (NRC 1996). Other National Research Council reports address risks of specific agents. Rodricks (1992) offers a readable introduction that emphasizes toxicologic approaches in *Calculated Risks*. The journal *Risk Analysis* focuses on the topic.

The Evolution of Risk Assessment

The formal characteristics of risk assessment have a brief history (NRC 1994a; Rodricks 1992). While many core concepts had been developed earlier, the origins of contemporary risk assessment can be traced to the 1970s when new environmental regulations called for information on risks in order to set policy. Even earlier, however, the need to protect the general public and workers had led to the development of methods for setting exposure limits that inherently involved risk estimation. To protect workers, particularly against short-term toxicity, exposure limits were set that were below levels known or considered likely to have adverse effects. For example, Threshold Limit Values (TLVs) were first set by the American Conference of Government Industrial Hygienists (ACGIH). For foods, acceptable daily intakes (ADIs) of pesticides and food additives were set based on animal assays. The no-observed-effect level (NOEL) in the assay, subsequently modified to the no-observed-adverse-effect level (NOAEL), was divided by a safety factor to yield the ADI for people. For foods, a safety factor of 100 was assumed. These approaches implicitly assume that there is a threshold level of exposure or dose that must be exceeded for an adverse effect to occur at an unacceptable frequency.

In the 1960s and 1970s, mounting concern about environmental carcinogens accelerated the use of risk assessment by federal agencies, including the Food and Drug Administration, the Environmental Protection Agency, and the Occupational Safety and Health Administration. The widening use of risk assessment, as regulators attempted to manage increasing numbers of chemicals, motivated the Food and Drug Administration to support the National

Research Council Committee, which wrote the Red Book. The committee had three principal objectives: (1) "to assess the merits of separating the analytic functions of developing risk assessments from the regulatory functions of making policy decisions," (2) "to consider the feasibility of designating a single organization to do risk assessments for all regulatory agencies," and (3) "to consider the feasibility of developing uniform risk assessment guidelines for use by all regulatory agencies" (NRC 1983).

The committee's response to this charge continues to set the framework for risk assessment and risk management. The committee recommended a clear conceptual distinction between risk assessment and risk management (Figure 5-1) and formalized the risk assessment process into the four-step paradigm (Table 5-2). Paramount for epidemiologists, the report further distinguished research from risk assessment. The report acknowledged that uncertainties affect risk assessments and that gaps in knowledge need to be filled by making choices among plausible options, termed "inference options." The committee also called for the development of uniform guidelines for selecting among inference options. The committee recognized that the inference option selected could carry policy implications.

Subsequent to the Red Book, use of risk assessment at the federal and state levels increased. Guidelines for carcinogen assessment and other types of toxicity were published by the Environmental Protection Agency (US Environmental Protection Agency [US EPA] 1986), which also developed guidelines for exposure assessment (US EPA 1992). Risk assessment was used as a priority-setting tool by the Department of Energy in implementing clean-up programs at its nuclear sites; and the Agency for Toxic Substances and Disease Registry applied risk assessment approaches to contaminated sites throughout the United States. The Environmental Protection Agency took a risk-based approach in attempting to assign priorities to the many environmental hazards that it faced. A 1987 report, *Unfinished Business*, provided the findings of agency staff on the relative importance of a listing of 31 hazards in four categories of risk: human cancer risk, human noncancer risk, ecological risk, and welfare risk (US EPA 1987). This type of ranking was needed to consider strategic options, and the report represented one of the first comprehensive exercises in risk ranking. In the 1990 follow-up report, *Reducing Risk: Setting Priorities and Strategies for Environmental Protection*, a committee addressed the data and methodologies needed for risk ranking (US EPA 1990). The committee's recommendations emphasized the pervasive need for information on risk in setting environmental policies.

The Clean Air Act Amendments of 1990 required a review by the National Academy of Sciences of methods used by the Environmental Protection Agency to estimate risk. The review, published in 1994 and entitled *Science and Judgment in Risk Assessment* (NRC 1994a), provides a summary of the state of the art in risk assessment as of the early 1990s. It recommended the continued use of risk assessment but called for an iterative approach that better blends risk assessment with risk management. The report identified many gaps in the data needed for risk assessment and in the methods and assumptions made by the agency in conducting its risk assessments. A chapter addressed use of observational evidence.

The Clean Air Act amendments also mandated the establishment of a Commission on Risk Assessment and Risk Management that would "make a full investigation of the policy implications and appropriate uses of risk assessment and risk management in regulatory programs under various Federal laws to prevent cancer and other chronic human health effects which may result from exposure to hazardous substances." The commission's report comments that risk assessment has become more refined analytically but notes that risk assessments done for regulation tend to give insufficient attention to risk reduction and improving health (The Presidential/Congressional Commission on Risk Assessment and Risk Management 1997). It proposes a new framework for risk management that places collaboration with stakeholders at the center. Risk assessment remains key, but risks should be placed into the broad context of public health, and comparisons should be made to other risks to the population.

A similar broadening of the Red Book framework was proposed in the 1996 report of a committee of the National Research Council: *Understanding Risk. Informing Decisions in a Democratic Society* (NRC 1996). This report extended the concept of risk characterization articulated in the Red Book. Like the draft report of the Commission on Risk Assessment and Risk Management, this report noted that a broad context needs to be set for risk characterization and recommended broad participation in risk characterization from all stakeholders. It called for an iterative process of analyses and deliberation and for determining the concerns and perceived risks of stakeholders as the risk assessment is initiated. A risk characterization, to be informative, may need to be expressed along multiple dimensions, and not be limited to a simple numeric expression of harm, e.g., the number of excess cancers. It should be aimed at informing the decision process and solving problems.

In the mid-1990s, we seem poised for a broadening use of risk assessment in developing public policies, particularly those involving environmental regulation. In fact, in 1994, the 104th Congress of the United States began with clamor for "regulatory reform," and most draft reform bills gave risk assessment a central role in the setting of regulations and in evaluating the costs and benefits of regulations. There was an accompanying call for "sound science" as the basis for risk assessments. Risk assessment has also assumed increasing importance as a regulatory tool at state and local levels, and internationally.

In spite of its brief history, risk assessment has already gained substantial notoriety; so, too, has the use of epidemiologic data for risk assessment purposes. Examples of controversial and debated applications of the method and the use of epidemiologic data include the Environmental Protection Agency's risk assessments for environmental tobacco smoke (US EPA 1992a) and for radon (US EPA 1992b), and the assessment of the risk of workplace exposure to environmental tobacco smoke conducted by the Occupational Safety and Health Administration (US Department of Labor and Occupational Safety and Health Administration [US OSHA] 1994). Consequently, there have been published evaluations of the utility of epidemiologic data for risk assessment purposes (Graham 1995) and attempts to develop guidelines for their use (Federal Focus Inc. 1996). These guidelines are covered in this chapter.

For epidemiologists, the lessons to be learned from this brief review should include recognition that risk assessment is now ensconced as a policy-making tool and that epidemiologic data may have a central role in setting policies that have substantial societal implications. Legislative trends indicate that risk assessment will likely gain prominence as a tool for translating epidemiologic research into public policy.

Epidemiology and Risk Assessment

The value of epidemiologic data for risk assessment has been widely discussed (Graham 1995). Pundits argue that epidemiologic data are rarely relevant and too often flawed by poor quality and uncontrolled biases (Graham 1995). Epidemiologic studies have also been deemed uninformative given the "weak associations" anticipated for typical levels of exposure to many environmental agents. Proponents of epidemiology, while acknowledging the limitations of observational studies, advance its strengths: the investigation of the effects of real exposures as received by the population; the characterization of effect across the full range of susceptibility in the population; and, above all, the direct relevance of epidemiologic evidence to public health (Hertz-Picciotto 1995; Burke 1995). The debate on the role of epidemiologic evidence in risk assessment has proceeded both generally and specifically, and risk assessment findings for individual agents, such as radon and environmental tobacco smoke, have been questioned. Guidelines for epidemiologic research to be used in risk assessment have been offered as one solution to strengthening the evidence base (Hertz-Picciotto 1995; Federal Focus Inc. 1996; Auchter 1995). The guidelines largely echo principles that are already tenets of the field.

Uncertainty and Variability

Two concepts central to the interpretation and application of a risk assessment are uncertainty and variability. Any assessment of risk involves developing an underlying model with attendant assumptions that cover gaps in knowledge. "Uncertainty" refers to this lack of knowledge (NRC 1994a). Examples of sources of uncertainty include extrapolation of findings from animals to humans, extrapolation from high-dose observable effects to the unobservable low-dose range, and use of models or assumptions to estimate population exposure indirectly, rather than with direct measurements. Analyses of uncertainty may be qualitative or quantitative. Qualitative analyses may involve expert judgments, whether accomplished informally or more formally using a systematic approach for achieving convergence among experts (National Council on Radiation Protection and Measurements [NCRP] 1996). Quantitative assessments of uncertainty may use sensitivity analyses—that is, varying model assumptions and assessing the consequences—or model-based approaches may be employed that characterize the contributions of various sources of uncertainty to overall uncertainty.

Variability, although distinct from uncertainty, may also cloud the interpretation of a risk assessment. There are many sources of variability that may affect a risk assessment (NRC 1994a). These include variability in exposures and susceptibility; together, these two sources of variability could lead to a wide range of risk in a population. Central estimates of risk, which do not address variation in risk across a population, may be misleading and may obscure the existence of a group at unacceptable risk that is hidden in the tail of the risk distribution. For example, Figure 5-2 shows the approximate distribution of radon levels in US homes. Assuming that risk and exposure to radon are related in a linear fashion, then the distribution of risk is highly skewed. The range of concentrations extends up to about 1,000-fold greater than the mean. Different risk management strategies may be appropriate for those homes around the average versus the very high homes.

For some regulatory programs, the Environmental Protection Agency has used the upper 95% bound of the confidence interval on risk estimates to guide standard setting and evaluate potential population impacts. This "conservative" approach acknowledges general sampling variability but may not fully account for all sources of variability. Factors that may determine the range of susceptibility include genetic background, sex, age, race and ethnicity, and exposures to other agents. The Environmental Protection Agency has published exposure assessment guidelines for use in risk assessment which acknowledge the variability of exposures across the population (US EPA 1992c).

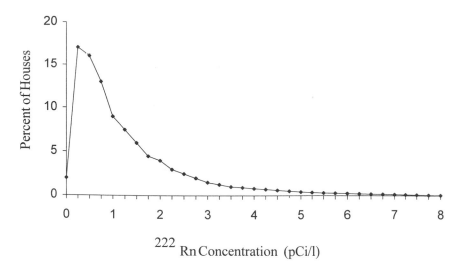

Figure 5-2. Distribution of indoor radon levels in US homes

Use of Epidemiologic Data in Risk Assessment

Hazard Identification

Hazard identification is the first step of a risk assessment, addressing the question of whether the agent or factor poses a risk to human health. This step is inherently integrative, as it may draw evidence from structure–activity relationships for chemical agents, in vitro evidence of toxicity, animal bio-assays, and epidemiologic data (NRC 1983). Epidemiologic data indicative of an adverse effect, when available, are strongly weighted in the evaluation of the weight of evidence to determine if an agent presents a hazard. Human data provide direct evidence of a hazard without the need to extrapolate from knowledge of toxicity in analogous agents or from another species. In fact, as we have gained a further understanding of the complexity of cross-species extrapolation from animal to man, such extrapolations are viewed with less certainty, unless buttressed by an understanding of human and animal path-ways of absorption and metabolism and of mechanisms of action. Further, epidemiologic studies evaluate the impact of exposures received by the population, including complex mixtures which may not be readily replicable in the laboratory. Epidemiologic research captures the consequences of inter-actions among agents, and investigations in populations may capture the full range of susceptibility. However, given the numbers of agents of concern, epidemiologic data have been available on only a small number of environmental contaminants, and there is more often reliance on toxicologic evidence in identifying a hazard. In addressing gaps in the database on an agent's toxicity, the Blue Book gives toxicologic data collection higher priority than epidemiologic data collection, justifying this ordering by the cost of epidemiologic data and the ambiguity of the findings of some observational studies.

In using epidemiologic data for the step of hazard identification, researchers' interpretation of the evidence is fully parallel to the assessment of the causality of an association between an exposure and an adverse health effect. There are no specific guidelines for interpretation of epidemiologic data in risk assessments that go beyond the conventionally applied criteria for causality. For cancer, guidelines for interpreting the strength of evidence have been published, for example, by the International Agency for Research on Cancer (WHO IARC 1972). However, these guidelines are not rigid criteria and, as with the widely applied criteria for causality, there may be disagreement on the proper classification of epidemiologic evidence for the purpose of hazard identification. For example, the interpretation of negative epidemiologic findings in the hazard identification process is a major source of disagreement.

Nonetheless, epidemiologic data have played a central role in some risk assessments, e.g., lung cancer/environmental tobacco smoke (US EPA 1992a) and lung cancer/indoor radon (US EPA 1992b). In its 1992 risk assessment, the Environmental Protection Agency classified environmental tobacco smoke as a class A carcinogen (i.e., a carcinogen for which definitive human carcinogenicity was available). The report noted that the data from active smokers, in combination with an understanding of mechanisms and dose–response relations, were sufficient for this classification. However, a principal basis for the classification was the result of a meta-analysis of the epidemiologic studies on lung cancer risk in never-smoking women married to smokers. The agency's analysis was also careful to consider potential sources of bias affecting the findings of the epidemiologic studies. In the example of radon, there is convincing evidence on human carcinogenicity from epidemiologic studies of radon-exposed miners (NRC 1988). All of the studies show strongly increased overall risks of lung cancer, approximately increased by three- to sixfold, and radon exposure alone causes lung cancer in laboratory models. Approximately 20 studies have shown excess lung cancer occurrence; the excess cannot be explained by confounding by smoking or other factors and the effect is strong. In assessing the risk of indoor radon, the agency has considered that the findings from epidemiologic studies of underground miners are sufficient for the hazard identification step.

Dose–Response Assessment

Once a hazard is identified, the second step—the dose–response assessment—is initiated to establish the quantitative relationship between dose and response. Dose, the quantity of material entering the exposed person, is not identical to exposure, which is defined as contact with a material at a potential portal of entry into the body: the skin, the respiratory tract, and the gastrointestinal tract (NRC 1991a). Typically, epidemiologic studies characterize the relationship between exposure, or a surrogate for exposure, and response; the dose–response relationship may be estimable if the relationship between exposure and dose can be established. For a risk assessment, description of the exposure–response relationship may be sufficient as exposure can be linked to response. In combination with data on the distribution of exposure, the risk posed to a population by an agent can be estimated without moving to establish the dose–response relationship.

For the purpose of risk assessment, characterization of the exposure–response relationship in the range of human exposures is needed. For a few agents, e.g., environmental tobacco smoke, data on risks are available in the exposure range of interest and risk to the general population can be estimated directly; for others, data from exposures above those received by the population may be available from worker groups, e.g., radon exposures of uranium miners, or from persons who have been accidentally exposed, e.g., radiation exposures of the survivors of the atomic bomb blasts in Hiroshima and Nagasaki. For such exposures above the range of usual environmental levels, exposure–response relationships estimated at the higher exposures are extended downward. Epidemiologic studies rarely include comprehensive data on exposure or dose during the biologically relevant interval and exposures are often estimated from incomplete data. Consequently, misclassification of exposure may bias the description of the exposure–response relationship. Simple generalizations concerning the consequences of measurement error cannot be made (Armstrong et al. 1992). Random error or nondifferential misclassification tends to blunt the exposure–response relationship but other effects may also occur (Dosemeci et al. 1990). Nonrandom errors or differential misclassification may increase or decrease the gradient of the exposure–response relationship.

In analyzing epidemiologic data to characterize the exposure–response relationship, there is a priori interest in determining if the exposure–response relationship is statistically significant—i.e., whether the null hypothesis of a flat exposure–response relationship can be rejected—and in characterizing the shape of the relationship. For the former, the significance of the trend in response with exposure is of interest, but not the significance of the effect within a stratum for the null hypothesis of no effect within the stratum.

Initially, the shape of the exposure–response relationship may be explored descriptively, but inevitably statistical models are used to quantitate the change in response with increasing exposure. To date, models have been used primarily to characterize the effects of carcinogenic agents; less effort has been directed at noncancer effects for which human data have been less abundant.

For cancer, a number of alternative models have been used to characterize the association between exposure and risk (Figure 5-3). Arguments for the biologic plausibility of some of the key alternatives can be made, and some of the alternative models have substantially different public health and regula-

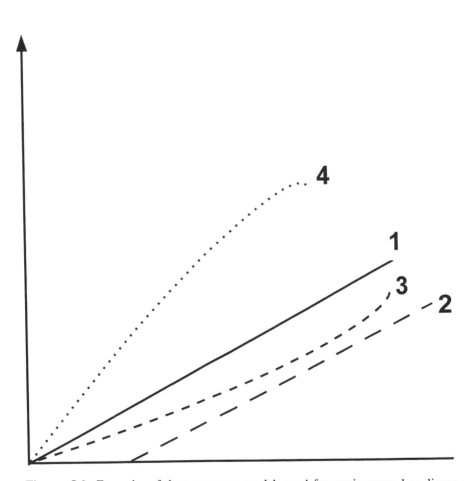

Figures 5-3. Examples of dose–response models used for carcinogens: 1 = linear nonthreshold mode; 2 = linear threshold model; 3 = sublinear nonthreshold model; and, 4 = supralinear nonthreshold model

tory implications. The models differ in the presence of a threshold of exposure that must be exceeded before cancer occurs and in the shape of the relationship between exposure and response. A threshold would be anticipated if repair processes could accommodate some level of damage or if the low levels of exposure had a salutary effect. For example, the identification of adaptive responses to radiation has led to speculation that there are "hormetic" effects of radiation at low levels which are actually beneficial (Luckey 1991). In addition to a linear relationship between exposure and response, sub- and supralinear alternatives may also be plausible.

A model of the exposure–response relationship might be estimated from epidemiologic data in order to extrapolate from higher exposures, where observations have been made, to lower levels, where population exposures occur, or to describe the exposure–response relationship quantitatively at typical exposures. In modeling epidemiologic data, a priori biologic considerations should determine the choice of the model. For example, a linear relationship without a threshold would be consistent with an exposure that caused irreparable genetic damage with a single "hit" from the agent. Genetic injury from alpha particles released by deposited radionuclides—"internal emitters"—is an example. For some agents, modeling approaches have been established that have a biologic rationale and historical precedent. For ionizing radiation, a linear no-threshold relationship has long been assumed, although there is the possibility of departure from linearity at the lowest level of exposure (NRC 1990; United Nations Scientific Committee on the Effects of Atomic Radiation [UNSCEAR] 1993). The assumption that there is not a threshold is also protective of public health, as it implies that no level of exposure is safe. For example, to develop a model for the lung cancer risk of indoor radon, data from studies of miners have been analyzed with Poisson regression models for the excess relative risk of lung cancer. These models describe the increment in relative risk with increasing exposure to radon progeny.

Epidemiologic data may also be fit with alternative models of the exposure–response relationship if there is uncertainty about the most appropriate shape. Model fit may be used to guide the selection of the "best" model. However, epidemiologic data are rarely sufficiently abundant to provide powerful discrimination among alternative models, and sample size requirements for comparing fit of alternative models having different public health implications may be very high (Land 1980; Lubin et al. 1990). For example, Lubin and colleagues (1990) calculated sample size requirements for testing if the exposure–response relationship for radon and lung cancer differed by 100% from that observed in underground miners. The calculations indicated that approximately 10,000 participants would be needed in a case-control study if sufficient power were to be achieved.

Biomarkers of exposure, dose, and response, and also of susceptibility, have been touted as possible solutions to the limitations of epidemiologic studies for characterizing the exposure–response relationship, particularly at low levels of exposure (Links et al. 1994; Mendelsohn et al. 1995). Use of biomarkers of exposure may reduce misclassification, while biomarkers of dose or response could potentially provide more proximate indicators of risk; biomarkers are also potential bridges for extending the results of animal studies to humans.

Exposure Assessment

For the purpose of risk assessment, information is needed on the full distribution of exposures in the population. Measures of central tendency may be appropriate for estimating overall risk to the population, but reliance on central measures alone may hide the existence of more highly exposed persons with unacceptable levels of risk. For example, the average concentration of indoor radon in US homes is about 1 picocurie per liter (pCi/l—a measure of radioactivity). About 5% of homes are above the guideline for action of 4 pCi/l and some homes have concentrations of 1,000 or more. Focusing solely on control measures to lower the average exposure would obscure the need to find the homes in the tail of the distribution which have unacceptable levels. The Environmental Protection Agency has recognized the need to characterize the upper end of the exposure distribution in its exposure assessment guidelines (US EPA 1992c). Driven largely by the needs of risk assessment, exposure assessment has matured: its underlying concepts have evolved and its methods have become more sophisticated. In fact, a field of exposure assessment has emerged, spawning a specific scientific society for exposure assessment—the International Society of Exposure Analysis—and the *Journal of Exposure Analysis and Environmental Epidemiology*. Key concepts of exposure assessment are presented in a 1991 National Research Council report (NRC 1991b).

Modern exposure assessment is based on a conceptual framework that relates pollutant sources to effects through the intermediaries of exposure and dose (Figure 5-4) (NRC 1991b, 1994a). The concept of total personal exposure is central; that is, for health risk assessment, exposures received by individuals from all sources and media need to be considered. For some agents, e.g., lead, exposures may arise from multiple sources, media of exposure, and activities. Thus, lead may enter the body through ingestion of lead-paint-contaminated house dust, consumption of lead-contaminated foods and beverages, and inhalation of airborne lead. The tools of the exposure assessor include questionnaires to describe activities, monitoring devices for environmental and personal sampling, and biomarkers. Too often, data on exposures

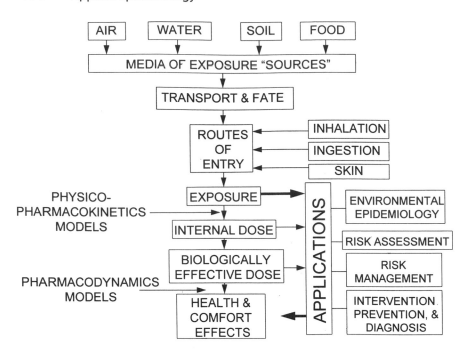

Figure 5-4. Representation of the pathways from sources and media of exposure to health effects. From *Human Exposure Assessment for Airborne Pollutonts: Advances and Opportunities,* Copyright 1991 National Academy of Sciences. Courtesy of the National Academy Press, Washington, D.C. Used with permission

are limited, and model-based approaches may be substituted for actual population-based data. Modeling approaches, based on assuming an exposure model and statistical distributions for key model parameters, can yield exposure distributions. However, absent validation, the results of such exercises are subject to substantial uncertainty.

To date, epidemiologic data have not played prominent roles in exposure assessment. However, epidemiologic-based surveillance and screening approaches have the potential to provide important insights into population exposures. For example, blood lead surveillance has been a critical part of understanding the risks of environmental lead. Population-based survey data may be available on exposures, often describing contact with sources, e.g., exposure to smokers as an indicator of exposure to environmental tobacco smoke (Jenkins et al. 1991), or levels of biomarkers, e.g., cotinine (Mendelsohn et al. 1995). However, the data collected for evaluating exposure–disease associations may not adequately meet the needs of risk assessment.

Risk Characterization

Risk characterization represents the final step in risk assessment. During this phase, the data on exposure are combined with the exposure–response relationship to estimate the potential risk posed to exposed populations. The risk characterization becomes the fulcrum for decision-making and the basis for communication with stakeholders (NRC 1996). Epidemiologic studies may provide a direct risk characterization if the findings can be linked to a specific population and the exposure assessment component of the study is sufficient. The population attributable risk, an indication of the burden of imposed morbidity or mortality, is an appropriate parameter for risk characterization, as would be years of life lost. This step puts the risk in perspective for risk managers and the public. The Red Book approach emphasized the presentation of the probability of harm. However, a recent National Research Council report (1996) has called for risk characterization to be broader and to consider social, economic, and political factors in describing risk and guiding risk management options. This report emphasized the need to engage stakeholders through a risk assessment so as to assure that the risk characterization addresses the full range of concerns. Epidemiology offers an effective tool for addressing the population impacts and public health relevance of a risk in a holistic and meaningful fashion for those exposed and those deciding upon risk management strategies.

Special Issues in Using Epidemiologic Data

Guidelines

Policy decisions and risk management strategies based upon risk assessments may have substantial societal implications. Consequently, approaches have been developed for standardizing the approach to risk assessment for specific classes of agents. These guidelines, such as those published by the Environmental Protection Agency, offer a framework for evaluating the available information, whether from epidemiologic or experimental research, and then using the data in the risk assessment process. The rising use of epidemiologic evidence in risk assessments with regulatory implications has led to concern that specific guidelines are needed for epidemiologic studies with regulatory implications. This section also addresses proposals for such guidelines.

Guidelines have been most extensively developed for determining carcinogenicity. Perhaps the longest-standing guidelines are those of the International Agency for Research on Cancer (IARC), which began a program in 1969 to evaluate the carcinogenic risk of chemicals to humans (WHO IARC 1972). The procedures of the agency only take the evaluation through the step of hazard identification, determining whether the evidence of carcingenicity is sufficient. The monographs on the chemicals do not attempt to quantify the risk, although dose–response relationships are considered as the causality of associations is assessed. The IARC working groups are charged with considering only epidemiologic studies of adequate quality and with considering the methodology of the study: definition of the study population, disease, and exposure; confounding and the selection of the comparison population; adequate description of the basic data; and use of proper analytic methods. The totality of the epidemiologic evidence is to be evaluated with criteria that emphasize the strength of the association, replication, dose response, and specificity. The guidelines also provide criteria for interpreting studies as showing a lack of carcinogenicity. In the final classification of a chemical, the strength of the evidence from both human and animal studies is considered and integrated for the overall evaluation.

One of the earliest attempts to develop regulatory guidelines was the report of the Interagency Regulatory Liaison Group (IRLG) (IRLG 1979). This wide-ranging report covered the types of input information needed to conduct a cancer risk assessment and offered recommendations for the evaluation of this information. It described the epidemiologic approach to studying carcinogens and indicated the need for attention to biologic plausibility, bias, confounding, and chance.

The Environmental Protection Agency has published a series of guidelines on cancer and other health endpoints. The Cancer Guidelines date to 1986, but proposed revisions have been published (US EPA 1986). The 1986 guidelines follow the structure of the IARC approach then in use and classified agents into five groups: group A (Human Carcinogen), group B (Probable Human Carcinogen), group C (Possible Human Carcinogen), group D (Not Classifiable as to Human Carcinogenicity), and group E (Evidence for Non-Carcinogenicity for Humans). The guidelines acknowledge the potentially unique contribution that human data can make but caution that epidemiologic data "are inherently capable of detecting only comparatively large increases in the relative risk of cancer." The criteria offered for assessing epidemiologic studies parallel those in the IARC guidelines. The agency's proposed new guidelines offer a markedly different classification scheme that replaces the five categories with verbal descriptors. Information on mode of action receives greater emphasis, reflecting the substantial evolution in the understanding of mechanisms of carcinogenesis. The guidelines offer 10 criteria for evaluating epidemiologic studies (Table 5-3). These criteria are fully

Table 5-3. Guidelines For Assessing Epidemiologic Studies (US Environmental Protection Agency's Cancer Guidelines)

1. Clear articulation of study objectives or hypothesis
2. Proper selection and characterization of the exposed and control groups
3. Adequate characterization of exposure
4. Sufficient length of follow-up for disease occurrence
5. Valid ascertainment the causes of cancer morbidity
6. Proper consideration of bias and confounding factors
7. Adequate sample size to detect and effect
8. Clear, well-documented, and appropriate methodology for data collection and analysis
9. Adequate response rate and methodology for handling missing data
10. Complete and clear documentation of results

consistent with usual practices of epidemiologists in conducting research studies. The guidelines' scheme for weighing human evidence follows closely the widely applied criteria for causality.

More general guidelines for the conduct of epidemiologic research with regulatory implications have been proposed. The Chemical Manufacturers Association has published guidelines for "good epidemiologic practices" that provide specifications for both design and documentation. The calls for rigorous and standardized documentation of protocols in these recommendations and those of the new Cancer Guidelines of the Environmental Protection Agency are warranted, and current practices may often not meet these guidelines. The general need for guidelines was the topic of a 1994 conference (Graham 1995). In follow-up of this conference a set of guidelines entitled "Principles for Evaluating Epidemiologic Data in Regulatory Risk Assessment" was published in 1996. These guidelines were based on a panel of 18 individuals who were convened by Federal Focus Inc., a nonprofit foundation established to "engage in research and educational activities pertaining to Federal government policy issues, particularly ones of inter-agency concern."

The Federal Focus guidelines offer principles for assessing the utility of an epidemiologic study for risk assessment, for evaluating epidemiologic reports on cause–effect relationships, and for using human and animal data in dose–response evaluation. Checklists are provided for evaluating the adequacy of studies for the hazard identification of a risk assessment. The listed items are appropriate but criteria are not offered for their use nor are any tests of their application shown. Recommendations emphasizing interaction between epidemiologists and risk assessors are also made to improve the use of epidemiologic evidence in risk assessment.

Additional guidelines, focused on the dose–response step, were recently offered by Hertz-Picciotto (1995). She proposed a three-tiered evaluation scheme based on five criteria (Table 5-4). Category 1 studies were considered as offering a direct basis for deriving a dose–response relationship. Studies in this category are to meet four of five criteria. The first criterion, having a moderate-to-strong association, may inappropriately exclude studies of agents for which more modest effects are anticipated on a biological basis. Criteria 3 and 4 are reflective of the extent of the data that may be needed to address risk assessment needs. Studies in categories 2 and 3 are less informative than those in category 1 and cannot contribute directly to the dose–response step. Like other approaches to evaluating epidemiologic studies, application of the criteria could prove difficult and a test of the proposed classification has not yet been made.

These newer proposed guidelines, from the Federal Focus panel and Hertz-Picciotto, have not yet been applied, nor have they been endorsed by professional societies. In fact, professional organizations in epidemiology have remained silent on the use of epidemiologic evidence in risk assessment. While the guidelines remain untested, they are indicative of the scrutiny applied to epidemiologic findings in the risk assessment context and represent a starting point for broader discussion on evaluation of epidemiologic studies used in risk assessment.

Meta-Analysis

Epidemiologic studies may have limited power to address the effects of exposures in a range that would be of concern for the general population Meta-analysis has been used to summarize data for the steps of hazard identification and dose–response assessment. It has been used increasingly as a tool for summarizing experimental and observational studies (Petitti 1994), and methods for epidemiologic data have been extensively reviewed (see Chapter 2) (Greenland 1987; Dickersin and Berlin 1992). For experimental data, meta-analysis of observational data provides a potentially more informative interpretation of the evidence when sampling variation and small studies have obscured the status of the evidence. Thus, statistical power for detecting an effect is gained and dose–response relationships can be described with greater precision. Meta-analysis has now been applied to a number of environmental agents including environmental tobacco smoke (US EPA 1992a), electromagnetic radiation (NRC 1996), nitrogen dioxide (Hasselblad et al. 1992), and indoor radon (Lubin and Boice 1997).

The use of meta-analysis for risk assessment has proved controversial in

Table 5-4. Classification Of Epidemiologic Studies For Risk Assessment by Proposed Use

Criteria	Proposed Use		
	1. Can Be Basis for Extrapolation	2. Can Be Used to Check Plausibility of Animal-Based Assessment	3. Can Contribute to Hazard Identification
Moderate to strong association	Necessary	Not necessary	Can add to weight of evidence
Strong biases ruled out or unlikely	Necessary	Should be met, at least partially	If met, strengthens hazard identification
Confounding controlled or likely to be limited	Necessary	Should be met, at least partially, or extent of bias estimated	If met, strengthens hazard identification
Exposures quantified for individuals	Necessary	Some qualification of exposure is needed	Usually not met
Monotonic dose-response relationship	Not necessary but odds certainty	Not necessary	May or may not be met
Summary of require-ments	First four criteria 1–4 should be met	Two of first three criteria 1–3 should be met	All other studies

Source: Hertz-Picciotto (1995).

the instance of environmental tobacco smoke, which is the mixture of side-stream smoke and exhaled mainstream smoke involuntarily inhaled by non-smokers. In evaluating the carcinogenicity of this mixture, the Environmental Protection Agency used meta-analysis to summarize the findings of case-control and cohort studies of environmental tobacco smoke and lung cancer (US EPA 1992a). By 1992, when the agency's risk assessment was completed, 31 studies had been reported. Effect estimates covered a relatively narrow range of effect, from none to an approximate doubling of risk. The effects were not statistically significant in a number of the studies. While the case-control studies were generally similar in design, they had been conducted throughout the world and were potentially subject to differing sources of bias. The agency's meta-analysis showed a significantly increased risk, about 25%, for lung cancer among nonsmoking women married to smokers. The agency's risk assessment of environmental tobacco smoke and the use of meta-analysis as a method for summarizing the evidence have been heavily criticized, largely in work supported by the tobacco industry (Biggerstaff et al. 1994; Tweedie and Mengersen 1995). One particular point of criticism has been the agency's use of 90% confidence intervals rather than 95% confidence intervals for summary estimates. This approach was based on the prior assumption of carcinogenicity of environmental tobacco smoke.

Meta-analysis has been used to characterize the relationship between exposure to indoor radon and lung cancer risk, as investigated in case-control studies in the general population. A number of case-control studies on indoor radon and lung cancer were initiated over the last decade to estimate the risk of indoor radon directly and to avoid the uncertainty arising from extrapolation of risks from underground miners to the general population. Sample size needs of these studies were not fully appreciated as they were designed (Lubin et al. 1990) and a number of studies have had null findings but wide confidence intervals on effect estimates. Lubin and Boice (1997) have recently completed a meta-analysis of eight case-control studies that were completed as of mid-1996. Although five of the individual studies were considered to be "negative," the overall effect of indoor radon on lung cancer was statistically significant and the dose–response relationship was fully compatible with observations in miners.

Pooled Analysis

Pooled analysis refers to the analysis of data from multiple studies at the level of the individual participant, unlike meta-analysis, which uses data aggregated at the study level. This type of approach has received less formal treatment in the literature, but it has proved informative in characterizing dose–response relationships for radiation and cancer and for evaluating modifiers of these relationships. A number of studies of radiation-exposed individuals, exposed from occupational and nonoccupational sources, include information on the exposures of the individual participants to radiation and also on exposures to some potential confounding and modifying factors. Pooled analyses on radiation risks have been published for nuclear workers (Cardis et al. 1995), underground miners (NRC 1988), and for women who received repeated fluoroscopy in the management of tuberculosis (Howe and McLaughlin 1996).

The analyses of data from cohort studies of radon-exposed underground miners are illustrative. The dose–response relationship observed in the underground miners has been extended to the general population for the purpose of estimating the lung cancer risk associated with indoor radon. Dose–response relationships can be obtained from individual studies but variation exists among the studies in the magnitude of the estimated excess risk. To characterize the dose–response relationship between indoor radon and lung cancer, the Biological Effects of Ionizing Radiation (BEIR) IV Committee obtained data from four epidemiologic studies, including about 22,000 subjects who had experienced 350 lung cancer deaths during follow-up. The data were analyzed with regression methods to characterize the dose–response relationship. A linear model was used and the risks were found to decline with increasing time since exposure and increasing age at observation. With the completion of additional studies, the data available for pooling expanded to 68,000 men and 2,700 lung cancer deaths drawn from 11 cohorts (Lubin et al. 1995). In the resulting model, lung cancer risk was further found to increase with lower exposure rates; i.e., at a given level of cumulative exposure those receiving exposures at lower rates have higher risk. Because the database included smoking information for a substantial number of participants, risks were also estimated separately for smokers and for nonsmokers. Pooled analysis of this database will be the basis for the new risk model to be published by the Biological Effects of Ionizing Radiation (BEIR) VI Committee (NRC 1994b). Meta-analyses of the case-control studies of indoor radon will eventually be followed by pooled analyses.

Training in Risk Assessment

As the application of risk assessment to decision-making continues to increase, so too does the need for professionals who can conduct assessments and apply risk information to decision making. A recent study of the environmental health infrastructure revealed a need to improve the capacity of a wide range of agencies to evaluate, manage, and communicate risks (Burke et al. 1995; 1996). Burke and colleagues examined the impact of federal health and environmental statutes on state regulatory agencies. The study revealed increasing requirements to apply risk-based regulatory strategies throughout the states. However, few states currently have adequate multidisciplinary capacity to conduct and implement risk-based decision-making. Clearly there is a broad need for improved professional training in the risk sciences and their application to policy in government and the private sector.

To address the growing need for training and education in risk sciences, it is important to consider the tremendous diversity of professionals involved in the many aspects of evaluating, managing, and preventing risks. The educational challenge facing public health institutions is twofold: there is a need to train *risk professionals* as well as *professionals in risk*. Risk professionals include those scientists from a variety of disciplinary backgrounds who may conduct research on hazards, biological effects, exposure, and the characterization and communication of risk. Professionals in risk may come from a diverse range of educational backgrounds and be filling a wide array of job descriptions, all involving use of risk assessment or other types of risk information. Examples of professionals in risk include regulators, elected officials, corporate executives, economists, engineers, physicians, lawyers, and journalists. While these professionals may never actually conduct a risk assessment, they are called upon increasingly to apply and interpret risk information. It is therefore essential that they develop an understanding of the basic concepts, strengths, and limitations of risk assessment.

Meeting the challenge of the education and training of the new risk workforce will require a strengthening of the academic infrastructure. Because risk assessment is multidisciplinary by nature, it has not been well developed within the traditional disciplined-based programs of higher education. This has resulted in a paucity of academic programs, little training support, and a lack of research funding. A 1993 report of the US Congress Office of Technology Assessment (US Congress 1993) pointed out:

> few incentives exist for long-term multi agency and multi disciplinary research on health risks, and very few resources are allocated to this work. Scientists from all the environmental health disciplines, such as toxicology, epidemiology, biostatistics, environmental chemistry, and clinical studies, make contributions to health risk assessments and are the mainstay of agency research to improve the risk assessment process. Nonetheless, those fields remain disparate, and collaborative studies remain the exception rather than the rule.

Successful implementation of risk-based decision-making and regulatory reform will require a strong academic base and new approaches to education and training. Epidemiologists who are engaged in risk assessment activities need grounding in exposure assessment and toxicology and an understanding of the regulatory and political scenes. Currently this background is gained primarily through individually tailored programs and work experience. Comprehensive programs are needed to complement training in specific public health disciplines, such as epidemiology. Few programs with this breadth are available and schools of public health are only now recognizing this need. The Center for Risk Analysis at the Harvard School of Public Health was a pioneering initiative in bringing risk assessment activities and education into an academic institution. Through its new Risk Sciences and Public Policy Institute, the Johns Hopkins School of Hygiene and Public Health is initiating a broad training program in risk assessment and its application. The training programs of the institute complement traditional discipline-based degrees in epidemiology with an overlay of additional courses and educational experiences in the risk sciences.

Other Considerations for Practitioners

Complex, nontechnical issues may also engage the practitioner involved in risk assessment. These issues may include the need to make decisions with policy implications in the conduct of a risk assessment, the potential for ethical issues to arise, and the difficulty of effectively communicating findings. Other chapters in this book address aspects of these topics (see Chapter 11), and the National Research Council has published a comprehensive report on risk communication (NRC 1989). The potential ethical challenges mirror those of public health practice more generally. Sponsoring entities, whether public or private, may have an interest in achieving a specific finding with a risk assessment and attempt to manipulate the outcome of a risk assessment. Given the implications of selected assumptions in a risk assessment, the risk assessment process may be subject to influence; the communication of the findings may also raise conflicts among interested parties. General ethical guidelines are applicable but these issues have received little specific treatment.

Risk assessment is a tool for organizing information about hazards to characterize the nature and probability of adverse effects. Uncertainty is inherent in the existing risk assessment process due to the limitations of existing data and the multitude of assumptions necessary through virtually every step. Despite its limitations, risk assessment is an increasingly important policy tool, shaping a wide range of regulatory and business decisions. Therefore the risk scientist or practitioner must be aware that there are unique challenges involving the characterization and communication of risk.

The determination that a substance, product, or pollutant poses a risk to a population may have enormous social and economic implications that often hinge upon whether the risk is "acceptable." The acceptability of risk is not purely a scientific question; it must incorporate the social, political, and economic context of the risk. The formulation of risk management decisions often involves an interface of science and politics which calls upon practitioners to integrate a broad range of considerations, including social values. Since epidemiology often provides the scientific basis for risk estimates, epidemiologists are increasingly called upon to participate in the shaping of risk management strategies. Therefore, it is important that epidemiologists develop an appreciation for the social context of risk decision-making and recognize the interests and information needs of the various stakeholders in the process. The active involvement of epidemiologists should include refinement of study methods to improve the utility of epidemiology in risk assessment and to meet the information needs of risk managers.

The challenge of communicating risks faces all practitioners of risk assessment and risk management. It is widely recognized that public perceptions of risk are often inconsistent with the scientific estimates of those same risks. For example, the public has been apathetic about the risks of indoor radon, yet incensed about the risk of low-level nuclear waste disposal. Since risk perceptions may play a larger role in decision-making than risk science, it is important that practitioners continue to refine the translation and communication of risk information. This should include the active involvement of epidemiologists to make study findings understandable; to work with the media to improve risk reporting; to inform policy-makers; and to improve the application of epidemiology in risk management.

Summary

In the United States, quantitative risk assessment has become widely used to translate the findings of epidemiologic and toxicologic research into public policy; this methodology is also being advanced in other countries. A trend now exists of including risk assessment in legislation related to environment regulation, and this predicts increasing use. Epidemiologic data may play a prominent role in risk assessment by providing information relevant to hazard identification, exposure assessment, and dose response. Attributable risk estimates may contribute to risk characterization.

Epidemiologists may contribute to risk assessment through their research findings or through active engagement in risk assessment and management. The potential implications of epidemiologic evidence in risk assessments have led to calls for guidelines for epidemiologic studies and have focused attention on limitations of epidemiologic data.

Epidemiologists conducting research on the environment, pharmaceutical agents, and other exposures that may be covered by regulation need to understand the methods of quantitative risk assessment and the uses of epidemiologic data in risk assessment. Training programs to introduce epidemiologists to risk assessment are just being developed. Undoubtedly, the future will see further engagement of epidemiologists in risk assessment.

CASE STUDIES

Assessing the Risks of Indoor Radon

Background
Radon is an invisible gas that occurs naturally when uranium decays. Radon is a human carcinogen that causes cancer of the lung. It damages lung cells via alpha particles emitted by radon progeny. Convincing evidence has been obtained from epidemiologic studies of underground miners, confirmatory animal studies, and an evolving understanding of mechanisms of carcinogenesis. Since the 1970s, it has been widely recognized that radon can be found in homes. Some homes were found to have extremely high level of radon (in the early 1980s). This precipitated the national concern that led to creation of the Radon Program of the Environmental Protection Agency. Levels of projected risk were large—approximately 14,000 lung cancer deaths per year in the United States attributable to indoor radon. How were those risks projected? Where do uncertainties lie in the risk projections?

Key Questions
In developing and implementing programs to manage indoor radon, answers to the following are needed.
1. What is the distribution of exposures received by the general population?
2. What risks result from these exposures?
3. What factors determine susceptibility to radon-caused lung cancer?
4. How certain is our understanding of the risks associated with indoor radon?
5. Can radon concentrations be reduced? To what extent?
6. What are the costs of reducing indoor radon concentrations?
7. Do the benefits favorably outweigh the costs?

Implications for Practice
Hazard Identification (Determining Whether Radon Causes Lung Cancer). Radon is a human carcinogen and "passes" the step of hazard identification. Where does the evidence come from?

1. Epidemiologic studies of underground miners, demonstrating strong and consistent excess occurrence of lung cancer
2. Animal studies showing that inhalation of radon alone by animals causes lung cancer
3. Mechanistic studies showing that alpha particles, the type of radiation ultimately released by radon, effectively damage DNA and cause cancer

As radon "passes" the hazard identification step we move on to exposure, dose response, and risk characterization.

Exposure Assessment (Describing the Exposure Distribution). Radon levels can be easily measured using relatively inexpensive passive devices. Concentrations have now been measured in representative samples of US homes and also in millions of commercially tested homes (Figure 5-2).

From the perspective of risk management, several features of the concentration distribution are relevant:

1. The average concentration is about 1 pCi/l.
2. The distribution is not symmetrical.
3. Most homes have very low levels, near the average.
4. Some homes have high levels, up to the thousands on this graph (Figure 5-2).

This information is used in the risk characterization step to project the risk of indoor radon. The projection inherently contains several messages about successful management of the risks:

1. If any exposure carries some risk, then much of the risk to the population will come from homes having low levels, near the average.
2. A strategy will be needed to find the homes with the highest levels.

Exposure–Response (Determining Whether Risk Varies With Exposure). The exposure–response relationship describes how risk of lung cancer varies with exposure to radon. In current risk assessments, the exposure–response relationship from studies of miners is used. The National Cancer Institute and a collaborating, international group of investigators have brought together data on 68,000 miners in 11 different studies, including studies of uranium, iron, tin, and fluorspar miners. These data have been pooled and analyzed with Poisson regression to develop a risk model.

A linear nonthreshold model fits the data well. The model allows for time- and age-dependent effects of exposure. A model for the exposure–response relationship is given below:

$$RR = 1 + \beta X \left(w_{5-14} + \theta_{15-24} w_{15-24} + \theta_{25+} w_{25+} \right) X \phi_{age} X \gamma_{WL}$$

where

$$\beta = 0.0611, \ \theta_{15-24} = 0.81, \ \theta_{25+} = 0.40$$

$$\phi_{age} = \begin{array}{ll} 1.00 & \text{for age} < 55 \text{ years} \\ 0.65 & \text{for } 55 \le \text{age} < 65 \\ 0.38 & \text{for } 65 \le \text{age} < 75 \\ 0.22 & \text{for } 75 \le \text{age} \end{array}$$

$$\gamma_{WL} = \begin{array}{ll} 1.00 & \text{for } WL < 0.5 \\ 0.51 & \text{for } 0.5 \le WL < 1.0 \\ 0.32 & \text{for } 1.0 \le WL < 3.0 \\ 0.27 & \text{for } 3.0 \le WL < 5.0 \\ 0.13 & \text{for } 5.0 \le WL < 15.0 \\ 0.10 & \text{for } 15.0 \le WL \end{array}$$

Where β is the overall exposure–response coefficient; w_{5-14}, w_{15-24}, and w_{25+} are exposures during time windows of 5–14, 15–24, $\ge$25 years previously; θ_{15-24} and θ_{25+} allow for change in effect in these windows; ϕ_{age} describes change in risk with age; and

γ_{WL} describes change in risk by exposure rate, the level of WL, or working level, a measure of concentration.

The model describes how risk changes with (1) exposure to radon progeny, w_{5-14}, $\theta_{15-24}w_{15-24}$, and $\theta_{25+}w_{25+}$; (2) the rate of the exposure γ_{WL}; (3) time since the exposure θ_{15-24} and θ_{25+} (note, θ_{5-14} is assumed to be 1); and (4) and age at risk, ϕ_{age}. The model is a relative risk model. The additional risk of lung cancer from radon adds to the background risk, represented by the value of "1." It is a linear model and does not have any threshold—the so-called "linear nonthreshold model." Risk from exposure decreases as the time since the exposure lengthens. There is lower risk for persons as they age, and the risk increases as the rate of exposure (the WL value) decreases; this means that the exposure is more harmful if delivered over a longer period of time. The exposure-rate effect is one source of uncertainty in extrapolating a model from miners to the general population.

Dose Response (Determining Whether Exposure Relates to Dose). Dose refers to the amount of the agent delivered into the body. In the case of radon, we refer to the dose of alpha radioactivity delivered to the cells in the airways of the lung which are affected and become malignant. The dose depends on the exposure and also on the size distribution of the particles in the inhaled air, the rate of breathing, the amount of inhaled air, and whether breathing takes place primarily through the nose or the mouth. The dose also depends on the characteristics of the exposed individual: age, sex, and the presence of any lung damage or disease, including that produced by smoking.

We can account for all of these factors using a model that physically represents the lung. The results of modeling the dose of radioactivity for miners and the population have been summarized into a single number:

$$K = \frac{(\text{Dose/exposure})_{\text{Home}}}{(\text{dose/exposure})_{\text{Mine}}}$$

If K is 1, then we do not need to make an adjustment as we extend the exposure–response relationship from studies of miners to the general population. To the extent that K is significantly higher or lower than 1, an appropriate adjustment can be made. In fact, K is approximately 1, so an adjustment is not needed (NRC 1991c).

Risk Characterization (Assessing the Risk to the Population). To characterize the risk of indoor radon for the United States, we combine the distribution of radon exposures with the predicted risk for the exposures. The needed information on exposure is available from the National Residential Radon Survey of 4,000 US homes done by the EPA. The risk model from the miners is used to estimate risk without adjustment for K, which is about 1. To extend the risk model to the entire general population, we need to make assumptions about the effect of radon on:

1. Women (only male miners have been studied)
2. Children (primarily adult miners have been studied)
3. Smokers
4. Non-smokers

Consider the most recent risk assessment for indoor radon, using the risk model from the pooled analysis of data from underground miners (Lubin et al. 1995). To project the risk of lung cancer for the general population, Lubin et al. used lung cancer mortality rates for the United States for 1985–1989 as background rates. They calculated the attributable numbers of lung cancer deaths for 1993; during that year there were about 149,000 deaths, 93,000 in men and 56,000 in women. Assuming that 70% of the deaths are in residents of single-family homes, we then estimate that 14,400 lung cancer deaths per year are attributable to radon—4,700 in never-smokers and 9,700 among smokers. These figures are the numbers of deaths theoretically preventable by lowering the concentration of radon to *background* levels, an unachievable target. A more informative risk characterization would also provide the numbers of deaths that can be prevented by various mitigation strategies. For indoor radon, Lubin and Boice (1989) have shown that there is a substantial difference between the number of deaths theoretically preventable (about 14,000) and the numbers of deaths that are preventable by current mitigation strategies (about 3,000).

Part of any risk analysis is an assessment of *uncertainty*. Consider the steps of the risk assessment and the assumptions that have been made in developing this risk characterization.

Steps:

1. Obtain population exposure estimate from the National Residential Radon Survey.
2. Analyze data from 11 cohorts of underground miners to develop risk model.
3. Evaluate exposure–dose relationships in homes and mines and calculate K.
4. Assume background lung cancer mortality rates for the general population.
5. Extend model to women and children.
6. Assume risks to smokers and nonsmokers.
7. Use lifetable method to project risks.

This is a multistep process with many assumptions and uncertainties (Table 5-5). How do we capture the uncertainty in our final estimates? What is the plausible range of attributable lung cancer deaths? Could the lower end of the range be as low as zero? These questions can be addressed using the methods of uncertainty analysis.

Chromium Contamination in Hudson County, New Jersey

Background

The case study of chromium contamination in the communities of Hudson County, New Jersey, illustrates the application of the risk assessment framework to a specific, community-based problem. From 1905 to 1976, Hudson County was a center for chromate chemical manufacturing. Chromite ore from around the world was processed to convert insoluble compounds to the more soluble hexavalent form, which was leached out with water. This process produced 1.5 pounds of waste slag for every pound of useful product. Over the period of operations it is estimated that between 2 and 3 million tons of waste were produced (Burke et al. 1991). Despite the potential toxicity of the waste, it was sold and given away for use as fill material and was widely used in construction at hundreds of residential and commercial sites throughout the county. During the 1980s it was recognized that the waste material may pose serious health risks to community members and workers in the vicinity of these sites.

Key Questions

1. Does chromium pose a risk to human health?
2. What are the pathways of exposure?
3. What is the magnitude of the risk?
4. How should risk be managed?

Table 5-5. Sources of Uncertainty in Assessing the Health Risks of Indoor Radon

	Error	Uncertainty
Epidemiologic studies of underground miners	Random and systematic errors in exposure estimates Random and systematic errors in lung cancer	Lack of information on tobacco smoking Lack of information on arsenic, diesel exhaust, and other potential carcinogens
Individual and pooled analysis of miner data	Precision of estimates of effect Precision of estimates of effects of effect-modifiers	Appropriateness of model assumptions Appropriateness of model specification
Extending the model to the general population		Model for higher-dose to lower-dose extrapolation Model for higher to lower dose-rate extrapolation Extending the model to the full lifespan Effect of age at exposure Effect of gender
Exposure	Errors in measurements of radon concentrations	Estimation of exposures with current concentration distribution
Exposure–dose relationship	Errors in measurement of activity-size distributions and equilibrium fraction	Lack of information of activity-size distributions on mines included in epidemiologic studies Lack of information on breathing patterns of miners in the past and the general population at present Appropriateness of deposition and clearance models Target cells for malignancy Effect of smoking on delivered dose
Risk characterization		Stability of background lung cancer rates

Implications for Practice

Hazard Identification. Adverse effects of exposure to chromium compounds in the occupational setting have been known since the 19th century. Chromium compounds were found to cause damage to the skin and mucosal surfaces, including skin ulcers, irritant and allergic dermatitis, and perforation of the nasal septum. Late toxic effects of high exposure include kidney and liver failure (WHO 1988). Epidemiological studies of workers exposed to chromium have shown an increased risk of lung cancer associated with exposure to the more biologically active hexavalent form. Early studies of highly exposed chromate workers identified relative risks as high as 80, but subsequent studies of later cohorts found reduced risks (Langard 1990). Hexavalent chromium has also demonstrated evidence of mutagenicity in bacterial and mammalian cell assays (Agency for Toxic Substances and Disease Registry [ATSDR] 1993).

The evidence from the hazard identification step clearly indicates a potential hazard for exposed workers and community members. A primary concern in Hudson County was thus increased risk of lung cancer in the potentially exposed communities.

Dose–Response Evaluation. Evaluation of the doses which cause acute and noncancer effects provides guidance in the risk assessment process. Published guidelines such as the no-observable-adverse-effect level (NOAEL) and the reference dose (RfD) provide the basis for determining if the chromium contamination may lead to adverse health effects in the community.

A primary concern is the carcinogenic hazard, since it is currently assumed that there is no threshold or safe level of exposure to agents which have been shown to cause cancer in humans. Extrapolating from the occupational studies, the EPA has estimated that chronic inhalation of hexavalent chromium at levels of 0.008 μg per cubic meter of air increases the population lifetime risk of lung cancer by one case for every 10,000 exposed individuals (US EPA 1984). Based upon this information, it was determined that the potential doses in Hudson County residents were within the range of concern.

Exposure Assessment. Hudson County is among the most densely populated areas of the United States. The waste material had been widely distributed throughout residential areas, workplaces, and public lands. Chromium levels in the soil at contaminated sites were as high as 53,000 parts per million. The contamination was found to be widespread, including soils, surface water, sediments, and groundwater. Potential exposure pathways included inhalation of suspended soil particles, direct contact with contaminated soil, dust, water, and surfaces; consumption of contaminated food; and ingestion of inspirable particles.

To evaluate exposure levels, the New Jersey Department of Health conducted an evaluation of urine chromium level in children and adults with possible exposure to the contaminated fill. Urine chromium levels for those in the potentially exposed areas were higher than for those from a comparison baseline sample. Children under 5 living near chromium sites were found to have increased urine chromium concentrations. Older children also showed evidence of exposure but less than the younger group. Workers at specific workplaces were also identified as having higher-than-baseline exposure levels (Fagliano and Savrin 1994).

Risk Characterization. The investigation of potential risks in Hudson County provided important public health guidance to support extensive short- and long-term remediation activities. Aggressive remediation of those sites which posed the greatest exposure risks has been undertaken and longer-term strategies for clean-up are being developed. The risk assessment approach provided important insights into the identification of those areas and populations at highest risk and shaped the public health response. This case study also demonstrates the limitations of risk assessment. Those at highest risk of lung cancer are most likely past residents who were exposed to higher levels of the contaminants. The contribution of chromium exposures to lung cancer occurrence in these persons cannot be readily estimated.

SUGGESTED READINGS

Graham JD, ed. The Role of Epidemiology in Regulatory Risk Assessment. New York, NY: Elsevier; 1995.

Hertz-Picciotto I. Epidemiology and quantitative risk assessment: a bridge from science to policy. Am J Public Health 1995;85:48–50.

National Research Council (NRC), Committee on the Institutional Means for Assessment of Risks to Public Health. Risk Assessment in the Federal Government: Managing the Process. Washington, DC: National Academy Press; 1983.

National Research Council (NRC), Committee on Advances in Assessing Human Exposure to Airborne Pollutants. Human Exposure Assessment for Airborne Pollutants: Advances and Opportunities. Washington, DC: National Academy Press; 1991.

National Research Council (NRC), Committee on Risk Characterization, and Commission on Behavioral and Social Sciences and Education. Stern PC, Fineberg HV, eds. Understanding Risk. Informing Decisions in a Democratic Society. Washington, DC: National Academy Press; 1996.

National Research Council (NRC) and Committee on Risk Assessment of Hazardous Air Pollutants. National Research Council (NRC), Committee on Risk Assessment of Hazardous Air Pollutants, eds. Science and Judgment in Risk Assessment. Washington, DC: National Academy Press; 1994.

Rodricks JV, Rodricks JV, eds. Calculated Risks. Understanding the Toxicity and Human Health Risks of Chemicals in Our Environment. London, England: Cambridge University Press; 1992.

REFERENCES

Agency for Toxic Substances and Disease Registry (ATSDR), Public Health Service. Toxicological Profile for Chromium. Atlanta, GA: U.S. Government Printing Office; 1993.

Armstrong BK, White E, Saracci R, Armstrong BK, White E, Saracci R, eds. Principles of Exposure Measurement in Epidemiology. New York: Oxford University Press; 1992.

Auchter TG. The reliable use of epidemiology studies in regulatory risk assessments. In: Graham JD, ed. The Role of Epidemiology in Regulatory Risk Assessment. New York: Elsevier; 1995.

Biggerstaff BJ, Tweedie RL, Mengersen KL. Passive smoking in the workplace:

classical and Bayesian meta-analyses. Int Arch Occup Environ Health 1994;66: 269–277.

Burke TA. The proper role of epidemiology in regulatory risk assessment: reaction from a regulator's perspective. In: Graham JD, ed. The Role of Epidemiology in Regulatory Risk Assessment. New York: Elsevier; 1995.

Burke T, Fagliano J, Goldoft M, Hazen RE, Iglewicz R, McKee T. Chromite ore processing residue in Hudson County, New Jersey. Environ Health Perspect 1991;92:131–137.

Burke TA, Shalauta N, Tran N. The Environmental Web: Impact of Federal Statues on State Environmental Health and Protection Services, Structure and Funding. Rockville, MD: U.S. Department of Health and Human Services; 1995.

Burke TA, Shalauta NM, Tran NL, Stern BS. The environmental web: a national profile of the state infrastructure for environmental health and protection. J Public Health Manage Pract 1997;3:1–12.

Cardis E, Gilbert ES, Carpenter L, Howe G, Kato I, Armstrong BK, Beral V, Cowper G, Douglas A, Fix J, Fry SA, Kaldor J, Lave C, Salmon L, Smith PG, Voelz GL, Wiggs LD. Effects of low doses and low dose rates of external ionizing radiation: cancer mortality among nuclear industry workers in three countries. Radiat Res 1995;142:117–132.

Dickersin K, Berlin JA. Meta-analysis: state-of-the-science. Epidemiol Rev 1992;14: 154–176.

Dosemeci M, Washolder S, Lubin JH. Does nondifferential misclassification of exposure always bias a true effect toward the null value? Am J Epidemiol 1990;132: 746–748.

Fagliano JA, Savrin JE. Chromium Medical Surveillance Project: Final Technical Report. Springfield, NJ: New Jersey Department of Health; 1994.

Federal Focus Inc. Principles for Evaluating Epidemiologic Data in Regulatory Risk Assessment. Washington, DC: Federal Focus; 1996.

Gordis L, ed. Epidemiology and Health Risk Assessment. New York: Oxford University Press; 1988.

Graham JD, ed. The Role of Epidemiology in Regulatory Risk Assessment. New York: Elsevier; 1995.

Greenland S. Quantitative methods in the review of epidemiologic literature. Epidemiol Rev 1987;9:1–30.

Hasselblad V, Kotchmar DJ, Eddy DM. Synthesis of environmental evidence: nitrogen dioxide epidemiology studies. J Air Waste Manage Assoc 1992;42:662–671.

Hertz-Picciotto I. Epidemiology and quantitative risk assessment: a bridge from science to policy. Am J Public Health 1995;85:48–50.

Howe GR, McLaughlin J. Breast cancer mortality between 1950 and 1987 after exposure to fractionated moderate-dose-rate ionizing radiation in the Canadian fluoroscopy cohort study and a comparison with breast cancer mortality in the atomic bomb survivors study. Radiat Res 1996;145:694–707.

Interagency Regulatory Liaison Group (IRLG), Working Group on Risk Assessment. Scientific bases for identification of potential carcinogens and estimation of risks. J Natl Cancer Inst 1979;63:241–268.

Jenkins P, Phillips TJ, Mulberg EJ. Activity patterns of Californians: use of and proximity to indoor pollutant sources. Atmos Environ 1992;26A:2141–2148.

Land CE. Estimating cancer risks from low doses of ionizing radiation. Science 1980;209:1197–1203.

Langard S. One-hundred years of chromium and cancer: a review of epidemiologic evidence and selected case reports. Am J Ind Med 1990;17:189–215.

Links JM, Kensler TW, Groopman JD. Biomarkers and mechanistic approaches in environmental epidemiology. Annu Rev Public Health 1994;16:83–103.

Lubin JH, Boice JD Jr. Estimating radon-induced lung cancer in the U.S. Health Phys 1989;57:417–427.

Lubin JH, Boice JD Jr. Lung cancer risk from residential radon: meta-analysis of eight epidemiologic studies. J Natl Cancer Inst 1997;89:49–57.

Lubin JH, Samet JM, Weinberg C. Design issues in epidemiologic studies of indoor exposure to radon and risk of lung cancer. Health Phys 1990;59:807–817.

Lubin JH, Boice JD Jr, Edling C, Hornung RW, Howe GR, Kunz E, Kusiak RA, Morrison HI, Radford EP, Samet JM, Tirmarche M, Woodward A, Yao SX, Pierce DA. Lung cancer in radon-exposed miners and estimation of risk from indoor exposure. J Natl Cancer Inst 1995;87:817–827.

Luckey TD, ed. Radiation Hormenesis. Boca Raton, FL: CRC Press; 1991.

Mendelsohn ML, Peeters JP, Normandy MJ, eds. Biomarkers and Occupational Health. Progress and Perspectives. Washington, DC: Joseph Henry Press; 1995.

National Council on Radiation Protection and Measurements (NCRP). A Guide for Uncertainty Analysis in Dose and Risk Assessments Related to Environmental Contamination. Bethesda, MD: NCRP. 14; 1996.

National Research Council (NRC), Committee on the Institutional Means for Assessment of Risks to Public Health. Risk Assessment in the Federal Government: Managing the Process. Washington, DC: National Academy Press; 1983.

National Research Council (NRC), Committee on the Biological Effects of Ionizing Radiation. Health Risks of Radon and Other Internally Deposited Alpha-Emitters: BEIR IV. Washington, DC: National Academy Press; 1988.

National Research Council (NRC), Committee on Risk Perception and Communication, Commission on Behavioral and Social Sciences and Education, and Commission on Physical Sciences and Mathematics and Resources. National Research Council (NRC), Committee on Risk Perception and Communication, Commission on Behavioral and Social Sciences and Education, et al., eds. Improving Risk Communication. Washington, DC: National Academy Press; 1989.

National Research Council (NRC), Committee on the Biological Effects of Ionizing Radiation. Health Effects of Exposure to Low Levels of Ionizing Radiation: BEIR V. Washington, DC: National Academy Press; 1990.

National Research Council (NRC), Committee on Advances in Assessing Human Exposure to Airborne Pollutants. Human Exposure Assessment for Airborne Pollutants: Advances and Opportunities. Washington, DC: National Academy Press; 1991a.

National Research Council (NRC). Frontiers in Assessing Human Exposures to Environmental Toxicants. Washington, DC: National Academy Press; 1991b.

National Research Council (NRC), Panel on Dosimetric Assumptions Affecting the Application of Radon Risk Estimates. Comparative Dosimetry of Radon in Mines and Homes. Companion to BEIR IV Report. Washington, DC: National Academy Press; 1991c.

National Research Council (NRC) and Committee on Risk Assessment of Hazardous Air Pollutants. National Research Council (NRC), Committee on Risk Assessment of Hazardous Air Pollutants, eds. Science and Judgment in Risk Assessment. Washington, DC: National Academy Press; 1994a.

National Research Council (NRC), Committee on Health Effects of Exposure to Radon (BEIR VI), Commission on Life Sciences. Health Effects of Exposure to Radon: Time for Reassessment? Washington, DC: National Academy Press; 1994b.

National Research Council (NRC), Committee on Risk Characterization, and Commission on Behavioral and Social Sciences and Education. Stern PC, Fineberg HV, eds. Understanding Risk. Informing Decisions in a Democratic Society. Washington, DC: National Academy Press; 1996.

Petitti DB. Meta-analysis, Decision Analysis, and Cost Effectiveness Analysis: Methods for Quantitative Synthesis of Medicine. New York, NY: Oxford University Press; 1994.

Rodricks JV, ed. Calculated Risks. Understanding the Toxicity and Human Health Risks of Chemicals in Our Environment. London, England: Cambridge University Press; 1992.

The Presidential/Congressional Commission on Risk Assessment and Risk Management. Framework for Environmental Health Risk Management. Final Report, Volume 1. Washington, DC: The Presidential/Congressional Commission on Risk Assessment and Risk Management; 1997.

Tweedie RL, Mengersen KL. Meta-analytic approaches to dose–response relationships, with application in studies of lung cancer and exposure to environmental tobacco smoke. Stat Med 1995;14:545–569.

United Nations Scientific Committee on the Effects of Atomic Radiation (UNSCEAR). Sources and Effects of Ionizing Radiation. Report to the General Assembly, with Scientific Annexes. New York: United Nations Press; 1993:1.

U.S. Congress, Office of Technology Assessment. Researching Health Risks. Washington, DC: U.S. Government Printing Office. OTS-BBS-570; 1993.

U.S. Department of Labor and Occupational Safety and Health Administration (OSHA). U.S. Department of Labor, Occupational Safety and Health Administration (OSHA), Eds. (29-CFR) Parts 1910, 1915, 1926, and 1928 Indoor Air Quality; Proposed Rule. Washington, DC: U.S. Government Printing Office; 1994.

U.S. Environmental Protection Agency (EPA), Office of Research and Development. Health Assessment Document for Chromium. Washington, DC: U.S. Government Printing Office; 1984.

U.S. Environmental Protection Agency (EPA). Guidelines for carcinogen risk assessment. Fed Reg 1986;51:33992–34003.

U.S. Environmental Protection Agency (EPA), Office of Policy Planning and Evaulation. Unfinished Business: A Comparative Assessment of Environmental Problems. Washington, DC: U.S. Government Printing Office; 1987.

U.S. Environmental Protection Agency (EPA), Scientific Advisory Board, Relative Risk Reduction Strategies Committee. Reducing Risk: Setting Priorities and Strategies for Environmental Protection. Washington, DC: U.S. Government Printing Agency; 1990.

U.S. Environmental Protection Agency (EPA). Respiratory Health Effects of Passive Smoking: Lung Cancer and Other Disorders. Washington, DC: U.S. Government Printing Office. EPA/600/006F; 1992a.

U.S. Environmental Protection Agency (EPA).Technical Support Document for the 1992 Citizen's Guide to Radon. Washington, DC: U.S. Government Printing Office; 1992b.

U.S. Environmental Protection Agency (EPA). Guidelines for exposure assessment. Fed Reg 57:22888–22938;1992c.

World Health Organization, International Agency for Research on Cancer (IARC). IARC Monographs on the Evaluation of Carcinogenic Risk of Chemicals to Man. Geneva, Switzerland: International Agency for Research on Cancer; 1972:1.

World Health Organization. Environmental Health Criteria 61: Chromium. Geneva, Switzerland: World Health Organization; 1988.

6

Epidemiologic Issues in the Design of Community Intervention Trials

THOMAS D. KOEPSELL

If epidemiology is the branch of science that seeks to understand the determinants of disease occurrence in populations, and if one such determinant is the effectiveness of organized efforts to prevent disease and promote health (Terris 1992a), then evaluation of these programs is a form of applied epidemiology.

This chapter concerns controlled evaluations of interventions aimed at entire communities in order to prevent disease or promote health. For present purposes, a community trial is defined as a study that involves at least one intervention site in which a community-wide health promotion or disease prevention program is implemented, and at least one control site without such an intervention that is studied concurrently, whether or not randomization is used to assign communities to treatment groups.

The design and analysis of community trials involves dealing not only with many of the generic methodological and practical issues that arise in most program evaluations but also with several special challenges that follow from aiming an intervention at an entire community rather than at selected individuals. The goal of this chapter is to orient the reader to these special issues, with an emphasis on principles and practical implications. Entry points will be provided into a rapidly growing and widely dispersed literature on evaluation of community interventions, where additional depth and details about these topics can be found.

Rationale for Community-Level Intervention

The high level of interest and investment in community trials over the last two decades has been fueled largely by the theoretical appeal of interventions aimed at intact social groups for prevention of disease and promotion of health. Because intervention at the community level has major implications for evaluation design, it will be helpful to review some of the key ideas behind this strategy.

Targeting Everyone May Prevent More Cases of Disease Than Targeting Just High-Risk Individuals

Rose (1985, 1992) has distinguished between two broad approaches to disease prevention in populations. Under a "high risk" strategy, risk-factor information about each individual is used to identify persons with the greatest chance of developing a preventable condition, and prevention efforts are then focused on those high-risk individuals. Under a "population" strategy, a preventive intervention is aimed at everyone in an attempt to produce a favorable shift in the overall risk-factor distribution in the population. Rose notes that for many diseases, the cases that occur in "high-risk" individuals may be only a small proportion of the total. Most fatal cases of coronary heart disease, for example, occur in people with "normal" cholesterol levels (Rose 1992), in whom dietary modification aimed at reducing cholesterol may lower the risk of coronary heart disease. Thus, a program aimed at both high- *and* low-risk individuals has the potential to prevent more cases than one aimed solely at high-risk individuals.

Environmental Modifications May Be Easier to Accomplish than Large-Scale Voluntary Behavior Change

It has long been recognized that community environment is an important determinant of disease risk (Terris 1992b). Modifying the physical, social, or legal/regulatory environment in which people live can be sometimes be more expedient and reach more people than attempting to induce voluntary behavior change on a mass scale. For example, requiring that children's sleepwear be manufactured from fire-retardant fabric may be a better way to prevent burns than teaching parents and small children about how to avoid ignition of sleepwear made from flammable fabric. Public or institutional policies, taking such forms as taxes on tobacco products, minimum legal drinking age, or subsidy of immunization services, can also create strong incentives or disincentives related to risk behavior (McKinlay 1993).

Risk-Related Behaviors Are Socially Influenced

Social learning theory holds that behavioral change is more readily achieved and maintained if norms and behavior in the peer group support the change

(Farquhar 1978). Community substance-abuse prevention programs, for example, have sought to change norms about illegal drug use among teenagers in order to influence individual behavior (Pentz et al. 1989).

Some Intervention Modalities Are Unselective by Nature

Fluoridation of the water supply to prevent dental caries automatically affects nearly everyone in a community. The word "mass" in "mass media" denotes the nonselective nature of public information dissemination that may be intended to change health-related attitudes and behavior (Flay 1987). Media campaigns about health topics typically seek to reach as large a share of the population within a media market as possible and can thus be regarded as community-level interventions.

Community Interventions Reach People in Their "Native Habitat"

Farquhar (1978) noted that people do not live in their doctors' offices, nor in the kinds of specialized environments created by large-scale, clinic-based lifestyle intervention trials such as the Multiple Risk Factor Intervention Trial (1982). Community interventions, in contrast, generally use intervention methods that apply in the "real-world" context of homes, workplaces, and neighborhoods.

Community Interventions Can Be Logistically Simpler and Less Costly on a Per-Person Basis

In contrast to the "high-risk" strategy described by Rose (1985), an intervention aimed at everyone in the community obviates the need to sort the population first into risk groups. Elimination of this step alone can reduce program complexity and cost (Farquhar 1978; Murray and Short 1995).

Examples of Community Trials

Community trials have involved a remarkable variety of settings, target populations, intervention strategies, outcomes, and approaches to evaluation. Four examples should help to illustrate this wide range of variation and provide specific contexts for later discussion of evaluation design issues.

The *Community Intervention Trial for Smoking Cessation* (COMMIT) sought to reduce the prevalence of heavy cigarette smoking in selected communities throughout the United States and Canada (Community Intervention Trial for Smoking Cessation [COMMIT] 1995a,b). In 1986, the National Cancer Institute invited applications from pairs of communities, requiring pair members to be from the same state or province and matched on approximate size and sociodemographic factors. Eleven pairs were chosen and randomized within pairs to intervention or control groups. Each intervention community received an average of $220,000/year for 4 years to mount a multifaceted program including public education through the media and community-wide special events, involvement of health care providers, activities at work sites and other community organizations, and resources to aid smokers in quitting. A process evaluation measured the nature and intensity of intervention activities of each type and smokers' exposure to them. An outcome evaluation used telephone surveys to monitor quitting in a cohort of about 1,100 smokers in each intervention and control community. Cross-sectional samples of smokers were also surveyed at baseline and follow-up to measure changes in smoking prevalence. The results showed no significant difference in quit rates among heavy smokers, but the quit rate among light to moderate smokers was about three percentage points higher in intervention sites compared to their matched controls ($p = 0.004$).

A randomized, double-blind, placebo-controlled community trial of vitamin A supplementation was carried out in rural Nepal in 1989–1990 (West et al. 1991). Twenty-nine local development units were studied, each with nine administrative wards, including about 28,000 children under 5 years of age. After obtaining written informed consent from the chairman of each development unit, the 261 wards were randomly allocated to treatment groups. Every 4 months, trained fieldworkers in each ward visited homes containing children under 5 years of age. In the intervention wards, children received a capsule containing 60,000 µg of retinol equivalent; in control wards, the children received an identical-appearing capsule containing 300 µg of retinol equivalent. Child deaths were identified both through vital records and at the time of 4-monthly follow-up visits. The trial, originally planned for 2 years, was halted early when results showed a statistically significant 30% reduction in child mortality in the vitamin A supplementation group.

In 1986, a community cardiovascular disease prevention program called Heart to Heart was mounted in the town of Florence, South Carolina (Goodman et al. 1995). The multicomponent intervention included media campaigns about smoking, physical fitness, and diet; public nutrition classes; information in supermarkets about food labeling; distribution of self-help resources for smoking cessation and weight control; a restaurant menu-labeling program; cholesterol and blood pressure screening at health fairs; and other activities. The town of Anderson, South Carolina, 200 miles away, served as a control community in which no special intervention activities were mounted. Telephone and questionnaire surveys were conducted in both sites in 1987 and 1991 to assess awareness of program components, knowledge about heart disease prevention, and key behavioral risk factors. A sample of individuals from each community also came to study clinics for measurement of blood pressure, lipid levels, and anthropometry. Although the two communities had been assigned en bloc to be intervention or control sites, individual respondents were used as the units of analysis. The results suggested modest but statistically significant benefits on the prevalence of high cholesterol and obesity, while changes in the prevalence of hypertension significantly favored the control community.

A publicly sponsored nurse-midwife program for low-income pregnant women was instituted in Boulder County, Colorado, to increase access to prenatal care and prevent adverse pregnancy outcomes (Lenaway et al. in press). To evaluate the program, birth-certificate data were analyzed for all singleton babies born alive to indigent mothers in Boulder County and in two neighboring control counties during a 16-month period. A random-effects logistic regression model was used to account for community-level allocation. The results showed significant reductions in the proportion of women who received inadequate prenatal care and in the proportion of infants with low 5-minute Apgar scores, and borderline reductions in the frequency of prematurity and low birth weight.

Key Terms and Concepts

Although most of this chapter will focus on more technical aspects of evaluation design, it is useful to begin by considering three broad issues that often arise in the context of community intervention studies and that can have major impact on program evaluation. The first two concern aspects of what we mean by a "community intervention."

What Is a Community?

Nutbeam (1986) defined a community as "A specific group of people usually living in a defined geographical area who share a common culture, are arranged in a social structure and exhibit some awareness of their identity as a group." Two features of this definition are worth noting. First, it places no restrictions on group size: groups as small as families or as large as nations could thus be regarded as "communities" of sorts. Many of the special methodological issues in evaluation of community interventions stem from allocation of intact social groups to different treatment conditions and do not depend strongly on group size. In practice, however, community interventions have typically been aimed at social groups ranging in size from workplaces to counties, as illustrated by all four of the examples above. Second, sharing a common culture, social structure, and awareness of group identity implies some degree of similarity and connectedness: Members of a community share certain characteristics and influence each other. This simple observation has important ramifications for design and analysis of community interventions, because it implies that measurements taken on different members of the same community are not necessarily statistically independent.

Who Controls the Intervention?

The "intervention" part of the term "community intervention" refers to a defined plan of action. A critical issue for evaluators, however, is, Who controls the action plan? Table 6-1 describes two poles of a continuum. At one extreme, a community intervention may be part of a grand social experiment, in which the evaluator/experimenter (and/or the funding agency) is in control. Major elements of the program—the focal risk behaviors or health conditions, specific target communities, intervention modalities, nature and extent of resources, timing, and duration—are determined by the goals of the research and by people who are not indigenous community leaders. The Nepalese vitamin A trial was near this end of the spectrum. The primary goal of such a social experiment is to gain generalizable knowledge about the effects of a certain kind of intervention in certain kinds of communities in order to permit future application of that knowledge in other similar communities. Direct benefit to study communities themselves may be a bonus, but it is of secondary importance. Some communities participate in such an experiment as

Table 6-1. Two Models of Community Interventions

	Social Experiment	"Grass Roots" Program
Origins	Outside community	Inside community
Funding	External	Internal or external source sought out by community
Primary goal	Generalizable knowledge about effectiveness	Solution of a perceived problem in the target community
Control over nature, timing, and target population	Evaluator/experimenter or funding agency	Community leaders
Number of invention communities	One or more	Usually just one

controls, gaining no direct benefit from participation besides sharing in the knowledge that results when the study is completed.

At the other extreme, an intervention may be community based in a very different sense. It may have "grassroots" origins, arising from the felt needs and priorities of people in a particular community. The primary goal of the intervention is to prevent or solve some perceived problem in that community. Resources required to mount the intervention are raised within the community itself through public funds or voluntary contributions, or help is sought from an external service-oriented government agency or philanthropy known to support that kind of program. Control over the program remains within the community; the evaluator is an observer, not an experimenter. The Boulder County nurse-midwife program fell near this end of the spectrum.

Many gradations between these extremes are possible. In the COMMIT study, for example, the National Cancer Institute set conditions under which communities could participate, controlled allocation to treatment groups, and established general guidelines for acceptable intervention programs. Nonetheless, tailoring and implementation of the action plan in each site was directed by a community board that could choose from a menu of intervention options and that had considerable flexibility in adapting them to local conditions and needs. Participating communities also supplemented COMMIT funding with contributed time and other resources generated from within.

Degree of external control over the intervention plays a major role in determining what kind of study design is feasible for program evaluation. Large-scale social experiments like COMMIT lend themselves to having multiple communities in the intervention and control groups and random allocation of communities to treatment groups. Programs with "grassroots" origins in a single community must typically be evaluated using less elaborate study designs and without the benefits of randomization.

What Is Community-Level Variation, and Why Does It Matter?

Imagine a hypothetical community trial in which a woefully underfunded and wholly ineffective smoking-cessation program in community A is compared with no intervention at all in community B. For simplicity, also assume that community A's program is evaluated based on a comparison of quit rates in a random sample of smokers in each of the two communities after the intervention in community A has been in place for a while. What is the probability of finding a statistically significant difference in quit rates between the two communities?

Given that the program in community A is ineffective, we might be tempted to think that this probability is simply α, the probability of a type I error when the null hypothesis is true, usually chosen to be 0.05. In fact, the chance of finding a significant difference is probably considerably higher than α. The reason is related to a very basic idea in epidemiology: namely, that diseases do not occur at random in populations but vary systematically in relation to personal characteristics, time, and (importantly) place. Often such geographic differences are the source of hypotheses, and often they remain unexplained, but there is generally no denying that they exist. Epidemiologists usually focus on disease occurrence, but the same observation applies to other health-related phenomena, including health behaviors. Diehr et al. (1993), for example, studied the prevalence of smoking, alcohol use, dietary fat consumption, and seatbelt use among 13 communities participating in a health promotion grants program before any intervention had been implemented. Many statistically significant differences among communities were found, and the variation between sites remained large and occasionally even increased after adjustment for a wide range of sociodemographic and health characteristics. LaPrelle et al. (1992) reported similar findings in a 10-community study on adolescent cigarette smoking.

Statistically, we can think of overall variability in some outcome measure, Y, in the large population formed by combining individuals across several study communities. The total variance of Y can be partitioned into two components: (1) the variance in Y between individuals *within* the same community, denoted σ^2 and assumed for simplicity to be the same for all communities; and (2) the variance in the community-specific mean value of Y *among* communities, denoted σ_C^2. The total variance of Y is $\sigma_C^2 + \sigma^2$.

In the community-trial literature, the phenomenon of community-level variation is discussed in two equivalent ways: (1) as *greater* variability in Y among community means than would be expected based on observed within-community variation—that is, $\sigma_C^2 > 0$; or (2) as *less* variability in Y within communities than would be expected from its total variation among individuals pooled across all communities—that is, $\sigma^2 < \sigma_C^2 + \sigma^2$, which just amounts to saying $\sigma_C^2 > 0$ in another way.

Depending on which perspective is taken, community-level variation may be quantified differently. One good measure of community-level variation is simply σ_C^2 itself. Another measure that appears commonly in the literature is the intraclass correlation coefficient (ICC), defined in our notation as

$$\frac{\sigma_C^2}{\sigma_C^2 + \sigma^2}$$

which expresses the size of σ_C^2 as a proportion of the total variation in Y. The ICC can also be interpreted as the degree of correlation in Y among individuals within the same communities. Donner (1981) describes a variance inflation factor, calculated from the ICC, that reflects the amount of increase in the variance of a treatment-group-specific mean over what would have been observed if individuals had been randomized.

Although epidemiologists involved in community trials must deal with community-level variation whether its causes are known or not, it helps to be aware of some generic mechanisms by which it can come about (Donner et al. 1990). One is self-selection: individuals often choose to reside in a given community because they have characteristics in common with other community residents and thus "fit in." Those characteristics may, in turn, be associated with the health behaviors of interest. Another mechanism is that residents of the same community share exposure to a common physical and sociocultural environment, which influences their behavior. Yet another mechanism is a type of contagion: just as infectious agents can be spread from person to person, so, too, may attitudes, norms, and behaviors be transmissible among people who are in regular contact, resulting in behavioral homogeneity. Heroin abuse, for example, has been investigated as a contagious disease (De Alarc'on 1969).

The situation becomes a little more complex when changes over time are also considered. Figure 6-1 shows two contrasting patterns of change in the prevalence of smoking in three hypothetical communities. In panel A, the vertical separation of the three community-specific lines implies community-level variation in smoking prevalence (a main effect of community), and there is an obvious downward trend in smoking prevalence over time in each site (a main effect of time). However, the time trends in the three communities are parallel (no community-by-time interaction). Panel B, in contrast, illustrates substantial community-by-time interaction variance: It is the degree of non-parallelism in the time paths observed for different communities, sometimes denoted as σ_{CT}^2. It, too, can arise for a variety of reasons, including different preexisting secular trends in different communities, sociocultural variation

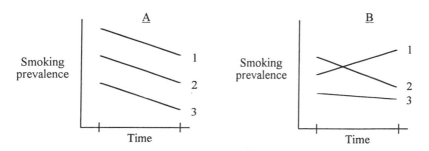

Figure 6-1. Illustration of community-by-time variation

among communities with regard to amenability to behavior change, and local current events that may act as cues to behavior change.

As described below, community-level variation plays an important role in the planning and analysis of community trials. Investigators are accustomed to estimating σ^2 when deciding on sample-size requirements for an ordinary clinical trial on individuals. In community trials, there are at least two kinds of sample sizes to consider (number of communities and number of individuals per community) and two kinds of variability to be estimated in study planning and accommodated during data analysis (σ^2 and either σ_C^2 or σ_{CT}^2, depending on the design). In addition, some study designs preclude accounting properly for community-level variation in the analysis. These designs are not well suited to evaluation of community-level interventions because they can lead to exaggerated claims of statistical significance and thus to erroneous conclusions about program effectiveness.

Overall Study Design

This section progresses from simpler to more complex study designs, noting the strengths and weaknesses of each for evaluating community interventions. More complete typologies of research designs in general can be found in Campbell and Stanley (1963) and in Cook and Campbell (1979). The designs differ in relation to the number of communities in each treatment group according to whether randomization matching is used to form comparison groups and the number and timing of observation occasions. The term "quasi-experiment" is often used to refer to intervention studies in which the comparisons used to evaluate program effectiveness are not based on random assignment.

Single-Community Designs

Technically, evaluation designs that lack at least one concurrently studied control community do not fit our definition of a community trial, so they will be mentioned only briefly. For evaluation of truly community-wide interventions, it is rarely possible to identify a satisfactory control group from within the intervention community, since those not exposed to the program despite being part of the target population are likely to be quite different from those who participated, and they are also likely to be relatively inaccessible to data collection (Ives et al. 1994). A *before–after* design is an option, but unless changes are truly dramatic, it may not be possible to conclude with confidence that the changes represent anything more than secular trends. A stronger alternative is the *interrupted time series* design (Cook and Campbell 1979), which involves multiple measurements of the outcome before and after an intervention and is therefore most feasible when an existing source of outcome data can be tapped. O'Carroll and colleagues (1991), for example, monitored monthly firearm- and nonfirearm-related homicides in Detroit before and after passage of a law requiring mandatory jail terms for illegally carrying a gun in public, to determine whether the new law had any effect. The interrupted time series design provides greater control over long-term secular trends than the before–after design.

Regression to the mean is also a threat to the validity of single-community designs, because the stimulus for mounting an intervention program may be perceptions that the health target of interest has become worse when in fact random variation over time may be partly or even entirely responsible.

One Intervention and One Control Community

This is the simplest controlled community trial design, and it has often been used. Examples include the North Karelia Project (Puska et al. 1983a), which compared cardiovascular disease and related behaviors between two Finnish provinces; the Pawtucket Heart Health Program (Carleton et al. 1995), which compared similar outcomes in Pawtucket, Rhode Island, with those in another New England town; and the Heart to Heart Project in Florence, South Carolina, mentioned earlier. In these studies and in most other applications of the design, at least one set of baseline measurements is taken in both sites. Changes over time in the control site are then used to estimate what changes would have been observed in the intervention site in the absence of an intervention. Any regional or national short- or long-term shifts in the outcome variables that happen concurrently with the intervention should apply to both communities.

The main limitation of this design is that it does not account for community-level variation. An observed difference in changes over time could represent an intervention effect, or it could simply represent "naturally occurring" community-by-time interaction variability for any of the reasons noted earlier. As in the Florence, South Carolina, project, data must typically be analyzed as though individual people had been allocated to intervention or control conditions, even though entire communities were the actual units of allocation. The result of this discordance between design and analysis is a nonconservative bias in tests of statistical significance, as has been pointed out frequently in the literature (Cornfield 1978; Zucker 1990; Koepsell et al. 1991; Murray et al. 1990a; LaPrelle et al. 1992). This effect may account for the statistically significant advantage found for the control group on hypertension control in the Heart to Heart evaluation, which is otherwise difficult to interpret. (p values for differences in either direction could have been affected.) The same problem applies in other designs with two or more interventions that have only one community per treatment group (Farquhar et al. 1977).

One Intervention Community and Multiple Control Communities

In principle, the best way to address the main limitation of the one-community-per-treatment-group design is to increase the number of communities per treatment group. Increasing the number of intervention sites may not be an option, especially if the program to be evaluated had "grassroots" origins in one particular community and resources are unavailable to replicate it simultaneously elsewhere. However, those constraints may not apply nearly as strongly to the control group, and there is a major advantage to studying more than one control community: namely, the ability to account for community-level variation.

Including multiple control communities can be especially attractive if key outcome information needed for evaluation can be obtained from existing sources. In the Boulder County, Colorado, nurse-midwife study, birth certificate data were as readily available from two neighboring counties as they were for one. Using both counties as controls permitted a proper analysis based on community-level allocation to treatment groups, and it obviated the need to choose one of them as the "best" control. Even when primary data collection is needed, serious consideration should be given to spreading observations among several control sites rather than concentrating them all in one site.

Multiple Intervention and Multiple Control Communities

The movement from one intervention community to two or more of them can be a big step. Intervention communities now become part of a larger social experiment, as exemplified by the COMMIT study. Major outside funding is often required, which imposes other expectations, reporting requirements, and timetables. Intervention communities must give up partial control in order to standardize intervention approaches among sites so that it is clear what is being evaluated.

The increase in scale and complexity, however, brings important benefits to society at large. Mounting intervention programs in several sites constitutes a form of internal replication: If a consistent effect is observed in multiple settings, we have a firmer basis for predicting what would happen if similar programs were mounted in other communities. If the intervention seems to work better in some sites than in others, this information can provide useful clues about the interaction between program features and community contextual factors. From a purely scientific viewpoint, this design offers the best opportunities to measure and account for community-level variation in both treatment groups, and thus leads to more trustworthy conclusions about program effectiveness.

Randomization

The identity of the intervention community is usually preordained in a "grassroots" community program, but in a social experiment involving multiple communities the evaluator may be empowered to assign certain communities to intervention and others to control conditions. The investigator must then decide whether to randomize the communities or to use some other allocation method. One argument sometimes offered against randomization is that, given a small number of communities, it will not be as effective in producing well-balanced groups as it normally is in a clinical-trial situation involving many individual patients. Another argument is that some possible outcomes of simple randomization may yield unacceptable contamination of the control group if, for example, an intervention and a control community share the same media market and the intervention will rely heavily on the mass media. Yet another objection is that cost and convenience will be adversely affected if intervention sites chosen at random are far from study headquarters, thus increasing travel time and cost.

Examined under close scrutiny, however, these objections are not compelling. The risk of unbalanced treatment groups is a consequence of the small number of communities available for assignment, which will remain a problem whether randomization is used or not. Moreover, several methods that can be used to guarantee balance when treatment groups are formed, such as matching of communities, can be used in conjunction with randomization, as illustrated by the COMMIT study (COMMIT Research Group 1991). Restricted randomization methods can be used to prevent unacceptable contamination while still choosing at random from among the many remaining possible outcomes of the allocation process. Requiring intervention sites to be near the evaluation center, which is often situated at an academic institution and/or in a large city, may ultimately expose the study to suspicion that these communities differed systematically from their comparators: they may be more urbanized or more receptive to working with outside investigators based in academia, for example. Ultimately, the benefits of random assignment are as important in community trials as they are in clinical trials: a firm basis for statistical hypothesis testing, some measure of control over determinants of outcome that are unknown or difficult to quantify, and avoidance of any suspicion of investigator bias in formation of treatment groups (Zucker et al. 1995; Green et al. 1995; Koepsell et al. 1995).

Opportunities to randomize communities are not necessarily limited to the planned social experiment, however. As described by Cook and Campbell (1979), some real-world situations can lend themselves to randomization. For example, several communities may be equally worthy competitors for funding from a regional or state funding source that cannot fund them all. Or it may not be possible to mount an intervention in all communities at once, in which case randomization can be used to choose which communities go first, allowing the later-intervention communities to be used as concurrent controls for the earlier-intervention ones.

Matching and Stratification

Communities can be allocated to treatment groups within pairs, as in COM-MIT (Gail et al. 1991) and the Minnesota Heart Health Program (Jacobs et al. 1986), or within strata, as in the Kaiser Community Health Promotion Grants Program (Wagner et al. 1991) and the Child and Adolescent Trial for Cardiovascular Health (CATCH), which allocated schools (Zucker et al. 1995). The advantages of doing so are potential reductions in bias and gains in precision. Bias may be reduced because both techniques render the two treatment groups similar overall with regard to the matching or stratification factors, and because comparisons between intervention and control communities are implicitly made within pairs or strata where comparability is greatest. Precision in estimating the intervention effect is also enhanced if the pooled within-pair or within-stratum variance in outcomes is less than the overall variance ignoring pairs or strata.

What factors should be used to form the pairs or strata? In principle, they should be factors that are known strong correlates of the outcome variable(s) under study. In practice, and in the absence of extensive prior knowledge about community-level correlates of outcomes, attention has focused on readily available population size and sociodemographic characteristics. Freedman et al. (1990) showed how matching on these factors in COMMIT appeared to enhance efficiency. Graham et al. (1984) described a multiattribute utility approach to matching when randomizing small numbers of aggregate units, which was used in a large school-based drug prevention trial in an attempt to balance the treatment groups simultaneously on school size, ethnic composition, socioeconomic status, and academic achievement (Dent et al. 1993).

Martin et al. (1993) considered the potential loss of study power when a small number of communities are matched on a poor correlate of outcome, due to the loss of degrees of freedom when pairs rather than individual communities are the units of analysis. Recently, however, Diehr et al. (1995b) showed by simulation that ignoring the matching in the analysis stage can be a legitimate approach when the matching factors are expected to be only weak correlates of outcome, and that doing so does not lead to an increase in the type I error rate. The mathematical statistical basis for this somewhat surprising finding has since been described by Proschan (1996).

Subject Selection

When primary data collection on a sample of community residents is necessary to track key behaviors or other outcomes over time, two broad alternatives are available for sampling participants. Under a *cohort* sampling approach, a sample of community residents is identified on the first survey occasion, and an attempt is made to recontact the same people on follow-up surveys. Under a *repeated cross-sectional* sampling approach, a fresh sample of respondents is drawn on each survey occasion.

The pros and cons of using cohort and repeated cross-sectional samples have been discussed elsewhere (Shea and Basch 1990b; Koepsell et al. 1992). Briefly, cohort samples are well suited to measuring individual-level behavioral change, which is often a main program goal, while repeated cross-sectional samples measure changes in prevalence at the community level, which may result from a mixture of behavior change and population turnover. Participation rates may be lower in cohort samples because of the greater expected respondent burden and the need to furnish identifying information for tracking purposes. Attrition affects only cohort samples, is a greater problem in populations with high in- and out-migration and/or with long study duration, and may be related to the outcomes under study, often with higher attrition among persons with worse health habits. Participation in repeated surveys may itself be a cue to behavior change (or change in reporting) among cohort members. Cohort members also get older while the community at large may not. Cross-sectional samples may include recent in-migrants to the community who have little or no exposure to the program. Most of these factors would apply to similarly chosen samples in intervention and control sites, however, and would thus not necessarily produce bias in estimating the effectiveness of the program.

Much attention has been paid to the different implications of the two sampling approaches for sample-size requirements and statistical power (Feldman and McKinlay 1994; Diehr et al. 1995a). A key parameter is the level of temporal correlation in the outcome of interest: When two measurements on the same person at two time points tend to be highly correlated, a cohort approach may require many fewer observations than a repeated cross-sectional samples approach. Feldman and McKinlay (1994) showed that such correlations varied widely among potential outcome variables for programs aimed at cardiovascular disease risk factors, from 0.43 for diastolic blood pressure to 0.97 for body mass index among women, suggesting that the best sampling approach may depend on the outcome variable. Dichr et al. (1995a) showed how the "optimal" sampling approach also depends on the degree of expected attrition in the cohort. Interesting "hybrid" sampling approaches, such as replenishing the cohort with new members as original members are lost, await further study.

Cohort and repeated cross-sectional sampling approaches are not mutually exclusive, and in fact several large community trials have used both (Jacobs et al. 1986; COMMIT 1995a,b; Wagner et al. 1991; Farquhar et al. 1990). Often the initial sample has served both as the first cross-sectional sample and as the cohort to be followed in subsequent survey waves.

Data Collection

Importance of a Causal Model

The notion of a community intervention for health promotion and disease prevention implies action at the level of a social unit in order to affect health outcomes at the level of individuals. At least implicitly, intervention designers have in mind a causal model that leads from program inputs to health outputs if the program works as intended. It is important for evaluation purposes that what Lipsey (1990) has termed this "small theory" of the intervention be made explicit early, often in the form of a diagram. Wagenaar et al. (1994), for example, presented a basic model of community intervention as used in the Communities Mobilizing for Change on Alcohol project, summarized in Figure 6-2. Other good examples appear in Puska et al. (1983), Pentz et al. (1989), Wagner et al. (1991), Worden et al. (1994), and Goodman et al. (1995). Shea and Basch (1990a) reviewed the causal models underlying five large community-based cardiovascular disease prevention projects.

The causal model identifies key constructs to be considered when formulating a data collection plan. In the Communities Mobilizing for Change on Alcohol project, for example, each of the constructs shown in Figure 6-2 was

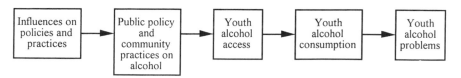

Figure 6-2. Simple casual model of a community intervention. *Source:* Wagenaar et al. (1994)

broken down into several dimensions: For example, the dimensions of alcohol consumption were drinking prevalence, drinking frequency, intoxication prevalence, intoxication frequency, quantity, drinking context, and drinking situation. Seven data collection strategies were then developed (e.g., archival data, surveys of school students, and merchant surveys), and each construct and dimension was explicitly linked to one or more of the seven data sources.

Besides helping to identify key information to be collected, a causal model can also be viewed as a set of hypotheses about program action, including the time sequence in which program-related changes should occur, which can later guide data analysis. The set identifies certain constructs as mediators between others that lie "upstream" or "downstream" from it (MacKinnon and Dwyer 1993). If the program later appears successful in influencing outcomes at the end of this causal chain, having measures of the intermediate steps aids interpretation by clarifying how those effects came about. Conversely, if little change in ultimate outcomes is observed, having measures of intermediate steps can help to diagnose where the causal chain was broken (Koepsell et al. 1992).

Process Evaluation

Process evaluation includes monitoring the extent to which an intervention is actually implemented as intended; its effects on phenomena that fall relatively early in the causal model, such as community activation and population exposure to the intervention; and other activities or events in the community unrelated to the program that may influence outcomes. Implementation evaluation seeks to quantify program activities and level of services delivered, describing how the intervention model actually played out in practice and thus providing an opportunity to detect what has been termed a "type III error": absence of any apparent intervention effect because the intervention was never adequately implemented (Goodman et al. 1994, 1995). Several approaches and data sources have been used, including maintenance of tracking files to document program events, organizations participating, materials disseminated, media coverage, and attendance; and surveys of key informants in community organizations (Assaf et al. 1987; Wickizer et al. 1993; Goodman et al. 1995). Qualitative research methods, including ethnography, may be helpful in describing changes in community culture that may not be easily quantifiable and in describing other contextual factors that may affect response to the intervention (Hunt 1994; Goodman et al. 1995; Israel et al. 1995). If community surveys are mounted, questions can be included to gauge target population awareness of and exposure to the program (COMMIT 1995a). Particularly careful and extensive process evaluations were carried out for the Heart to Heart project (Goodman et al. 1995), for the Child and Adolescent Trial for Cardiovascular Health (Stone et al. 1994) and for COMMIT (Corbett et al. 1990), illustrating several useful approaches.

In some instances, information from the process evaluation has been intentionally fed back to program staff in order to facilitate midcourse improvements (Goodman and Wandersman 1994). This kind of feedback can help the program meet its service goals, but it also blurs the distinction between intervention and evaluation and may put research and service objectives into competition. If data fed back from this kind of formative evaluation are used to guide and modify the intervention, then the formative evaluation itself may arguably need to be regarded as an integral part of the intervention package: An otherwise similar intervention approach used in another community but without an ongoing flow of data from the formative evaluation component would not necessarily work as well.

Individual-Level Outcome Data

As illustrated by Figure 6-2, the ultimate goals of community-based interventions are often improvement of health behavior and health outcomes in members of the target population. An evaluation that lacks data on those endpoints would thus be at best incomplete and at worst misleading as to its conclusions about program effectiveness. The four introductory examples described earlier illustrate the wide range of data-collection alternatives, ranging from repeated in-person interviews and examinations in the Nepalese vitamin A study to extensive telephone surveys in COMMIT and in the Florence, South Carolina, Heart to Heart project to use of archival birth certificate data in the Boulder County midwife program.

The choice of a data-collection strategy for health behavior and health outcome information is likely to be a major determinant of total evaluation cost and thus influences the feasibility of an overall evaluation design. A careful review of existing potential data sources is therefore advisable before concluding that primary data collection is needed. In the Boulder County example, availability of birth certificate data on prenatal care and pregnancy outcomes for several Colorado counties made it possible to carry out the program evaluation as an in-house project without external funding while still reaping the crucial advantages of studying more than one community per treatment group.

Primary data collection may, however, be unavoidable for some outcomes. Methods for estimating sample-size requirements are discussed below. Because it will often be impossible to blind survey respondents to their treatment-group membership, methodological issues may arise about the validity of self-reported information about behavior or other outcomes (Koepsell et al. 1992; Patrick et al. 1994). Sometimes these threats to validity can be circumvented by using physiologic measures, such as cotinine or carbon monoxide for smoking behavior, or blood pressure and cholesterol for cardio-vascular disease prevention (Farquhar et al. 1990). In addition, if a cohort sample approach is used, there may be concern about whether repeated interviews about health behavior themselves constitute a co-intervention. Some studies (COMMIT 1995a; Worden et al. 1994) have chosen to do less-intensive data collection for part of the sample to allow this possibility to be assessed.

Community-Level Indicators

Another useful approach to assessing the effects of community interventions involves a class of outcome measures variously termed "community-level indicators" or "environmental indicators" (Cheadle et al. 1992). These measures are derived from observations of aspects of the community environment related to the target behaviors or conditions, aggregated to the community level. Examples related to smoking include the proportion of restaurants that offer nonsmoking seating, the existence of community ordinances prohibiting smoking in public buildings, and the prevalence of cigarette vending machines in stores and restaurants that are situated near schools. Cheadle et al. (1992) conceptualized several types of community-level measures, which differ according to their obtrusiveness (conspicuousness of the observation process), reactivity (likelihood that measurement itself could lead to changes in outcomes), and unit of observation (such as work sites, restaurants, or the community as a whole). They also described specific techniques for using grocery-store product displays to evaluate community-based nutrition programs (Cheadle et al. 1990, 1995) and surveys of restaurants to assess the health-promotion environment related to availability of low-fat menu items and of nonsmoking seating (Cheadle et al. 1994). Community-level comparisons between availability of healthful products in a sample of grocery stores and self-reported healthy dietary behavior in surveys of individuals in those communities showed positive and statistically significant (if sometimes modest) correlations (Cheadle et al. 1991).

While community-level indicators do not measure individual-level health behavior as directly as do surveys, they offer at least two attractive features. First, obtaining new data on them is usually substantially less costly than conducting large-scale primary data collection on individuals. Second, they can be expected to be less prone to bias due to inability to blind.

Data Analysis

Analysis and interpretation of data from a community trial can be complex and challenging. The investigator can expect to face not only such relatively familiar issues as confounding and effect modification, but also less familiar ones, including multilevel longitudinal data, causal modeling, and complex survey sampling plans. Accordingly, this is an excellent context for collaboration with biostatistical colleagues. This section will seek only to provide an orientation to analytic approaches with emphasis on dealing with community-level variation.

Analysis Approaches to Avoid: Ignoring Community-Level Variation

As noted earlier, the issue of community-level variation can be regarded equivalently in two ways: as an extra source of random variation above and beyond individual-to-individual variation, or as a problem of correlated or clustered data. A short and accessible paper by Cornfield (1978) provides an excellent introduction to the problem. It concludes with the following advice: "Randomization by cluster accompanied by an analysis appropriate to randomization by individual is an exercise in self-deception . . . and should be discouraged." Analyses based on ordinary chi-square, Pearson correlations, or *t*-tests or on familiar multivariate techniques such as standard least-squares multiple regression, one-way analysis of variance or covariance, or logistic regression are well known to lead to nonconservatively biased tests of significance, sometimes substantially so (Whiting-O'Keefe et al. 1984; Zucker 1990; Donner and Klar 1996; Murray et al. 1996; LaPrelle et al. 1992).

Unfortunately, reviews by Donner et al. (1990) and by Simpson et al. (1995) indicate that failure to account for clustering in the design and analysis stages is all too common in prevention trials involving group randomization. Among 16 such trials published in four leading medical journals from 1979 to 1989, only eight properly accounted for cluster allocation in the analysis; the other eight used analysis methods that implicitly assumed that individuals rather than clusters had been randomized, and seven of them yielded "statistically significant" results that must be viewed with suspicion (Donner et al. 1990). A subsequent review of studies published in 1990–1993 found that nine of the 21 trials identified failed to account for cluster randomization in the analysis (Simpson et al. 1995). While these reviews covered only randomized studies, the problem applies with equal force to corresponding nonrandomized designs. The high prevalence of this erroneous practice has unfortunately led some authors to justify an incorrect analysis by citing its use in previous studies, thus perpetuating the error across studies as a sort of pesky statistical virus.

Donner and Klar (1996) also examined the practice of using initial statistical testing to determine whether the degree of clustering is statistically significant and, if not, powering or analyzing group-randomized trials as though individuals were randomized. They note that those initial significance tests have low power and that the study design itself should lead investigators to assume the existence of intracluster correlation rather than seeking to disprove its existence with statistical testing. Many valid techniques are now available to account properly for allocation by cluster, and there is little justification for not using them.

Analysis Based on Community Means

One way to avoid violation of statistical independence assumptions is to aggregate individual-level observations to the community level and then use the community-level means or proportions as the primary data to be analyzed. This approach follows the classic Fisherian advice to "analyze as you randomize" (Fisher 1935). It is a simple and valid method for study designs in which the number of individuals studied per community is approximately the same across communities. The main test of statistical significance for an intervention effect may reduce to a simple t-test, comparing the means of the community-level means between intervention and control groups. Simulation work by Donner and Klar (1996) suggests that the two-sample t-test yields trustworthy significance levels even when there are as few as three communities per treatment group. Under the central limit theorem, the community-level means will tend toward a normal distribution even if individual-level observations are not normally distributed, and the t-test appears to be robust to moderate violation of the normality assumption (Donner and Klar 1994).

There are, however, two shortcomings to this analytic approach. First, if the number of individuals observed per community differs substantially across communities, a homoscedasticity assumption behind the t-test is violated: Other things being equal, estimated community-level means based on many individual observations are subject to less sampling variability than those based on fewer observations. Second, individual-level covariates are not taken into account. An individual's sociodemographic characterisics, for example, may be strong determinants of the behavioral outcome of interest, and sociodemographic mix often varies among communities. Methods of analysis that adjust for individual-level covariates can thus enhance the comparability of communities and improve power by removing an extraneous source of variation.

Adjustment of Individual-Level Analysis for Clustering

Another family of analytic methods described by Donner and colleagues (1981; 1987; 1993; 1994) involves use of inflation factors to correct the nonconservative bias in a t-test or chi square carried out on the individual-level data. In the simplest case, for clusters of fixed size n, the inflation factor for the variance of a treatment-group-specific mean is $[1 + (n-1)\rho]$, where ρ is the intraclass correlation coefficient (Donner et al. 1981). These methods have been extended to clusters of unequal sizes (Donner et al. 1981), construction of confidence intervals (Donner and Klar 1993), binary outcomes (Donner et al. 1981, 1994), and stratified data (Donald and Donner 1987). They do not, however, account directly for individual-level covariates.

Two-Stage Analysis to Account for Individual-Level Covariates

Investigators on the COMMIT (Gail et al. 1991) and CATCH (Zucker et al. 1995) studies proposed closely related two-stage analysis approaches. In the first stage, an individual-level statistical model is developed to predict some outcome variable using conventional tools that ignore clustering, such as ordinary least-squares multiple regression for continuous outcomes or logistic regression for binary outcomes to obtain a set of community-specific residuals. At the second stage, these residuals (or adjusted community-level means) are used as elementary data points in comparing the two treatment groups. Zucker et al. (1995) proposed use of analysis of variance or of covariance at the second stage, which may also include community-level covariates. In COMMIT, which involved 11 pairs of communities, a permutation test was applied at the second stage to minimize assumptions about the distribution of true community means within treatment groups (Gail et al. 1991; Green et al. 1995). A limitation of the permutation-test approach is that it would be unable to reject the null hypothesis with very few communities per treatment group.

Individual-Level Analysis for Correlated Data

Another set of statistical approaches fits the community-trial situation very well, allowing a valid analysis of individual-level observations without requiring an independence assumption. The mixed-model analysis of variance (or covariance) is the oldest among these (Murray et al. 1989; Koepsell et al. 1991; Murray and Wolfinger 1994a). It involves specifying an additive model for the outcome variable, with main-effect terms for treatment group, community, and time; group-by-time and community-by-time interaction effects; and an individual-level error term (Koepsell et al. 1991). The model is "mixed" because some of the terms (treatment group, time, and group-by-time interactions) correspond to fixed effects, while the others (community, community-by-time interaction, and individual) correspond to random effects. When there are no individual-level covariates and the same number of individuals studied across communities, the F-test for a treatment effect from this model reduces to exactly the same F-test that would be obtained from an analysis of community-level means. Although classical methods of estimation for the mixed model required balanced designs (equal number of individuals across communities), modern computer software uses other estimation methods, including restricted maximum likelihood, which can accommodate unbalanced study designs and both individual- and community-level covariates (Murray and Wolfinger 1994a). Simulation studies suggest that this method is sufficiently robust to yield valid significance tests even with binary outcome data (Hannan and Murray 1996).

Other relatively new statistical approaches allow valid use of familiar regression-analysis techniques on clustered data, using both cluster-level and subunit-level covariates (Liang and Zeger 1993; Breslow and Clayton 1993). Regression analysis based on generalized estimating equations is particularly flexible because it can accommodate normal, binary, or count-type outcome variables (Liang and Zeger 1993), although Donner (Murray et al. 1994b) notes that the validity of significance tests is assured only with a fairly large number of clusters.

Analysis of the One-Community-per-Treatment-Group Design

A study design involving only one community per treatment group puts the data analyst in a serious bind, because community-level variation is completely confounded with treatment-group status. An analysis that ignores the group allocation and treats the data as though individuals had been randomized runs the risk of exaggerating claims of statistical significance and violating Cornfield's cautionary advice (1978). Mickey et al. (1991) have suggested obtaining and applying external estimates of community-level variation, in the form of a "design effect" or variance inflation factor calculated from available data on other communities in the region. While this is a step in the right direction, it may overcorrect if the external communities on which data are available are not as closely matched to the intervention site as a set of deliberately chosen controls would have been. It may also be unclear how many degrees of freedom should be used for significance testing.

Ultimately the investigator in this situation must hope for a fairly dramatic intervention effect that will be convincing even when no proper test of significance can be done. It may be helpful to consider the criteria that epidemiologists often use to infer causal associations from nonexperimental data in order to guide interpretation of the findings.

Sample Size and Power Estimation

If primary data collection will be required, estimation of sample size require-ments is an important part of evaluation design in order to balance the com-peting aims of sufficient power to detect an intervention effect and efficiency in the face of limited resources. The task is more difficult than for simpler study designs in which individuals are randomized due to the need to account for community-level variation and perhaps other design features. Several authors have described the information and assumptions needed and provide helpful formulas and graphical aids. Donner et al. (1981) addressed simple group-randomized studies with continuous or binary outcomes and group-randomized designs with stratification (Donner 1992). Donner and Klar (1996) published a short computer program in the SAS programming lan-guage to estimate statistical power. Hsieh (1988) also considered these designs and provided power curves for determining number of clusters required as a function of number of individuals studied per cluster and estimated intraclass correlation. Shipley et al. (1989) addressed matched-pair designs with ran-domization by group. Koepsell et al. (1991) described methods for power and sample-size estimation when comparing patterns of change over time between intervention and control sites. Murray et al. (1994c) presented formulas for the smallest detectable intervention effect given specified values of various design parameters. Gail et al. (1991) described how computer simulations were used to estimate power in COMMIT in anticipation of an analysis based on permutation tests.

All of these approaches require advance estimation of community-level variation in the form of intraclass correlation coefficients, variance compo-nents, or design effects. When secondary data will be used, historical infor-mation may be available to provide estimates of community-level variation specific to the proposed study communities; otherwise, external information sources will be needed. Fortunately, several research teams have now pub-lished such estimates, most of them obtained from ongoing or completed community intervention trials, specifically to aid design of future studies. Table 6-2 lists several of these sources. Feng and Grizzle (1992) noted that intraclass correlations can often be estimated only imprecisely from studies with relatively few groups randomized. They suggested a simulation ap-proach to sample-size estimation, varying the estimated intraclass correlation coefficient over a plausible range.

Investigators are often concerned to find that the projected power of a planned community trial is low for a feasible number of communities and individuals per community. This conclusion has much to do with the extra source of variation and the small number of degrees of freedom available for

Table 6-2. Selected Published Sources for Estimates of Cluster-Level Variation

First author (year)	Outcome	Unit of Study
Murray (1990)	Smoking and drug use in adolescents	School
Koepsell (1991)	Smoking	Community (usually county)
Mickey (1991)	Mortality from ischemic heart disease, stroke, cancer of the lung, colon, or breast	County, state
Hannan (1994)	Media exposure, attitudes about heart disease prevention, physical activity, physiological and behavioral risk factors for coronary heart disease	City
Feldman (1994)	Height, weight, body-mass index, blood pressure, cholesterol	City
Murray (1994c)	Smoking in adolescents	School
Fortmann (1995)	Triglyceride, cholesterol, blood pressure, Framingham risk score for coronary heart disease	City
Murray (1995c)	Alcohol use in young adults	Community

testing the statistical significance of an intervention effect. Possible coping strategies in this situation include:

1. Look for ways to increase the number of study communities, even if the number of individuals studied per community must be reduced to do so. For a simple parallel-groups study design with outcomes measured on a single occasion, c communities in each of two treatment groups, and n individuals studied per community, power is inversely related to the variance of a treatment-group-specific mean, which is:

$$\frac{\sigma_C^2 + \sigma^2/n}{c}$$

where σ_C^2 denotes community-level variance and σ^2 denotes individual-level variance. Increasing n decreases the value of this expression only up to a point, after which σ_C^2 dominates the numerator. Increasing c is always effective. Even if cost and feasibility preclude increasing the number of intervention communities, increasing the number of control communities may be both feasible and desirable from a power standpoint.

2. Consider a matched-community study design if many communities are available for study. Although there remains much uncertainty about what the best matching factors should be, matching on community characteristics that are likely strong correlates of the outcome variable has the theoretical potential to reduce the effect of community-level variation. In the COMMIT trial,

matching on population size and sociodemographic characteristics seemed to help efficiency (Freedman et al. 1990).

3. Obtain and use baseline data in intervention and control communities. Information from completed trials suggests that communities often "track," just as individuals do, with correlated baseline and follow-up community means. Analyses that assess intervention effects by comparing patterns of change over time between intervention and control sites let each community serve as its own control. Statistically, this means that intervention effects are tested against community-by-time variance, which is often much smaller than community-to-community variance at a single time point.

4. Consider a cohort sampling approach for individual participants. As discussed earlier, this is a multifaceted trade-off that involves issues besides statistical power. But for outcomes that are relatively stable within individuals over time (such as body-mass index and serum cholesterol) and for study settings and durations that would yield low attrition in panels of individuals followed over time, cohort samples can offer significant power advantages (McKinlay 1994).

Summary

Intervention at the community level for disease prevention and health promotion has considerable theoretical appeal, but formal evaluations of these programs have yielded very mixed results. We have much more to learn about where, when, and how they can be effective. Because community interventions are being applied to an ever wider range of target conditions and populations, often with noble goals and high hopes but limited resources, it is important that new programs be evaluated.

The concept of community-level variation presents a special challenge in the design and analysis of community intervention studies. It can be viewed as an added source of variation in health behaviors or outcomes that affects estimation of an intervention effect, or as correlation of health-related characteristics among individuals in a community. In either event, it must be estimated from historical data or from external sources in order to estimate study power or sample-size requirements, and it must be accommodated in the data analysis strategy to avoid overestimating program effectiveness. Fortunately, several valid analytic approaches are available. Study designs that involve only one intervention site and one control site cannot separate intervention effect from community-level variation, and they should be avoided in preference for designs involving more communities.

The rigor and comprehensiveness of evaluation must often be balanced against feasibility and cost. Strategies to enhance efficiency include emphasizing more communities over more observations per community, exploiting secondary data sources, exploring community-level indicators of outcome, choosing carefully between cohort and repeated cross-sectional samples when primary individual-level data are needed, and gathering baseline data in intervention and control sites in order to allow changes over time to be tracked. Whenever possible, randomization should be used in assigning communities to treatment groups.

Evaluation of community interventions can be a challenging and stimulating form of applied epidemiology. By helping to reach valid conclusions about which programs work well and which fall short, epidemiologists can play an important role in enhancing community health in the face of limited resources.

CASE STUDIES

HIV Prevention in Rural Tanzania

Background

Human immunodeficiency virus (HIV) infection and AIDS are a global pandemic, but the population of sub-Saharan Africa has been hit particularly hard. The World Health Organization estimated that over 10 million adults in the region were infected with HIV by mid-1994 (WHO 1994). Heterosexual transmission is the main route of exposure. The prevalence of HIV seropositivity has been found to be highest in cities, sometimes with prevalences over 20%, but most of the population at risk lives in rural areas (Hayes et al. 1995). Prevention efforts aimed at behavioral change have been hampered by geographic dispersion of the population, low literacy, and lack of resources.

The risk of heterosexual transmission of HIV is thought to be increased in the presence of other sexually transmitted diseases (STDs), perhaps in part because of disruption of mucous membrane barriers (Pepin et al. 1989). Many other STDs that are common in sub-Saharan Africa, including chancroid, syphilis, gonorrhea, chlamydia urethritis, and trichomoniasis, can be treated effectively with antibiotics. Hence control of curable STDs may offer a way to reduce the incidence of HIV infection.

An international public health team designed an intervention to improve control of STDs in the Mwanza region of Tanzania (Hayes et al. 1995). Its components included increased training on treatment of STDs for staff of government health centers, a supply of antibiotics, community health education on recognition and treatment of STDs, and a regional referral center for difficult-to-manage cases.

Key Questions

1. Given the nature of the intervention, what overall evaluation design would provide the most convincing evidence for or against its effectiveness?

Because the STD control program was aimed unselectively at everyone in a community served by a government health center, a comparative evaluation is needed to involve intervention in some communities while using other communities as concurrent controls. Twelve health centers and the communities served by them were selected and arranged in six matched pairs according to proximity to a main road or to the shores of Lake Victoria, geographical area, and level of clinic use for STDs as assessed from clinic records. Within each matched pair, one community was selected at random for early intervention; its counterpart became a control community for 2 years, after which it also received the intervention.

2. How could contamination of the control communities be prevented?

Study communities were widely dispersed over a large geographic area in rural Tanzania, minimizing the likelihood that a person with an STD in a control community would travel to an intervention community for treatment. Place of residence was recorded in clinic records, permitting the extent of use by out-of-area patients to be assessed.

3. What kind of data should be collected to gauge effectiveness of the program?

Because prevention of HIV infection was the program's primary goal, the incidence of HIV infection was assessed in a cohort of 1,000 adults aged 15–54 chosen by a cluster sampling method from each study community (Grosskurth et al. 1995). Serologic testing at baseline provided an estimate of prevalence; repeat serologic testing of the same individuals 2 years later provided incidence data that could be compared between intervention and control sites. Implementation of the program was monitored in part through supervisory visits to each health center. Supplementary samples of 100 consecutive women attending prenatal care clinics and of 100 randomly chosen men from each community were used to assess the incidence and prevalence of STD infection.

4. How many survey participants were needed to provide adequate statistical power?

Sample-size calculations focused on the primary end-point, incidence of HIV infection. A recent study in a neighboring region suggested 1% annual incidence, which was assumed to hold for control communities in the study area. It was assumed that an effective intervention would reduce incidence by half. Data on extent of community-level variation in incidence of HIV infection were unavailable, so sample-size calculations were repeated over a range of assumed values. A conservative choice led to studying 1,000 cohort members per community. Estimates from the baseline survey later showed that observed community-level variation in seroprevalence, which may provide a reasonable guide to community-level variation in incidence, was close to the value assumed.

Implications for Practice

This brief example illustrates several key issues for researchers and practitioners. Chief among them is the importance of early specification and implementation of a rigorous evaluation plan. In this instance, the investigators seized upon the fact that resources were too scarce to intervene in all communities at once as an opportunity to randomize communities to early versus late intervention. Their evaluation design should provide excellent information about the effectiveness of this approach to HIV prevention and enhance applicability of the findings to other sites in sub-Saharan Africa.

Cardiovascular Disease Prevention in a Low-Income Urban Area

Background

Despite recent declines in cardiovascular disease (CVD) mortality, heart disease remains the leading cause of death in the United States. The burden of CVD falls especially heavily on persons with low educational attainment and from racial minorities (McCord and Freeman 1990; Shea et al. 1991). Early evidence from large, well-funded, community-based CVD prevention programs suggested favorable effects on behavioral risk factors (Farquhar et al. 1977; Puska et al. 1983a) and on CVD mortality (Puska et al. 1983b). However, it remains unclear whether a community-based intervention approach for CVD could work as well in disadvantaged urban areas with fewer resources.

In 1988, the New York State Department of Health funded eight CVD prevention programs in communities around the state, one of them in the Washington Heights–Inwood area of Manhattan (Shea et al. 1992, 1996). In contrast to earlier CVD prevention programs with major federal funding, this program involved a far more modest intervention budget and a clear shift in emphasis from research toward community service. Less than 10% of the program's budget was set aside for evaluation.

Key Questions

1. How would funding-agency priorities affect overall evaluation design?

Communities took part in a competitive grant application process, with selection of sites on the basis of need and merit. This process and tight budget constraints precluded the ability to study well-defined control communities concurrently. Moreover, no funds were available to monitor the incidence of cardiovascular disease events in study sites. Accordingly, the evaluation focused on implementation, process evaluation, and impact on behavioral risk factors for CVD. These compromises sacrificed the ability to determine whether the programs actually prevent CVD, with the possible exception of fatal CVD as monitored through available mortality statistics.

2. How could program-related activities be systematically monitored and quantified?

In the Washington Heights–Inwood site, a database system was created to keep simple counts of events, participants, and materials distributed (Shea et al. 1992). These included number of risk-factor screening and health-promotion events, number of radio and television "spots" about the program, number of volunteers who participated, and number and characteristics of participants when available. Additional qualitative feedback was obtained from a Community Advisory Board.

3. How were changes in CVD-related health behavior tracked?

At the state level, a telephone survey was mounted using a modified form of the Behavioral Risk Factor Survey (BRFS) developed by the Centers for Disease Control (Remington et al. 1988). It was conducted at baseline and planned for 5 years later, with oversampling in the eight study communities and planned comparison with BRFS data for the rest of the state. This strategy had several limitations, including relatively lower telephone coverage in disadvantaged study communities, reliance on self-report, difficulty in estimating and accommodating community-level variation in the statewide control sample, and limited power. Because of cost and changing funding-agency priorities, plans for the follow-up telephone survey had to be abandoned. For some program components, however, a community-level indicator approach was successfully used. Availability of low-fat milk, for example, was monitored by conducting on-site surveys in 98% of the 251 bodegas and in all 25 supermarkets in the Washington Heights–Inwood community (Wechsler et al. 1995). Choice of low-fat milk at lunchtime was also monitored at low cost through area schools and showed sharp increases (Shea et al. 1996).

Implications for Practice

As is common in smaller-scale community interventions, the investigators noted that the low evaluation budget left many questions unanswered about behavior change, CVD incidence, and program cost-effectiveness. They noted: "Although the cost of evaluative research to address these issues is high, it is no higher than the cost of clinical trials of medical interventions (the population benefits of which are likely to be no greater than those of community health education) or than the cost of not knowing what is effective." As similar interventions are undertaken in the future, it is critical to ensure that adequate evaluation resources are available to determine program effectiveness.

SUGGESTED READINGS

Cheadle A, Wagner E, Koepsell T, Kristal A, Patrick D. Environmental indicators: a tool for evaluating community-based health-promotion programs. Am J Prev Med 1992;8:345–350.

Community Intervention Trial for Smoking Cessation (COMMIT): I. Cohort results from a four-year community intervention. Am J Public Health 1995;85:183–192.

Cornfield J. Randomization by group: a formal analysis. Am J Epidemiol 1978;108: 100–102.

Donner A, Klar N. Statistical considerations in the design and analysis of community intervention trials. J Clin Epidemiol 1996;49:435–439.

Koepsell TD, Martin DC, Diehr PH, et al. Data analysis and sample size issues in evaluations of community-based health promotion and disease prevention programs: a mixed-model analysis of variance approach. J Clin Epidemiol 1991; 44:701–713.

Murray DM, McKinlay SM, Martin D, et al. Design and analysis issues in community trials. Eval Rev 1994;18:493–514.

REFERENCES

Assaf A, Banspach S, Lasater T, McKinlay S, Carleton R. The Pawtucket Heart Health Program: II. Evaluation strategies. Rhode Island Med J 1987; 70:541–546.

Breslow NE, Clayton DG. Approximate inference in generalized linear mixed models. J Am Stat Assoc 1993;88:9–25.

Campbell DT, Stanley JC. Experimental and Quasi-Experimental Designs for Research. Boston: Houghton Mifflin; 1963.

Carleton RA, Lasater TM, Assaf AR, Feldman HA, McKinlay S. The Pawtucket Heart Health Program: community changes in cardiovascular risk factors and projected disease risk. Am J Public Health 1995;85:777–785.

Cheadle A, Psaty B, Wagner E, et al. Evaluating community-based nutrition programs: assessing the reliability of a survey of grocery store product displays. Am J Public Health 1990;80:709–711.

Cheadle A, Psaty BM, Curry S, et al. Community-level comparisons between the grocery store environment and individual dietary practices. Prev Med 1991;20: 250–261.

Cheadle A, Wagner E, Koepsell T, Kristal A, Patrick D. Environmental indicators: a tool for evaluating community-based health-promotion programs. Am J Prev Med 1992; 8:345–350.

Cheadle A, Psaty B, Curry S, et al. Community-level assessment of the health promotion environment in restaurants. Am J Health Promotion 1994;9:88–91.

Cheadle A, Psaty BM, Diehr P, et al. Evaluating community-based nutrition programs: comparing grocery store and individual-level survey measures of program impact. Prev Med 1995;24:71–79.

COMMIT Research Group. Community Intervention Trial for Smoking Cessation (COMMIT): summary of design and intervention. J Natl Cancer Inst 1991;83: 1620–1628.

Community Intervention Trial for Smoking Cessation (COMMIT): I. Cohort results from a four-year community intervention. Am J Public Health 1995a;85:183–192.

Community Intervention Trial for Smoking Cessation (COMMIT): II. Changes in adult cigarette smoking prevalence. Am J Public Health 1995b;85:193–200.

Cook TD, Campbell DT. Quasi-Experimentation: Design and Analysis Issues for Field Settings. Boston: Houghton Mifflin; 1979.

Corbett K, Thompson B, White N, Taylor M for the COMMIT Research Group. Process evaluation for the Community Intervention Trial for Smoking Cessation (COMMIT). Int Q Community Health Educ 1990–1;11:291–309.

Cornfield J. Randomization by group: a formal analysis. Am J Epidemiol 1978;108: 100–102.

De Alarc'on R. The spread of heroin abuse in a community. Community Health Bristol 1969;1:155–161.

Dent CW, Sussman S, Flay BR. The use of archival data to select and assign schools in a drug prevention trial. Eval Rev 1993;17:159–181.

Diehr P, Koepsell T, Cheadle A, Psaty BM, Wagner E, Curry S. Do communities differ in health behaviors? J Clin Epidemiol 1993;46:1141–1149.

Diehr P, Martin DC, Koepsell T, Cheadle A, Psaty BM, Wagner EH. Optimal survey design for community intervention evaluations: cohort or cross-sectional? J Clin Epidemiol 1995a;48:1461–1472.

Diehr P, Martin DC, Koepsell T, Cheadle A. Breaking the matches in a paired t-test for community interventions when the number of pairs is small. Stat Med 1995b; 14:1491–1504.

Donald A, Donner A. Adjustments to the Mantel-Haenszel chi-square statistic and odds ratio variance estimator when the data are clustered. Stat Med 1987;6:491–499.

Donner A. Sample size requirements for stratified cluster randomization designs. Stat Med 1992;11:743–750.

Donner A, Birkett N, Buck C. Randomization by cluster. Sample size requirements and analysis. Am J Epidemiol 1981;114:906–914.

Donner A, Donald A. Analysis of data arising from a stratified design with the cluster as unit of randomization. Stat Med 1987;6:43–52.

Donner A, Brown KS, Brasher P. A methodological review of non-therapeutic intervention trials employing cluster randomization, 1979–1989. Int J Epidemiol 1990;19:795–800.

Donner A, Klar N. Confidence interval construction for effect measures arising from cluster randomization trials. J Clin Epidemiol 1993;46:123–131.

Donner A, Klar N. Methods for comparing event rates in intervention studies when the unit of allocation is a cluster. Am J Epidemiol 1994;140:279–289.

Donner A, Klar N. Statistical considerations in the design and analysis of community intervention trials. J Clin Epidemiol 1996;49:435–439.

Farquhar JW. The community-based model of life style intervention trials. Am J Epidemiol 1978;108:103–111.

Farquhar JW, Wood PD, Breitrose H, et al. Community education for cardiovascular health. Lancet 1977;1:1192–1195.

Farquhar JW, Fortmann SP, Flora JA, et al. Effects of communitywide education on cardiovascular disease risk factors. The Stanford Five-City Project. JAMA 1990; 264:359–365.

Feldman HA, McKinlay SM. Cohort versus cross-sectional design in large field trials: precision, sample size, and a unifying model. Stat Med 1994;3:61–78.

Feng Z, Grizzle JE. Correlated binomial variates: properties of estimator of intraclass correlation and its effect on sample size calculation. Stat Med 1992;11:1607–1614.

Fisher RA. The Design of Experiments. Edinburgh: Olver and Boyd; 1935.

Flay BR. Efficacy and effectiveness trials (and other phases of research) in the development of health promotion programs. Prev Med 1986;15:451–474.

Flay BR. Mass media and smoking cessation: a critical review. Am J Public Health 1987;77:153–160.

Fortmann SP, Flora JA, Winkleby MA, Schooler C, Taylor CB, Farquhar JW. Community intervention trials: reflections on the Stanford Five-City Project Experience. American Journal of Epidemiology 1975;142(6):576–586.

Freedman LS, Green SB, Byar DP. Assessing the gain in efficiency due to matching in a community intervention study. Stat Med 1990;9:943–952.

Gail MH, Byar DP, Pechacek TF, Corle DK for the COMMIT Study Group. Aspects of statistical design for the Community Intervention Trial for Smoking Cessation (COMMIT). Controlled Clin Trials 1991;13:6–21.

Goodman RM, Wandersman A. FORECAST: a formative approach to evaluating community coalitions and community-based initiatives. J Community Psychol 1994; Special issue:6–25.

Goodman RM, Wheeler FC, Lee PR. Evaluation of the Heart to Heart Project: lessons from a community-based chronic disease prevention project. Am J Health Promotion 1995;9:443–455.

Graham JW, Flay BR, Johnson CA, Hansen WB, Collins LM. Group comparability: a multiattribute utility approach to the use of random assignment with small numbers of aggregated units. Eval Rev 1984;8:247–260.

Green SB, Corle DK, Gail MH, et al. Interplay between design and analysis for behavioral intervention trials with community as the unit of randomization. Am J Epidemiol 1995;142:587–593.

Grosskurth H, Mosha F, Todd J, et al. A community trial of the impact of improved sexually transmitted disease treatment on the HIV epidemic in rural Tanzania: 2. baseline survey results. AIDS 1995;9:927–934.

Hannan PJ, Murray DM, Jacobs DR Jr, McGovern PG. Parameters to aid in the design and analysis of community trials: intraclass correlations from the Minnesota Heart Health Program. Epidemiol 1994;5:88–95.

Hannan PJ, Murray DM. Gauss or Bernoulli? A Monte Carlo comparison of the performance of the linear mixed-model and the logistic mixed-model analyses in simulated community trials with a dichotomous outcome variable at the individual level. Eval Rev 1996;20:338–352.

Hayes R, Mosha F, Nicoll A, et al. A community trial of the impact of improved sexually transmitted disease treatment on the HIV epidemic in rural Tanzania: 1. Design. AIDS 1995;9:919–926.

Hsieh FY. Sample size formulae for intervention studies with the cluster as unit of randomization. Stat Med 1988;8:1195–1201.

Hunt GP. Ethnography and the pursuit of culture: the use of ethnography in evaluating the Community Partnership Program. J Community Psychol 1994;special issue:52–60.

Israel BA, Cummings KM, Dignan MB, et al. Evaluation of health education programs: current assessment and future directions. Health Educ Q 1995;22:364–389.

Ives DG, Traven ND, Kuller LH, Schulz R. Selection bias and nonresponse to health promotion in older adults. Epidemiology 1994;5:456–461.

Jacobs DR Jr, Luepker RV, Mittelmark MB, et al. Community-wide prevention strategies: evaluation design of the Minnesota Heart Health Program. J Chronic Dis 1986;39:775–788.

Koepsell TD, Martin DC, Diehr PH, et al. Data analysis and sample size issues in evaluations of community-based health promotion and disease prevention programs: a mixed-model analysis of variance approach. J Clin Epidemiol 1991;44:701–713.

Koepsell TD, Wagner EH, Cheadle AC, et al. Selected methodological issues in evaluating community-based health promotion and disease prevention programs. Annu Rev Public Health 1992;13:31–57.

Koepsell TD, Diehr PH, Cheadle A, Kristal A. Invited commentary: symposium on community intervention trials. Am J Epidemiol 1995;142:594–599.

LaPrelle J, Bauman KE, Koch GG. High intercommunity variation in adolescent cigarette smoking in a 10-community field experiment. Eval Rev 1992;16:115–130.

Lenaway D, Koepsell TD, Vaughan T, van Belle G, Shy K, Cruz-Uribe F. Evaluation of a public-private certified nurse midwife maternity program for indigent women. Am J Public Health (in press).

Liang K-Y, Zeger SL. Regression analysis for correlated data. Annu Rev Public Health 1993;14:43–68.

Lipsey MW. Theory as Method: Small Theories of Treatment. AHCPR Conference Proceedings. Research Methodology: Strengthening Causal Interpretations of Nonexperimental Data. Sechrest L, Perrin E, Bunker J, eds. DHHS pub. no. (PHS) 90-3454;1990:33–51.

MacKinnon DP, Dwyer JH. Estimating mediated effects in prevention studies. Eval Rev 1993;12:144–158.

Martin DC, Diehr P, Perrin EB, Koepsell TD. The effect of matching on the power of randomized community intervention studies. Stat Med 1993;12:329–338.

McCord C, Freeman HP. Excess mortality in Harlem. N Engl J Med 1990;322:173–177.

McKinlay JB. The promotion of health through planned sociopolitical change: challenges for research and policy. Soc Sci Med 1993;36:109–117.

McKinlay SM. Cost-efficient designs of cluster unit trials. Prev Med 1994;23:606–611.

Mickey RM, Goodwin GD, Costanza MC. Estimation of the design effect in community intervention studies. Stat Med 1991;10:53–64.

Multiple Risk Factor Intervention Trial Research Group. Multiple risk factor intervention trial. Risk factor changes and mortality results. JAMA 1982;248:1465–1477.

Murray DM, Hannan PJ, Zucker D. Analysis issues in school-based health promotion studies. Health Educ Q 1989;16:315–320.

Murray DM, Hannan PJ. Planning the appropriate analysis in school-based drug-use prevention studies. J Consult Clin Psychol 1990;58:458–468.

Murray DM, Wolfinger RD. Analysis issues in the evaluation of community trials: progress toward solutions in SAS/STAT MIXED. J Community Psychol 1994a; Special issue:140–154.

Murray DM, McKinlay SM, Martin D, et al. Design and analysis issues in community trials. Eval Rev 1994b;18:493–514.

Murray DM, Rooney BL, Hannan PJ, et al. Intraclass correlation among common measures of adolescent smoking: estimates, correlates, and applications in smoking prevention studies. Am J Epidemiol 1994c;140:1038–1050.

Murray DM, Short B. Intraclass correlation among measures related to alcohol use by young adults: estimates, correlates, and applications in intervention studies. J Stud Alcohol 1995;56:681–694.

Murray DM, Hannan PJ, Baker WL. A Monte Carlo study of alternative responses to intraclass correlation in community trials. Is it ever possible to avoid Cornfield's penalties? Eval Rev 1996;20:313–337.

Nutbeam D. Health promotion glossary. Health Promotion 1986;1:113–127.

O'Carroll PW, Loftin C, Waller JB Jr, et al. Preventing homicide: an evaluation of the efficacy of a Detroit gun ordinance. Am J Public Health 1991;81:576–581.

Patrick DL, Cheadle A, Thompson DC, Diehr P, Koepsell T, Kinne S. The validity of self-reported smoking: a review and meta-analysis. Am J Public Health 1994;84:1086–1093.

Pentz MA, Dwyer JH, MacKinnon DP, et al. A multicommunity trial for primary prevention of adolescent drug abuse. Effects on drug use prevalence. JAMA 1989;261:3259–3266.

Pepin J, Plummer FA, Brunham RC, Piot P, Cameron DW, Ronald AR. The interaction of HIV infection and other sexually transmitted diseases: an opportunity for intervention. AIDS 1989;3:3–9.

Proschan MA. On the distribution of the unpaired t-statistic with paired data. Stat Med 1996;1059–1063.

Puska P, Salonen JT, Nissinen A, et al. Change in risk factors for coronary heart disease during 10 years of community intervention programme (North Karelia project). Br Med J 1983;287:1840–1844.

Remington PL, Smith MY, Williamson DF, Anda RF, Gentry EM, Hogelin GC. Design, characteristics, and usefulness of state-based behavioral risk factor surveillance: 1981–1987. Public Health Rep 1988;103:366–375.

Rose G. Sick individuals and sick populations. Int J Epidemiol 1985;14:32–38.

Rose G. The Strategy of Preventive Medicine. New York: Oxford University Press; 1992.

Shea S, Basch CE. A review of five major community-based cardiovascular disease prevention program. Part I: rationale, design, and theoretical framework. Am J Health Promotion 1990a;4:203–213.

Shea S, Basch CE. A review of five major community-based cardiovascular disease prevention program. Part II: intervention strategies, evaluation methods, and results. Am J Health Promotion 1990b;4:279–287.

Shea S, Stein AD, Basch CE, et al. Independent associations of educational attainment and ethnicity with behavioral risk factors for cardiovascular disease. Am J Epidemiol 1991;134:567–583.

Shea S, Basch CE, Lantigua R, Wechsler H. The Washington Heights-Inwood Healthy Heart Program: a third generation community-based cardiovascular disease prevention program in a disadvantaged urban setting. Prev Med 1992;21:203–217.

Shea S, Basch CE, Wechsler H, Lanigua R. The Washington Heights-Inwood Healthy Heart Program: a 6-year report from a disadvantaged urban setting. Am J Public Health 1996;86:166–171.

Shipley MJ, Smith PG, Dramaix M. Calculation of power for matched pair studies when randomization is by group. Int J Epidemiol 1989;18:457–461.

Simpson JM, Klar N, Donner A. Accounting for cluster randomization: a review of primary prevention trials, 1990 through 1993. Am J Public Health 1995;85:1378–1383.

Stone EJ, McGraw SA, Osganian SK, Elder JP, eds. Process evaluation in the multi-center Child and Adolescent Trial for Cardiovascular Health (CATCH). Health Educ Q 1994;21(Suppl 2):1–143.

Terris M. The Society for Epidemiologic Research (SER) and the future of epidemiology. Am J Epidemiol 1992a;136:909–915.

Terris M. Concepts of health promotion: dualities in public health theory. J Public Health Policy 1992b;13:267–276.

Wagenaar AC, Murray DM, Wolfson M, Forster JL, Finnegan JR. Communities Mobilizing for Change on Alcohol: design of a randomized community trial. J Community Psychol 1994;Special issue:79–101.

Wagner EH, Koepsell TD, Anderman C, et al. The evaluation of the Henry J. Kaiser Family Foundation's Community Health Promotion Grant Program: design. J Clin Epidemiol 1991;44:685–699.

Wechsler H, Basch CE, Zybert P, Lantigua R, Shea S. The availability of low-fat milk in an inner-city Latino community: implications for nutrition education. Am J Public Health 1995;85:1690–1692.

West KP Jr, Pokhrel RP, Katz J, et al. Efficacy of vitamin A in reducing preschool child mortality in Nepal. Lancet 1991;338:67–71.

Whiting-O'Keefe QE, Henke C, Simborg DW. Choosing the correct unit of analysis in medical care experiments. Med Care 1984;22:1101–1114.

Wickizer TM, Von Korff M, Cheadle A, et al. Activating communities for health promotion: a process evaluation method. Am J Public Health 1993;83:561–567.

Worden JK, Mickey RM, Flynn BS, et al. Development of a community breast screening promotion program using baseline data. Prev Med 1994;23:267–275.

World Health Organization. The current global situation of the HIV/AIDS epidemic. WHO Weekly Epidemiol Rec 1994;69:191–192.

Zucker DM. An analysis of variance pitfall: the fixed-effects analysis in a nested design. Educ Psychol Measurement 1990;50:731–738.

Zucker DM, Lakatos E, Webber LS, et al. Statistical design of the Child and Adolescent Trial for Cardiovascular Health (CATCH): implications of cluster randomization. Control Clin Trials 1995;16:96–118.

7

Screening in the Community

BENEDICT I. TRUMAN
STEVEN M. TEUTSCH

Screening for disease in the community to promote health and prevent disease is one of the practical applications of epidemiology delineated by Terris and reiterated in Chapter 1 of this text. Green and Kreuter (1991) distinguish a "community intervention" from an "intervention in a community." A community intervention is community-wide and aims to achieve a small but pervasive change in most of the population. An intervention in a community aims to accomplish more intensive or profound change in a subgroup of the population, usually within selected settings (e.g., workplace, hospital or clinic, place of worship, or school). We use the same logic to distinguish between "community-wide screening" and "screening in the community."

Screening for disease is defined as the examination of asymptomatic members of a defined community to classify them as either likely or unlikely to have the target disease or health condition. Persons who appear likely to have the target disease are referred for definitive diagnosis and treatment (Morrison 1992). Persons who appear unlikely to have the disease are educated to be vigilant for early warning signs and symptoms and encouraged to seek early diagnosis and treatment, if necessary. Educating persons who have "normal findings" may positively influence future health behaviors and encourage follow-up by primary care providers (Mittelmark et al. 1993).

Early detection and effective treatment are expected to result in substantial reductions in morbidity, mortality, and disability from targeted health conditions in a screened population. For example, screening for early detection and treatment of hypertension has contributed to an estimated 50% reduction in age-adjusted mortality from stroke in the United States since 1972 (National High Blood Pressure Education Program [NHBPEP] 1993; Garraway and Whisnant 1987; Casper et al. 1992). Similarly, early detection by mammography (with or without clinical breast exam) and effective treatment of breast cancer are expected to reduce mortality rates by as much as

30% over ≥10 years in a screened population of women 50–69 years of age (U.S. Preventive Services Task Force [USPSTF] 1996).

In addition to its role as a population-based prevention strategy, screening for selected target conditions is equally important as a clinical preventive service. Primary care practitioners, during a clinical visit for episodic health care, can deliver this service to asymptomatic persons of all ages and in all risk categories (USPSTF 1996). This screening strategy also is referred to as "case-finding" or "in reach" (Sackett et al. 1991; Lantz et al. 1995). Screening of persons and of populations is expected to play an important role in the attainment of the year-2000 national health promotion and disease prevention objectives (US Dept of Health and Human Services [USDHHS] 1991). For example, mortality objectives have been set for coronary heart disease; cancers of the breast, cervix, colon, and rectum; and other conditions for which screening is relevant. Progress toward achieving year 2000 objectives for mortality and related screening-procedure uptake is being monitored and publicized by means of annual reports (National Center for Health Statistics [NCHS] 1996b). For example, the rate of death among women from breast cancer (age adjusted per 100,000 US standard population in 1970) has declined from 23.0 in 1987 to 21.6 in 1993, nearing 20.6 (the year 2000 target). In addition, the proportion of females ≥50 years of age who have received clinical breast examination and mammogram in the preceding 1–2 years has increased from 25% in 1987 to 55% in 1993, nearing the year 2000 target of 60%.

In recent years, screening has been more commonly associated with the control of chronic conditions such as heart disease (e.g., blood pressure and cholesterol), cancer (e.g., mammography, Pap test, and testicular examination), and congenital abnormalities (screening among newborns). However, important applications of screening for the prevention and control of infectious diseases have a long history and current importance in traditional public health practice. For example, the US Preventive Services Task Force (USPSTF) has recommended selective screening in high risk populations for several infectious conditions (e.g., human immunodeficiency virus [HIV], tuberculosis, chlamydia, rubella, syphilis, and gonorrhea) in the context of a clinical periodic health examination (USPSTF 1996). As with chronic conditions, early detection and treatment of cases of infectious disease improves the clinical outcome of persons affected by disease. In addition, early detection and successful treatment of infectious diseases interrupts transmission of infection to other members of the community (Morrison 1992).

The integration of screening at the individual, setting, and community levels can be illustrated conceptually (Figure 7-1). At the individual level, health care providers interact with patients in a clinic to address their needs for preventive services (e.g., vaccinations, counseling to encourage health-promoting behaviors, and screening for selected health conditions). The community liaison, based in the clinic, "reaches in" to encourage patients receiv-

Community

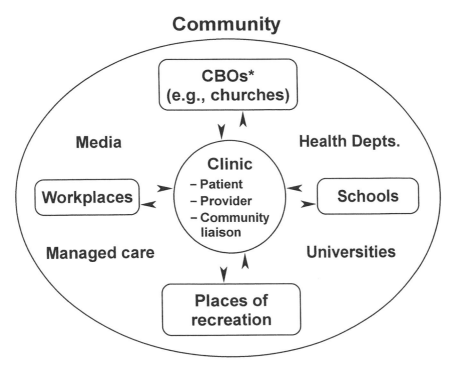

Figure 7-1. Conceptual framework relating screening at the individual, settings, and community levels. *A CBO is a Community Based Organization.

ing care to use available preventive services and "reaches out" into a specific community setting to help persons who are not receiving care to gain access to the preventive services they need. In each community setting (a place of worship, workplace, or school), health promotion and disease prevention goals are pursued in collaboration with clinicians and other health-related institutions. Health departments, universities, managed-care plans, the media, and other institutions provide leadership and support for community-wide interventions to promote health and prevent disease.

This chapter reviews basic concepts and principles associated with (1) screening to control disease; (2) adopting and implementing practice guidelines on screening; and (3) developing, implementing, and evaluating public health screening programs.

Concepts and Principles

Public health practitioners, clinicians, and other members of community coalitions who are contemplating organized screening for disease control in different settings should be familiar with the concepts and principles that lend rationality and coherence to the required operational tasks. The operational tasks to be accomplished in developing and implementing organized screening programs in the community include (1) defining the target population, (2) setting priorities among target diseases or health conditions, (3) selecting appropriate screening tests or examinations, and (4) assessing the effectiveness of community screening programs. For each of the four operational tasks, concepts, and principles associated with screening for disease in the community are described in this chapter and illustrated with examples from the annals of everyday public health and clinical practice.

Defining the Target Population

Defining the target population for a screening program involves describing the settings and the characteristics of the collection of persons who would be eligible for screening (Last 1995). This should be the first step in planning a population-based screening program because screening programs should be tailored to meet the needs of a defined target population. In practice, however, screening programs are developed and implemented in response to the availability of an effective screening test for a particular health condition. Concepts and principles for selecting a target population are defined at the beginning of this chapter to reinforce the advantages of thinking about ends before means. Important concepts related to defining the target population include community, settings, mass versus selective screening, risk stratification, and high-risk versus population strategies.

Community. A community is "a group of individuals organized into a unit, or manifesting some unifying trait or common interest; loosely, the locality or catchment area population for which a service is provided, or more broadly, the state, nation, or body politic" (Last 1995). Green and Kreuter have refined the definition of community to distinguish between the structural and functional dimensions of the concept. They state that, structurally, a community is a neighborhood, township, city, county, district, or metropolitan area demarcated by geographic and often political boundaries; and functionally, a community is a place where "members have a sense of identity and belonging, shared values, norms, communication, and helping patterns." Further, they continue, "unrestrained by place, a functional community of interest or constituency of concerned citizens also may exist, scattered across one or more geopolitical jurisdictions" (Green and Kreuter 1991).

Several important considerations are warranted when defining a target population for screening within the community. First, the size and characteristics of the target population should be tailored to the availability and appropriateness of the resources available to provide advice, referral, and follow-up for participants (Rose 1992; Wilson and Jungner 1968). Second, the characteristics of the target population should be similar to those of the populations in which the screening test has been accurate and early detection and follow-up have been proven effective (USPSTF 1996). And third, governmental public health agencies often must define target populations within geopolitical boundaries and constituent groups prescribed by a legislative mandate. Nongovernmental public health agencies often have more flexibility in defining target populations that cut across the boundaries of governmental mandates. Thus, coalitions between governmental and nongovernmental agencies offer the greatest flexibility in ensuring that a successful screening program reaches the widest possible target population (Grad 1990; Institute of Medicine [IOM] 1988).

Settings. Mullen and Evans reviewed the importance of settings in health promotion and disease prevention (Mullen et al. 1995). They defined settings as major social structures or institutions that provide channels and mechanisms of influence for reaching defined populations. These institutions are characterized by patterns of formal and informal membership and communication and involve frequent and sustained interaction among members. Potential settings for screening programs include community units (e.g., neighborhoods, counties), workplaces, schools, places of worship, and health care settings. Settings often vary in their capacity to reach populations differentiated by age, gender, socioeconomic status, race, ethnicity, or combinations of such characteristics.

Settings are important to screening policy, programs, and research because they obviate the need to create new social structures, are organized for purposes more deeply binding than the single mission of health improvement, and create efficiencies in time, resources, access to selected populations, and potential for social influences (Mullen et al. 1995).

Mass and Selective Screening. In mass screening, the entire target population, regardless of level of risk for the target condition, is eligible to be screened (Last 1995). For example, in a screening program to detect hypertension, all residents of county X, regardless of age, may be deemed eligible for screening. In selective screening, the target population is refined to include only those persons who meet a predetermined set of eligibility criteria. Such eligibility criteria may include age, sex, race, ethnicity, comorbid conditions, or a combination of risk factors. For example, to prevent end-stage renal disease (ESRD) among residents of county X, a highly selective screening program for hypertension may restrict eligibility to black men with non-insulin-dependent diabetes mellitus (NIDDM) because risk is very high for this population group. Sackett has used the term "case finding" to characterize the strategy of selective screening when the target population is restricted to persons who visit a physician for intercurrent illnesses or other purposes unrelated to the condition being screened for. For example, the physicians in a managed care plan may decide to screen for hyperlipidemia or hypertension among all enrollees 40 years or older who are seen for any reason during a 2-year period (Sackett et al. 1991).

Selective screening and care usually are more cost effective than mass screening (Rose 1992). Opportunities for the application of cost-effective mass screening are likely to be confined to special conditions (e.g., neonatal screening) or in selected settings. For example, screening by chest radiography to rule out or detect active tuberculosis (TB) in jails with high turnover, some homeless shelters, and among immigrants and refugees recently arrived from countries with a high incidence or prevalence of TB might be considered an application of mass screening in selected settings (CDC 1995b). This latter example illustrates that the distinction between mass and selective screening is sometimes blurred.

Risk Stratification. The risk for occurrence of a health event (condition or disease) in an individual (or population) is the probability that the event will occur within a stated time period (Last 1995). Risk stratification is a process of classifying the members of a population into levels of risk (i.e., high, medium, or low) for the occurrence of a target health condition on the basis of risk factors (e.g., genotype, demographic characteristics, environmental exposure, or personal behavior) that are epidemiologically associated with that event (Kelsey et al. 1996). Often, risk stratification is essential to defining a target population for selective screening. For example, subgroups at higher risk for death from breast cancer include black women of all ages (20% higher mortality rate than white women) and black women ≥65 years of age (73% higher mortality rate than black women ages 45–64 years) (Brownson et al. 1993; Beckles et al. 1994).

A useful distinction exists between the *high-risk* and *population strategies* of preventive medicine (Rose 1992). The high-risk strategy of screening for hypertension to prevent stroke would entail the early detection and treatment of black or elderly residents of state X with diastolic blood pressure of ≥90 mmHg or systolic pressure ≥140 mmHg. Black or elderly residents would be targeted for screening because hypertension and stroke are more common in these groups than in their counterparts (USPSTF 1996).

The population-wide strategy for preventing stroke by blood pressure reduction would seek to shift the entire continuous population distribution of diastolic (or systolic) blood pressures toward lower values. Thus, some researchers have estimated that a nationwide moderation of salt intake would lower the blood pressure distribution by about 5% and prevent as many as

25% of all strokes (Stamler et al. 1989; Law et al. 1991). Population-wide strategies (e.g., nationwide reduction of salt intake to reduce prevalence of hypertension) are potentially more effective than high-risk screening and treatment strategies (e.g., early detection of black or elderly persons with hypertension) for the prevention of some conditions (e.g., stroke). However, the two types of strategies are complementary (i.e., they require different types of resources), potentially synergistic, and often can be implemented together (Rose 1992).

Setting Priorities Among Diseases and Conditions

After identifying a particular reference population in need of intervention, organizers of community screening programs must decide what health conditions or diseases should be given priority for new or expanded efforts. Potential criteria for ranking conditions or diseases in order of priority include disease burden; availability of one or more effective screening tests; availability of effective treatment and follow-up for cases detected early; cost-effectiveness, initial costs, and availability of resources for treatment and follow-up; community consensus about preferences, urgency, and equity; and historical precedent (i.e., experiences with screening programs already in place) (USDHHS 1991; USPSTF 1996).

The relative weight given to each criterion varies among communities and decision-makers and often must be negotiated among the involved parties. Some practitioners believe that the relationship between the rarity (prevalence) of a candidate disease and the proportion of false positives (persons without the target condition who test positive, given fixed sensitivity and specificity) is the most important principle of screening. This principle explains why selective screening strategies and risk-based strategies are often preferable to mass screening. Moreover, sequential screening to reduce false positives in the case of a rare disease increases in importance when the adverse consequences of a false positive test are severe and costly. In the final analysis, therefore, conditions of low morbidity and mortality (e.g., lower back pain) tend to be unsuitable candidates for screening even when highly prevalent. Similarly, conditions of high morbidity and mortality (e.g., HIV) tend to be better candidates for screening efforts, even when they are rare (low prevalence).

Important epidemiologic concepts and principles that relate to setting priorities among health conditions eligible for screening are natural history and clinical stages of disease and burden of suffering (e.g., incidence, prevalence, mortality, and case-fatality rates; quality of life; and cost of illness). Often, a public health agency must decide whether expansion of the activities of an existing screening program is preferrable to starting a new screening program for another condition. In this instance, the same concepts and principles are germane to evaluating the effectiveness of the screening program that has already been implemented; past performance becomes relevant to the issue of expansion.

Natural History of a Disease. The natural history of a disease in a population is a sequential record over time of pathogenesis from initiation by one or more causal agents through clinical manifestations as signs and symptoms, the usual circumstances of its presentation and diagnosis in routine medical care, the rate of progression and response to treatment, and ultimate health outcomes. The term "natural history" also is sometimes used in the practice of epidemiologic surveillance to refer to trends in morbidity from a disease over time (Last 1995).

Lead Time. Figure 7-2 illustrates the natural history of a hypothetical case of hypertension, which is a target of screening both as a preventable disease and a risk factor for cardiovascular disease. Biologic onset is the point at which interactions between human host gene products, exposure to causal environmental agents, and behavioral risk factors lead to the initiation of a pathologic process (e.g., carcinogenesis, atherosclerosis, or physiologic dysfunction). The earliest point of detection of preclinical or asymptomatic disease is the point in disease progression at which an available screening test becomes effective. The usual point of diagnosis, in the absence of a screening program, is the point at which affected persons seek medical care for symptoms or signs

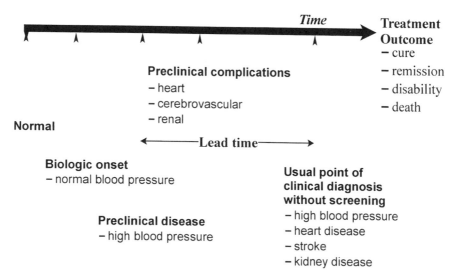

Figure 7-2. Natural history of a hypothetical case of hypertension

of complications (e.g., pain, bleeding, or a mass) or a motivated clinician initiates a diagnostic procedure for some other reason (Morrison 1992; Sackett et al. 1991). Lead time is the interval from the earliest point of detection by a screening test to the usual point of diagnosis in the absence of screening.

The natural history of a disease determines its suitability for screening. In addition, effective screening and treatment alter the natural history of a disease in both individual cases and in populations by improving health outcomes. The opportunity to control a disease by means of screening and treatment will arise only if the disease progresses through an asymptomatic phase during which it is usually undiagnosed but detectable. Moreover, early treatment must prolong life or reduce morbidity more effectively than later treatment to make intervention worthwhile (Morrison 1992). In the absence of a screening program, the point of usual clinical diagnosis is determined by the interaction of levels of popular awareness of symptoms and signs, provider awareness and incentives to act, care-seeking behavior of the population, and access to medical care (Morrison 1992).

Clinical Stage (or Severity of Illness). The clinical course of a disease is that part of its natural history that begins at diagnosis and ends at recovery, death, or disability (Sackett et al. 1991). The short-term objective of screening is to shift the distribution of cases detected by screening toward less advanced clinical stages or severity of illness at diagnosis when prognosis after treatment is better. For example, the short-term goal of breast-cancer screening in a community is to increase the proportion of cases detected by screening that are localized or limited to regional spread (CDC 1996b; Kosary et al. 1996). Similarly, the short-term goal of screening for high blood pressure is to detect persons with hypertension, particularly those with more severe disease, and to reduce blood pressure to safer levels. The clinical stages of breast cancer and hypertension are illustrated in Tables 7-1 and 7-2, respectively.

Burden of Suffering. The burden of suffering in a population from a health condition or disease is an indication of its public health importance. Measures of disease burden include incidence rate, prevalence rate, mortality rate, case-fatality rate, quality of life, and cost of illness. High *incidence rate* (IR) (defined in Chapter 2) usually indicates a need for screening services. Effective screening and treatment for a disease, however, also alter its incidence rate in the screened population (Morrison 1992). Thus, trends in the IR of the disease may be useful in evaluating the uptake and effectiveness of a screening program. During periods of increasing use of a new screening test for a disease, the incidence rate of disease may increase, decrease, level off as uptake of the test becomes optimal, and finally decrease as preclinical cases are exhausted. For example, the age-adjusted breast-cancer incidence rate among women (of

Table 7-1. Clinical Staging of Breast Cancer by the TNM and SEER Systems and Mammography Coding by the Karolinska System

Stage Grouping (TNM System)[a]	SEER System[b]	Karolinska Mammography Coding System (Nonpalpable Cancers)[c]
Stage 0 (carcinoma in situ)	Unstaged	0 = no breast 1 = normal mammogram 2 = abnormal—cancer not suspected 3 = abnormal—cancer suspected 4 = probable cancer 5 = definite cancer
Stage I (T≤2 cm; no nodes; no distant metastasis)	Localized	
Stage IIA (T≤5 cm; ± axillary nodes; no distant metastasis)	Regional	
Stage IIB (T2–5+ cm; axillary nodes; no distant metastasis)	Regional	
Stage IIIA (T any size; + axillary nodes; no distant metastasis)	Regional	
Stage IIIB (T any size + extension to chest wall or skin; + internal mammary nodes; no distant metastasis)	Regional	
Stage IV (T any size; nodes; distant metastasis)	Distant	

[a]*Source:* Kinne (1991): T = primary tumor size at greatest diameter; N = node; M = metastasis.
[b]*Source:* Kosary et al. (1996): Surveillance, Epidemiology, and End Result. Localized is an invasive neoplasm confined to the organ of origin. Regional is a neoplasm that has extended beyond the organ of origin directly into the surrounding organs, tissues, and/or regional lymph nodes. Distant is a neoplasm that has spread to parts of the body remote from the primary tumor either by direct extension or by discontinuous metastasis.
[c]*Source:* Svane et al. (1993): Mammograms classified into codes 3–5 (<3%) are recalled for follow-up studies including fine needle aspiration, cytology, and/or biopsy.

all races) increased 32 % during 1980–1987, partly resulting from increases in early diagnosis and use of mammography as a screening examination (Miller 1993). During 1987–1992, breast-cancer incidence remained relatively stable (NCHS 1996a).

A high prevalence rate (defined in Chapter 2) also is a measure of need for screening. In the absence of widespread screening for a disease, the population prevalence rate reflects the detection of symptomatic or clinical cases and the effectiveness of treatment in preventing death and achieving cure. In the presence of screening, the prevalence rate also depends on the periodicity of repeat screening, the mix of clinical and preclinical cases, and rates of death and cure. Because screening aims to detect preclinical disease, the prevalence rate of diagnosed preclinical disease increases as the uptake of screening increases in a population (Morrison 1992). The population prevalence of the target condition is a factor that determines the predictive value positive (PVP) of a screening test (see section on predictive value of a positive test). If sensitivity and specificity are constant, the higher the prevalence rate, the higher the PVP (Morrison 1992).

High mortality rate from a potentially lethal condition is perhaps the best indicator of need for a screening program. The population mortality rate or death rate from a disease is analogous to the incidence rate, except that the event being counted in the numerator is death instead of onset of disease (Kelsey et al. 1996). Death rate is one of the most useful measures of the value of a screening program that aims to prevent or delay death by early detection and intervention to favorably alter the natural history of the disease (Morrison 1992). Screening for hypertension aims to reduce the population mortality from stroke and heart disease (NHBPEP 1993), and screening for breast cancer aims to reduce the population mortality rate from that condition (CDC 1996a). The case-fatality rate (CFR) is the mortality or death rate among persons diagnosed with the disease. This rate is the complement $(CFR = 1 - SR)$ of the survival ratio (SR)—the proportion of diagnosed cases who are alive at the end of a defined time period since diagnosis (usually 5 years) (Morrison 1992). The CFR and SR overestimate the effect of screening and treatment in screened populations (compared with unscreened populations) because of lead time and prognostic selection or length biases (see section on choosing effective screening tests). Therefore, they are

Table 7-2. Clinical Staging of Hypertension for Adults Age 18 Years and Older[a]

Category	Systolic (mmHg)	Diastolic (mmHg)
Normal[b]	< 130	< 85
High normal	130–139	85–89
Hypertension[c]		
Stage 1 (mild)	140–159	90–99
Stage 2 (moderate)	160–179	100–109
Stage 3 (severe)	180–209	110–119
Stage 4 (very severe)	≥210	≧120

[a]Not taking antihypertensive drugs and not acutely ill. When systolic and diastolic pressures fall into different categories, the higher category should be selected to classify the individual's blood pressure status.

[b]Optimal blood pressure with respect to cardiovascular risk is SBP <120 mmHg and DBP <80 mmHg. However, unusually low readings should be evaluated for clinical significance.

[c]Based on average of two or more readings taken at each of two or more visits following an initial screening. Note: In addition to classifying stages of hypertension based on average blood pressure levels, the clinician should specify presence or absence of target-organ disease and additional risk factors.

Source: National High Blood Pressure Education Program (1993).

unsuitable outcome measures of the efficacy or effectiveness of screening programs.

The primary long-term goal of screening is to prevent or postpone death from a particular target condition. Life recouped by postponing death varies in both quantity (years) and quality (absence of impairment or disability). *Quality of life measures*, population health-status measures that combine the quality or desirability of a health state with its duration, are discussed in Chapter 8. A variety of survey instruments have been developed to collect the data needed to construct quality of life indexes (e.g., Quality of Well-Being [QWB] Scale) (Dasbach and Teutsch 1996). The number of quality-adjusted years of life saved by a screening program often is used as the effect measure when comparing screening programs that affect both morbidity and mortality, aim to improve social or physiologic functioning as a primary objective, or lead to outcomes measured in dissimilar natural units of morbidity or mortality. For example, a quality of life measure would be a more suitable outcome measure for comparing the relative cost-effectiveness of two screening programs for neural tube defects (to prevent mental retardation and death) and perinatal HIV infection (to prevent opportunistic cancers and infection, and death), respectively (Dasbach and Teutsch 1996).

In addition to measures of morbidity and mortality, the population burden of illness can be assessed in terms of the economic cost of a target disease for which screening is being considered. Health conditions with higher cost-burdens are usually given higher priority for developing and implementing screening technology. Approaches to assessing the economic cost of illness are discussed in Chapter 9 (Haddix et al. 1996; Luce et al. 1996).

Choosing Effective Screening Tests

Screening in the community for a priority health condition depends on the availability of a screening test that is reliable, accurate, acceptable to participants (i.e., patients and clinicians), and affordable in relation to its benefits (Wilson and Jungner 1968; Morrison 1992). Thus, screening for breast cancer is feasible because mammography, an effective screening test, is available. However, screening for lung cancer (an equally important health condition) is considered infeasible because neither early detection nor effective treatment is available (USPSTF 1996). Important epidemiologic concepts that relate to the accuracy of a screening procedure are sensitivity, specificity, predictive value of positive and negative test results, and lead time. In addition, cost-effectiveness and cost-benefit are important concepts that underlie judgments about the affordability of a screening procedure in relation to its benefits.

The ideal screening test would have high values of sensitivity, specificity, and positive predictive value and would tend to maximize the yield of true positives and minimize the yield of false positives. However, there are often trade-offs to be made between sensitivity and specificity in optimizing the yield of screening tests, especially those based on a cut-point applied to a continuously distributed variable (e.g., blood pressure). When the cut-point is decreased to increase sensitivity, the specificity will simultaneously decrease and vice versa. Strategies for balancing benefits and costs of screening include adjusting the criterion level for positivity, adjusting the frequency of screening, sequential testing (combining two or more different tests in sequence), and targeting high-risk groups with high prevalence of preclinical disease (Morrison 1992).

Sensitivity. The sensitivity of a screening test is the proportion of persons with the condition (based on a gold-standard test) who test positive. Alternatively, sensitivity is equal to number of true positives divided by the sum of true positives and false negatives (Table 7-3). Sensitivity is the property of a screening test that enables cases to be detected early (true positives). Thus, sensitivity is an important determinant of the disease-control value of a screening program. More sensitive tests tend to identify cases earlier and thus may increase the lead time that screen-detected cases gain (see section on natural history of disease). Thus, to be successful at reducing morbidity or mortality, a screening test must be highly sensitive (i.e., detect a high proportion of preclinical cases with sufficient lead time for treatment to improve outcome) (Morrison 1992).

Specificity. The specificity of a screening test is the proportion of persons without the condition who test negative. Thus, specificity is equal to the number of true negatives divided by the sum of true negatives and false positives (Table 7-3). Alternatively, specificity (1 minus % of false positives among nondiseased) is negatively related to the frequency of false positives in

Table 7-3. Measures of Accuracy of a Screening Test

Measure of Accuracy	Definition	Formula[a]
Sensitivity	Proportion of persons with condition who test positive	$a/a + c$
Specificity	Proportion of persons without condition who test negative	$d/b + d$
Positive predictive value	Proportion of persons with positive test who have condition	$a/a + b$
Negative predictive value	Proportion of persons with negative test who do not have condition	$d/c + d$

[a]Legend: a = true positive; b = false positive; c = false negative; d = true negative

Source: USPSTF (1996).

a screened population (Morrison 1992). High specificity is the property of a screening test that minimizes the number of false-positive tests and their adverse consequences that must be followed up. Conversely, a test with low specificity will lead to many false positives, requiring follow up, and may consume substantial resources. Thus, specificity has a major influence on the costs, acceptability, and feasibility of a screening program. Routine use of the prostate-specific antigen test (PSA) is a good example of a test with low specificity and a high burden of cost and side effects as a result of follow-up of false positives.

Predictive Value Positive (and Negative). The predictive value of a positive (PVP) screening test is the proportion of persons with a positive test who have the condition. PVP is equal to the number of true positives divided by the sum of true positives and false positives; or 1 minus % of false positives among screen positives (Table 7-3). The predictive value of a negative screening test is the proportion of persons with a negative test who do not have the condition (Morrison 1992; USPSTF 1996).

Reliability. The reliability of a test is its capacity to give the same result—positive or negative, whether correct or incorrect—on repeated application in a person with a given level of disease. Reliability depends on variability in the manifestations of preclinical disease being sought (e.g., daily fluctuation in blood pressure), the method of measurement, and the skill with which the observer makes the measurements. Measures of reliability include intra- or interobserver variability (Morrison 1992). A screening test of low reliability usually will not be sufficiently sensitive or specific to be useful in practice. Moreover, high reliability does not guarantee high sensitivity or specificity. However, a test that is highly sensitive is highly reliable among persons who have disease; and a test that is highly specific is highly reliable among persons who do not (Morrison 1992).

Multiple Testing Strategies. Multiphasic screening combines screening for multiple conditions on the same occasion (e.g., blood pressure, blood lipids, blood glucose, height, and weight among attendees of a county fair) (Sackett et al. 1991). The opportunity to screen for multiple conditions on a single occasion has obvious advantages in terms of convenience for the participants and potential efficiency for the organizers. However, the advantages of convenience and efficiency often are negated by the disadvantages of complex logistics, inadequate follow-up, and dilution of motivation for change when multiple problems are detected in the same person (Mittelmark et al. 1993). Integrated methods of early detection for coronary heart disease (CHD) include screening for high blood pressure and for elevated serum cholesterol and assessing behavioral risk factors (e.g., tobacco use, dietary fat intake, and physical activity level). Simultaneous screening for these risk factors as a prelude to multiple risk factor interventions is now well established in the practice of both high-risk and community-based approaches to primary prevention of CHD (Smith and Pratt 1993).

Sequential Testing Strategies. Sequential testing combines two different screening tests in sequence. The second test is done only if the first test is positive. For example, the combination of an abnormal digital rectal exam (DRE) and elevated prostate-specific antigen (PSA) test, in sequence, increased the PVP to 49% (positive on both tests), compared with 20% for PSA with negative DRE and 28%–35% for PSA alone (USPSTF 1996). More importantly, a repeatedly reactive EIA (enzyme immunoassay) test requires a sequentially administered positive Western blot test to confirm infection with the HIV (CDC 1992). Sequential testing is a technique for increasing the accuracy (PVP) of a screening procedure. However, an unknown number of persons with disease whose results are negative on the first test and are of unknown status on the second test will be missed. The alternative decision rule of admitting to diagnostic testing all persons who are positive on either test would trade off the PVP advantage of sequential testing in exchange for picking up the missed cases (Morrison 1992).

Assessing the Effectiveness of Screening Procedures

Decisions to initiate, modify, or terminate a community screening effort should be based on empirical evidence of actual or expected effectiveness. The effectiveness of a screening procedure or program is the improvement of health outcome that a prevention strategy can produce in typical community-based settings (Teutsch 1992). Actual effectiveness is determined by measuring the changes in health outcomes attributable to a program that has been implemented. Expected effectiveness is an estimate (made before implementation) of the impact of a planned program. Often the estimate is based on extrapolation from the experiences of a similar program in another community.

The following seven criteria for deciding if a community screening program is worth implementing (or continuing) have been suggested: (1) the effectiveness of a similar program based on a randomized trial; (2) the efficacy of treatment and/or prevention for the primary disorder and its complications; (3) the current burden of suffering from the target condition; (4) availability of an effective screening test; (5) high expected coverage or uptake in the target population; (6) adequate health system capacity to cope with referrals for diagnosis and follow-up; and (7) high expected compliance with subsequent advice and interventions among screened persons who test positive

(Cadman et al. 1984). Applying the criterion of "expected compliance" often requires an assessment of the extent to which members of the community perceive the proposed screening program as a priority need.

Epidemiologic concepts associated with assessing the effectiveness of a screening procedure include efficacy versus effectiveness (including compliance, penetrance, or intervention uptake), study design including randomized controlled trial, prevented fraction, cost-effectiveness, and cost-benefit. Those concepts and principles for their application are discussed below.

Efficacy. Efficacy is the improvement in health outcome that a screening procedure can produce under ideal circumstances (Teutsch 1992). Ideal circumstances are usually encountered in the context of well-financed randomized controlled trials involving highly motivated volunteers, sophisticated technology, and highly skilled specialists in both subject matter and study methods. Efficacy sets an upper limit of what might be expected in terms of effectiveness—performance under usual circumstances of limited resources (finances and expertise) and variable motivation of participants. Effectiveness is influenced by levels of compliance—the extent to which participants are exposed to the planned intervention and uptake or penetration of the intervention in the target population.

Study Design Including Randomized Controlled Trial (RCT). The design of studies to assess the effectiveness of a screening procedure can include RCTs, cohort studies, and case-control studies. Most experts agree that a properly executed RCT, if feasible, provides the best quality of evidence of the efficacy (or effectiveness) of a screening procedure (Sackett 1991; Shapiro in press; USPSTF 1996). Some experts have argued that a properly executed RCT is a minimum requirement for deciding to implement community screening (Sackett 1991).

In an RCT (field or community intervention trial) to assess the efficacy (or effectiveness) of a screening procedure, the investigator randomly allocates participants to be screened or not screened for the target condition. The investigator then follows the participants over time to assess the effect of screening on health outcomes (mortality or morbidity) from the target condition. Random allocation of participants to groups that will be screened and unscreened aims to reduce selection bias associated with nonrandom allocation. In a blinded RCT, the participants (if feasible), assessors of outcome, or both (double-blinded) do not know the allocation status of each participant. This technique aims to reduce information bias which can accrue when assessments of outcomes are influenced by knowing whether or not a particular participant was screened (Rothman 1986; USPSTF 1996):

Prevented Fraction. The Prevented fraction (PF) of a health problem is the proportion of its incidence in a given time period that can be avoided by implementing an intervention in that population. The PF can be computed from either of the two equations (Gargiullo and Rothenberg 1995; Rothenberg and Hahn 1996):

1. $PF = P_s(1 - RR)$ [where P_s = proportion of population screened; RR = ratio of mortality rates among screened (numerator) and unscreened women]; or,
2. $PF_s = 1 - RR$ [where PF_s = prevented fraction among screened women].

For example, during 1963–1984, an RCT among enrolled members of the Health Insurance Plan of Greater New York (HIP) showed that periodic screening with mammography and clinical examination of the breast resulted in 30% and 25% (prevented fractions) reductions in mortality from breast cancer after 10 and 18 years of follow-up, respectively, among women who were 40–64 years of age at entry (Shapiro et al. 1988). The preventable fraction is an estimate of the prevented fraction before the intervention has been implemented. It is based on the assumption that the results of studies like the HIP trial can be extrapolated with confidence to similar populations.

Both the strength and effectiveness (relative risk or risk ratio) of the screening procedure and, in particular its prevalence or uptake, are to some extent under the control of the public health program. Thus, the PF provides a direct measure of the portion of expected morbidity or mortality the program can promise to prevent before implementation or claim credit for delivering after implementation (Rothenberg and Hahn 1996).

Cost-Effectiveness and Cost-Benefit. As described in Chapter 9, the cost-effectiveness of a screening procedure summarizes information on cost and outcomes, allowing different screening procedures to be compared on the basis of their worth and priority to the participants, a community, or some other constituency. The related concept—*cost-benefit*—also translates health benefits into dollars (Haddix et al. 1996). Because resources for health improvement are limited and all effective screening interventions cannot simultaneously be implemented in most practical situations, cost-effectiveness analysis supports decisions about which screening procedures are more or less desirable and which opportunities to screen should be pursued in preference to others that are less worthwhile (USPSTF 1996).

Potential Hazards of Screening. Earlier diagnosis without benefit occurs when lead time is increased but early treatment does not improve the quantity or quality of life. Moreover, long lead time without benefit increases the risk for adverse consequences from labeling well persons as diseased and from initiating treatments in response to that labeling. *Lead-time bias* refers to bias introduced in a study that assesses the effect of a screening test on mortality by comparing survival rates in cases detected early with those detected later. *Length-time bias* refers to bias introduced into a similar study because of preferential detection of slowly progressive disease. Lead-time bias, length-time bias, and the tendency for the "worried-well" to volunteer always make screening appear to improve survival, even when early treatment does not reduce mortality or morbidity (Sackett et al. 1991).

Although screening is beneficial in many situations (Table 7-4), it can also be harmful when applied inappropriately. Several researchers and practitioners have identified situations in which inappropriate early detection of disease in asymptomatic persons can be harmful to both individuals and populations (Sackett et al. 1991; Rose 1992; Miller 1993). First, screening for a rare condition, even with a test that is highly sensitive and specific, can lead to a substantial number of false-positive diagnoses that are costly to manage.

Table 7-4. Conditions for Which Screening Is Recommended, USPSTF 1996

Health Outcome	Test(s)	Population(s)	Age Group (years)
Obesity	Height/Weight	General	All
CVD[a]/HBP	Blood pressure	General	All
CVD[a]	Cholesterol	General / HR6[d]	25–64 / 65 +
Injury/Liver disease	Alcohol overuse	General	11 +
Colorectal cancer	FOBT[b] Sigmoidoscopy	General	25 +
Breast cancer	Mammography /CBE[c]	General	50 + (female)
Cervical cancer	Pap smear	General	11 + (female)
Chlamydia	—	General / HR4	11–24 / 11–64
Gonorrhea	—	HR2	11–24, 25–64
Syphilis	—	HR1 / HR9	11–64 / 65 +
HIV	—	HR2 / HR3	0–10 / 11 +
HgbSS/ PKU/	Hgb/Phenylalanine/	General/General	Birth/Birth
Hypothyroidism	T4&TSH	General	Birth
Anemia	Hgb/Hct	HR1 / HR/P (female)	0–10 / 11 +
Lead poisoning	Blood lead	HR7	0–10
Rubella	—	General (female)	11–24, 25–64
Tuberculosis	PPD	HR1/HR3 /HR6 /HR7	65 +/ 0–24 /25–64
Hearing	—	General	65 +
Vision	—	General	0–10, 65 +

[a]Cardiovascular disease

[b]Fecal Occult Blood Test

[c]Clinical Breast Exam HgbSS = hemoglobinopathies

[d]HR = high risk group variously defined.

Source: U.S. Preventive Services Task Force [USPSTF] (1996).

Second, the treatment for persons diagnosed early may be ineffective or may do more harm than good. Third, if follow-up treatment is ineffective or harmful, screening substitutes "sick time" for "healthy time" by labeling apparently healthy persons as diseased. Fourth, when ineffective screening is implemented on a large scale, it diverts resources from more worthwhile activities, undermines the professional credibility of public health practitioners, and makes rigorous evaluation of potentially better interventions more difficult. Finally, inappropriate screening can burden the clinical-care system with unnecessary follow-up, excess legal liability exposure, and increased medical-care costs.

Adopting Practice Guidelines on Screening

Often practitioners and developers of organized screening programs do not have the time, expertise, and resources needed to assess the merits of a proposed screening effort. Therefore, most practitioners rely on advice offered by credible organizations in the form of practice guidelines. Practice guidelines offer advice to clinicians, public health practitioners, managed-care organizations, and the public on how to improve the effectiveness and impact of clinical and public health interventions. Guidelines translate the findings of research and demonstration projects into accessible and usable information for public health practice. Guidelines for community- and clinic-based screening are published by many governmental and nongovernmental agencies, including associations of medical and health professionals. For example, guidelines on community screening for hypertension have been published periodically by the National High Blood Pressure Education Program since 1972 (NHBPEP 1993). And since 1989 the USPSTF has published a guide to clinical preventive services including recommendations for primary care practitioners on screening for 53 health conditions or risk factors in the context of a periodic health examination of asymptomatic persons (USPSTF 1996).

A guide for community preventive services is currently under development. The Centers for Disease Control and Prevention (CDC), in collaboration with other PHS agencies, will provide institutional and staff support to the recently created Task Force on Community Preventive Services. The guide is intended to complement the US Preventive Services Task Force Guide to Clinical Preventive Services by focusing on community-based prevention and control strategies. The guide will be based on best available scientific evidence and current expertise regarding essential public health services and effective methods of delivering those services. It will issue recommendations on the most effective and cost-effective community preventive services and methods for their implementation. This information is intended to help public health practitioners make informed choices on the most effective public health strategies, policies, and programs for their communities. An electronic database of the guide, including supporting evidence, is among the expected products of this activity.

When making decisions about screening in the community, most organizers and program sponsors adopt and then adapt authoritative recommendations from agencies that routinely develop or endorse practice guidelines. A potential user adopts a guideline by deciding to accept and implement the recommended practices. Often the guidelines are modified or adapted prior to implementation to meet the particular needs of practitioners and participants in each setting. The issues associated with adopting screening guidelines for use in a specific setting include desirable attributes of practice guidelines, adapting published guidelines to local needs, and dealing with controversial and conflicting guidelines.

Desirable Attributes of Practice Guidelines

The Institute of Medicine (IOM) asserts that clinical practice guidelines that possess eight desirable attributes are more likely to be perceived as trustworthy, usable, and effective in achieving desired health outcomes. According to the IOM, good practice guidelines have the following characteristics:

- *Valid:* supported by strong scientific evidence linking recommendations to outcomes
- *Reliable or reproducible:* prepared using procedures and decision rules that would lead different experts to the same conclusions based on the same evidence
- *Applicable:* useful in populations that potential users would consider relevant to their practices
- *Flexible:* allowing for practitioner judgment and patient preferences
- *Clear:* presented in unambiguous language and easy-to-follow logic
- *Multidisciplinary:* prepared with input from relevant disciplines and stakeholders
- *Up to date:* reflecting the most recent evidence
- *Documented:* published along with explicit statements on assumptions, process, rationale, evidence, and decision rules

The IOM has published a document to be used in assessing the quality of published practice guidelines on the basis of these eight attributes (Field and Lohr 1992).

Adapting National Guidelines to Local Needs

Most published guidelines concerning screening for disease in the community are developed by governmental or private organizations with nation-wide or international constituencies. Organizers of screening programs with more limited coverage (e.g., states, counties, managed-care plans, or workplaces in a particular industry) often are forced to adapt or modify national guidelines to fill gaps in content, meet specific local objectives, live within resource constraints, educate practitioners and serve as a ratifying mechanism that helps win acceptance, and neutralize the effects of conflicts among national guidelines supported by different organizations. For example, the Group Health Cooperative of Puget Sound (a large health maintenance organization based in Seattle Washington) uses its experience over the preceding years to adapt national screening guidelines for use in their risk-based breast cancer screening program (Taplin et al. 1990). The 1990 screening algorithm and its implications for the distribution of women eligible for screening by mammography frequency, risk level, and risk criteria are illustrated in Table 7-5.

In addition to the potential benefits previously outlined, local adaptation of national guidelines also has potential hazards. Local adaptation without justification based on scientific evidence of effectiveness may serve to protect professional habits and local customs for the benefit of the organization and to guard economic self-interest by endorsing unnecessary care or care that others could provide or provide more economically. To guard against such hazards to effective screening, the IOM recommends that local adaptation of carefully developed and documented "national guidelines" should provide explicit rationales that relate to well-defined local conditions or objectives and that

Table 7-5. Group Health Cooperative of Puget Sound's Breast Cancer Risk Algorithm and Screening Protocol

Mammography Frequency	Risk Level	Risk-Level Criteria	Relative Risk	Percentage Women[b]
Annual	1	Previous breast cancer or atypia on biopsy results; at least two first-degree relatives with breast cancer[a]	4–14	1
Every 2 years	2	One first-degree relative with breast cancer; ≥50 years of age and ≥2 MRFs	1.9–3.5	15
Every 3 years	3	≥50 years of age and ≥1 MRF; or ≥50 years of age and ≥1 MRF	1.2–1.9	66
Not recommended	4	<50 years of age and no MRF	1.0	17
	Total			100

Source: Taplin et al. (1990).

[a]First-degree relative, mother, sister, or daughter; second-degree relative, grandmother, or aunt.

[b]Among Group Health Cooperative women >40 years of age who completed the risk factor questionnaire by 1987 ($n = 55\ 875$) but excluding women with a history of breast cancer ($n = 1\ 460$) or for whom information was missing ($n = 1\ 704$). MRF, minor risk factors. Second-degree relative with breast cancer; menarche age ≤10 years or menopause ≤30 years; previous negative breast biopsy.

consider the strength of the case for the original guidelines (Field and Lohr 1992).

Dealing With Controversial and Conflicting Guidelines

Leitch has reviewed recent controversies in breast-cancer screening—particularly in the context of screening guidelines for women 40–49 years of age. Her review illustrates the following two traditional strategies for dealing with controversial and conflicting guidelines: relying on a consensus recommendation and relying on expert advice advocating a particular preference (Leitch 1995). In addition, this example is used to illustrate the general principle of "shared decision-making" between clinician and patient (or client) in the context of screening. Shared decision-making means providing information in an unbiased way (often with instructional aids [e.g., videos] that help clients clarify their own risks and values) and attempting to elicit patient preferences based on the information provided.

Guidelines regarding breast-cancer screening have been issued by several organizations, including the American Cancer Society (ACS), American College of Radiology, American Medical Association, American College of Obstetricians and Gynecologists (ACOG), American Academy of Family Physicians, American College of Physicians, Canadian Task Force on the Periodic Health Examination, National Cancer Institute (NCI), and the US Preventive Services Task Force. In 1988, because of concerns that conflicting guidelines were confusing physicians and impeding screening for breast cancer, 12 of these organizations met to develop consensus recommendations. As a result of this meeting, they issued a joint statement on mammography guidelines, agreeing that mammography should be performed at intervals of 1–2 years for women 40–49 years of age.

Since 1988, the consensus on the value of screening among women 40–49 years of age has eroded. The results of eight randomized trials of breast-cancer screening have been published including two separate meta-analyses that arrived at conflicting conclusions based on the same studies. In 1993, the Fletcher meta-analysis concluded that screening mammography after 5–7 years of follow-up was not beneficial for women 40–49 years of age (Fletcher et al. 1993). In 1995, the Smart meta-analysis concluded that screening mammography reduced breast cancer mortality by 16–24% after 7–18 years of follow-up among women 40–49 years of age at study entry (Smart et al. 1995). As of 1996, more than five organizations continue to recommend annual screening for women 40–49 years of age, two organizations recommend against it, and two have issued neutral recommendations neither for nor against screening in this age group.

Leitch has offered the following advice to physicians who are functioning as advocates and who must counsel patients about breast-cancer screening. She advises, in part, that they:

1. Make recommendations to patients based on the best available data.
2. Inform patients about their personal risks for breast cancer and the controversies surrounding the screening guidelines.
3. Be honest about the effects of economics on setting breast-cancer guidelines.
4. Help patients understand that policy makers must be more concerned with the general good than with the good of any individual.

In contrast, the USPSTF, comprised mainly of primary care practitioners, advises their peers (primary care practitioners) that:

For women aged 40–49, there is conflicting evidence of fair to good quality regarding clinical benefit from mammography with or without CBE, and insufficient evidence regarding benefit from CBE alone; therefore recommendations for or against routine mammography or CBE cannot be made based on the current evidence. There is no evidence specifically evaluating mammography or CBE in high-risk women under age 50; recommendations for screening such women may be made on other grounds, including patient preference, high burden of suffering, and the higher PVP of screening, which would lead to fewer false positives than are likely to occur from screening women of average risk in this age group. (USPSTF 1996)

Translating Guidelines Into Programs

A screening program is an organized deployment of resources (i.e., financial, human, material, and technological), policies, and procedures for early detection and treatment of a target disease or health condition in a defined population. Usually a program is guided by explicit objectives and related activities. To be effective, screening programs must include integrated components or phases devoted to (1) outreach, testing, and referral (phase 1) and (2) diagnosis, treatment, and follow-up (phase 2). Although they must operate seamlessly to be effective, both phases of a screening program can each be evaluated separately. Indicators of success in phase 1 relate to frequency of positive tests, proportion of positives confirmed, frequency of false positives, morbidity and costs of false positives, and average lead time gained per case. Indicators of success in phase 2 include (1) improvement in morbidity, mortality, disability, and quality of life and (2) adverse effects and costs of diagnosis and treatment (Morrison 1992).

The USPSTF has recommended that primary care practitioners screen asymptomatic persons for the target conditions listed in Table 7-4. The health outcomes, screening procedures, target populations, and broad age groups, respectively, are listed in each column (USPSTF 1996). The priority conditions on that list provide the context for the following discussion of opportunities and challenges facing the major organizations that are likely to be involved in community coalitions to translate screening guidelines into programs. Those organizations include departments of health, managed care plans, community-based coalitions, and workplace coalitions.

Public Health Departments

Historically, public health departments have had a primary responsibility for meeting the screening needs for certain conditions (e.g., lead poisoning, sexually transmitted diseases [STDs], tuberculosis, and other health conditions associated with poverty). More recently, health departments also have increased screening for breast and cervical cancer, hypertension, and other cardiovascular risk factors, mainly among vulnerable populations with limited personal resources and access to private providers (Aday 1993).

Opportunities. Starfield has suggested that, in the future, public health departments might more often be required to provide outreach (including home visiting) and coordination of services in vulnerable populations residing in geographic areas with high concentrations of health problems (Starfield 1996). Although health departments at the national, state, and local levels will continue to share the responsibility for screening in the community with clinical medical-care facilities, some commentators have predicted increasing responsibilities for health departments in the functional areas of assessment and policy development (using interagency coalitions and community-wide social influences) and decreasing responsibilities in the area of service assurance (IOM 1988; Baker et al. 1994;).

Challenges Health departments at all three levels of government face the major challenge of doing more with less—increasing responsibilities in the face of budget cutbacks and reductions in staffing (Baker et al. 1994). In the HMO setting, Eddy has suggested that opportunities for doing more with less result from one of the following two categories of resource transfers: (1) transferring resources from an overused intervention of lower value to an underused intervention of higher value at comparable cost and (2) transferring resources within the same intervention from a target group where the preventable fraction of the burden of disease is smaller to a target group where the preventable fraction is larger at comparable cost. He illustrates the between-intervention resource transfer with an example involving the transfer of resources from an intervention to prevent adverse reactions from radiographic contrast media to a breast-cancer screening program for hard-to-reach women 50–75 years of age; and he illustrates the between-target group resource transfer from breast cancer for women < 50 years of age at low risk to women 50–75 years of age at high risk (Eddy 1994). The challenge for health departments is to seek out and implement that kind of resource transfer where they exist.

Managed-Care Organizations

Managed care is a strategy designed to increase efficiency, assure accountability, and promote quality in the financing and delivery of health care. Most managed-care organizations (MCOs) fall into one of three major patterns of organization: (1) staff-model health maintenance organizations (HMOs), which employ salaried providers; (2) network or independent practice associations (IPA), which contract with independent practitioners in private practice; and (3) group practice HMOs, which contract with physician-group practices that devote a substantial percentage of their practice to HMO patients. MCOs actively manage patient care and control or influence the medical treatment decisions of their providers including those health care professionals who are not employed but are under contract to provide services to enrollees according to the terms of a particular health plan (Gold et al. 1995).

HMOs are expected to play a major role in the delivery of preventive services (e.g., screening for disease) for several reasons (CDC 1995a). HMOs are rapidly becoming a major source of health care for most Americans, have historically included preventive services (e.g., screening), are responsible for defined or enrolled populations, and have enthusiastically embraced the recommendations of the USPSTF to define preventive services benefits (Woolf et al. 1996). Moreover, the preventive services measures developed by the National Committee for Quality Assurance (NCQA) to track health plan performance, the Health Plan Employer Data and Information Set (HEDIS), partly were based on the USPSTF recommendations. Specific measures include indicators of plan-specific effectiveness of care with respect to screening for breast cancer, cervical cancer, colorectal cancer, diabetic eye disease, hypertension, and chlamydia (NCQA 1996).

Opportunities. Clinicians, policy-makers, and public health practitioners see an opportunity to strengthen both primary care and public health in the promise of managed care to emphasize preventive services (e.g., screening for disease). To realize those opportunities, effective partnerships must be developed between public health and managed care, and second generation MCOs must strive to meet the standards of accountability for primary care: first contact access, continuity of care, comprehensiveness, coordination, community orientation, cultural sensitivity, and family-centeredness. Many of the first-generation, staff-model HMOs have already made important strides in that direction (CDC 1995a; Starfield 1996).

Challenges. In addition to the issue of accountability for meeting primary care standards, Starfield has identified other challenges associated with minimizing the potential adverse consequences of (1) high levels of cost sharing and enrollee turnover, (2) overreliance on perceived patient satisfaction as an indicator of quality, (3) increasing specialty orientation under the guise of "case management" in certain areas (e.g., mental health), and (4) usurping the traditional role of public health in terms of population-based prevention (Starfield 1996).

Community-Based Coalitions

Community coalitions (also discussed in Chapter 12) involving official health agencies, academic health centers, places of worship, and other community-based organizations have emerged as an essential part of any community-wide effort to improve health in many parts of the world including the United States (Green and Kreuter 1991). Levine and co-workers have described an ongoing community-based partnership in East Baltimore, Maryland, a community of 150,000 whose residents are predominantly African-American (Levine et al. 1994). The partnership involves a coalition of churches which have organized into an umbrella organization known as Clergy United for Renewal of East Baltimore (CURE), the Johns Hopkins Academic Health Center (the schools of medicine, nursing, and public health, and the Johns Hopkins Hospital), the Baltimore City Health Department and school system, and Health Care for the Homeless.

The appeal of places of worship as settings for health promotion and disease prevention is based on experience suggesting that such settings are receptive to health-related programs, have access to large numbers of persons from all socioeconomic and ethnic groups, have effective communication and meeting facilities, and are oriented to volunteerism (Lasater et al. 1990; 1991; DePue et al. 1990). Since its creation in 1989, the Heart, Body, and Soul Program has evolved in scope to include programs targeted against heart disease, smoking, obesity, violence, crime, substance abuse, and tuberculosis, as well as the promotion of youth education, completion of schooling, and career development. Examples of the effectiveness of this approach include significantly improved rates of identification, care, and control of hypertension, as well as concomitant decreases in related morbidity and mortality and significant improvement in smoking cessation (Levine et al. 1979, 1990; Morisky et al. 1983; Stillman et al. 1993).

Opportunities. Levine sees the replication of partnerships like the East Baltimore coalition in similar communities across the country as an opportunity to make substantial progress in decreasing the gap in the health status between underserved, minority populations and the majority of Americans. He points out that about 75% of the 126 academic health centers in the nation are located in communities of underserved minority populations similar to East Baltimore (Pew Health Professions Commission 1993); the mission of such centers is to gain new knowledge through research to enhance the health of the public, as well as to train health professionals to provide the best quality care to all citizens; and with federal and state government help and local leadership much more can be accomplished (Levine et al. 1994).

Challenges. Achieving long-term success in East Baltimore and elsewhere is a substantial challenge because of the difficulty of maintaining high levels of enthusiasm and effort among participants of demonstration projects over time and competition for philanthropic resources among potential coalition partners to address a long list of intractable problems (e.g., smoking, hypertension, hyperlipidemia, substance abuse, violence, and various cancers).

Essential characteristics of this model of coalitions that are likely to meet those challenges include community-based leadership and ownership of specific programs, training and utilization of indigenous community health workers, joint planning for a sequenced strategy of addressing various health problems, interdisciplinary community practice and training opportunities for faculty and students, built-in evaluation, and broad community development and long-term maintenance of effective strategies.

Workplace Coalitions

Work sites have become more important settings for health promotion and disease prevention activities in recent years. In 1992, the proportion of US private-sector organizations with 50 or more employees that offered at least one preventive screening service had increased to 52% from 30% in 1985 (Fielding and Piserchia 1989; USDHHS 1993). In both 1985 and 1992, larger work sites ($\geq$750 employees) were nine times as likely to offer cancer screening and three times as likely to offer hypertension control programs than were smaller work sites (<100 workers).

Stokols and co-workers state that integrating medical care and preventive services (for employees and their dependents) that are delivered inside and outside the workplace is a major challenge (Stokols et al. 1995). Such integration, they argue, is essential in the face of societal changes (e.g., managed care, corporate downsizing, part-time employment, desktop computing, and telecommuting), which are altering the structure, incentives for, and locations of work, as well as the organization and provision of health-care services.

Summary

This chapter provides a contemporary overview of issues relevant to practitioners as they design, implement, and evaluate screening programs. To facilitate their application, key concepts and principles were grouped under each of four operational tasks that practitioners must accomplish to be successful. Thus, concepts of community, settings, mass versus selective screening, risk stratification, and high-risk versus population strategy are important in defining the target population for screening. Concepts of the natural history of disease (preclinical and clinical stages of disease) and burden of suffering (including morbidity, mortality, and case-fatality rates, and cost and quality of life) are important in setting priorities among target diseases or health conditions for screening. Sensitivity, lead time, specificity, reliability, predictive value positive, and multiphasic and sequential screening are important concepts when selecting appropriate screening tests or examinations. Finally, efficacy, length bias, prevented fraction, cost-effectiveness and cost-benefit are essential concepts when assessing the impact of a screening program in a population.

Organizers of community screening programs rely on screening practice guidelines issued by authoritative bodies with national or international constituencies for guidance in setting local priorities and objectives for screening in the community. Adopting and adapting national guidelines to meet local needs often requires strategies for dealing with conflicting and controversial guidelines issued by different deliberative groups. Evidence-based screening guidelines (e.g., those published by the USPSTF) are available to guide the development of screening programs. To ensure their effectiveness, locally developed or adapted guidelines should possess the desirable attributes of guidelines as suggested by the IOM.

To be most effective, guidelines for screening practice (both national and locally adapted) must be translated into screening programs with dedicated resources and clearly defined target populations and objectives. To be effective, screening programs must include integrated components devoted to outreach (or in-reach), testing, referral, diagnosis, treatment, and follow-up. The integration of program elements related to volunteerism, public health, and clinical practice present both opportunities and challenges for the major institutional entities that are likely to be involved in community coalitions to translate screening guidelines into programs. Such agencies and individuals include the media, academia, managed-care organizations, occupational-health and community-based coalitions, and health departments.

In the future, several key issues are likely to increase in importance as we search and advocate for more effective and widespread use of screening in the practice setting. Other issues beyond those already discussed under the subheading "opportunities and challenges" include screening for genetic markers of disease susceptibility (e.g., genes for susceptibility to breast cancer, cystic fibrosis, hemochromatosis, and HIV/AIDS); using artificial-intelligence systems to automate the processing and interpretation of screening tests (e.g., neural networks for reading pap smears); and reconciling measures of screening effectiveness assessed in studies using different units of analysis (e.g., individual, family, and community).

CASE STUDIES

Hypertension Control and Medicaid-Managed Care

Background

Hypertension (defined as a diastolic blood pressure of ≥ 90 mmHg or a systolic pressure of ≥ 140 mmHg) and diabetes are leading risk factors (independent and interacting) for cardiovascular disease (CVD) and its complications (i.e., stroke, kidney failure, blindness, myocardial infarction, and sudden death) (USPSTF 1996). Randomized placebo-controlled trials have demonstrated the benefit of antihypertensive treatment and control of coexisting risk factors (e.g., smoking, hyperglycemia, dyslipidemia, and obesity) in preventing CVD and its complications.

Elderly adults, the poor, and black persons are at higher risk than their counterparts for uncontrolled hypertension and premature death from its resulting complications (NHBPEP 1993). In addition, these groups are dependent on Medicare and Medicaid programs, which have begun to enroll increasing numbers of their beneficiaries in managed-care plans. To determine whether managed care (MC) and fee for service (FFS) differed significantly in either the process or outcomes of care, Medicaid beneficiaries (including the elderly) in county X were randomized to prepaid care (35% of enrollees) and fee-for-service care (65%) (Coffey et al. 1995). No significant differences between MC and FFS were observed; yet, the researchers noted that "a substantial number of clients in both MC and FFS were overweight, had poorly controlled blood pressure or blood glucose, and reported receiving limited advice from and few referrals for help in adjusting their diet or lifestyle." Because county X places a high priority on hypertension screening and follow-up and on preventing complications from diabetes in the elderly, the health commissioner asked the director of the hypertension and diabetes prevention and control programs to prepare an action plan for responding to the problem.

Key Questions

1. Why are the study findings relevant to the county's hypertension screening and diabetes control programs?

By modulating its size, scope, content, and emphasis, the county hypertension screening program can play a critical role in helping the clinical care system (MC and FFS) to ensure adequate capacity for follow-up and optimal levels of patient compliance with clinical advice.

2. How should the county balance its efforts to find and refer new hypertensives with efforts to help MC and FFS providers be more effective with hypertensives (with or without diabetes) already under care?

County X can use decision analysis, cost-effectiveness analysis, and informal methods of integrating expert judgment, precedent, and consensus about roles among collaborating agencies, alone or in combination, to decide on the optimal balance between two essential program components of a hypertension screening program (NHBPEP 1993; Petitti 1994).

3. What indicators might the MC plans use to assess the quality of care for hypertension and hypertension with coexisting diabetes?

The Health Plan Employer Data Information Set (HEDIS 3.0), a set of standardized plan-specific performance measures, is available (NCQA 1996) (also see Chapter 10).

Implications for Practice

A journal article, whose findings might appear tangential to hypertension screening on the surface, has forced county X to reassess the rationale, effectiveness, and efficiency of its programs. Despite large reductions in mortality from coronary heart disease and stroke, these diseases are the first and third leading causes of death in the United States. The doctors, administrators, and other staff in both MC and FFS settings must become more aware and collaborate with others who can help them improve this situation. Researchers within health departments, academic centers, and the federal government are presented with new research questions related to optimal resource allocation and operational efficiency. The goal of such research is to achieve a better quality of life for elderly persons who have hypertension and diabetes.

Prevention and Control of Colorectal Cancer

Background

Each year, 134,000 Americans are diagnosed with and 55,000 die from colorectal cancer. Only 37% of new cases are in localized stages in which the affected persons have the best chance of survival (Wingo et al. 1995). Familial polyposis, inflammatory bowel disease, male gender, and black race increase the risk of excess mortality from colorectal cancer.

Each year, city Y (population: 700,000; 70% African-American) experiences 450 new cases and 200 deaths from colorectal cancer. A 1985 study of mass screening using the fecal occult blood test (FOBT) in the metropolitan area (3.6 million including city Y) estimated the cost at $15,000 (1990 dollars) per case of colon cancer diagnosed and $7,611 per polyp discovered (Trehu and Cooper 1992). A large drug store chain had distributed 100,000 FOBT kits (free of charge) to customers; of the 10,000 stool samples tested at a single hospital, 306 (3%) were positive for fecal occult blood; of the 272 FOBT-positive persons who had diagnostic studies, 14 cancers (5%) and 28 polyps (9%) were detected. The researchers concluded that "Given the high cost, low sensitivity and specificity, and lack of evidence for reduced morbidity and mortality, we believe mass screening for fecal occult blood should not be recommended at this time."

More recently, a large, randomized controlled trial (RCT) in the United States estimated that screening with FOBT reduces mortality from colorectal cancer by 33% at 13 years postrandomization (Mandel et al. 1993). Most experts now recommend annual screening with FOBT for persons ≥50 years of age or periodic flexible sigmoidoscopy (every 3–5 years by some experts) as an alternative to FOBT (USPSTF 1996).

City Y's health commissioner has asked the director of its cancer prevention and control program to develop a set of alternative options for a colorectal cancer screening program, perhaps modeled after the comprehensive breast and cervical cancer early detection program, including community outreach to educate and motivate women to be screened, screening (mammography and Pap tests) and referral services, provider education, and community coalitions to mobilize and deploy state and local resources in support of program objectives (CDC 1996).

Key Questions

1. What alternatives to mass screening with FOBT for colorectal cancer may be considered among the options?

Alternatives include mass screening with sigmoidoscopy, targeted screening of persons at high risk by means of FOBT and/or sigmoidoscopy, and targeted screening of persons at highest risk by means of barium enema and colonoscopy (USPSTF 1996).

2. What major features of city Y's Breast and Cervical Cancer Screening Program might serve as a model for developing a colorectal cancer screening program?

Community outreach, screening and referral, provider education, and community coalitions are among the program elements that are transferable.

3. How do mammography (with or without clinical breast exam [CBE]) and FOBT (with or without sigmoidoscopy) compare in terms of positive predictive value positive (PPV)?

Estimates of the positive predictive value of screening tests vary with study design, patient age, clinical outcomes, and the diagnostic gold standard. Positive predictive value (PPV) ranges from 11% to 18% for mammography (with CBE), 2% to 11% (for carcinoma), and 20% to 30% (for adenomas) using FOBT in persons >50 years of age.

Implications For Practice

Recent studies have provided new evidence that screening reduces mortality from colorectal cancer. However, mortality reduction was demonstrated in an RCT in which 32% of the annually screened population underwent a diagnostic colonoscopy during a 13-year follow-up. Because colonoscopy is relatively expensive, uncomfortable, and may have potential adverse effects, city-wide screening may require evidence of cost-effectiveness, wider professional and public consensus, and incremental implementation, if justifiable. The efficacy of using colonoscopy and barium enema as screening procedures in asymptomatic persons at high risk has not been determined by credible RCTs. The cost-effectiveness of mass screening with FOBT has not been rigorously assessed. Screening programs with lower PPV usually have higher proportions of false positives, higher costs per cancer detected, and lower acceptability.

SUGGESTED READINGS

Cadman D, Chambers L, Feldman W, Sackett D. Assessing the effectiveness of community screening programs. JAMA 1984;251:1580–1585.

Mullen PD, Evans D, Forster J, et al. Settings as an important dimension in health education/promotion policy, programs, and research. Health Educ Q 1995;22: 329–345.

Richart RM. Screening: the next century. Cancer 1995;76:1919–1927.

Rose G. The strategy of preventive medicine. New York: Oxford University Press; 1992.

Starfield B. Public health and primary care: a framework for proposed linkages. Am J Public Health 1996;86:1365–1369.

Teutsch SM. A framework for assessing the effectiveness of disease and injury prevention. Morb Mortal Wkly Rep 1992;41(No. RR-3):i-iv, 1-12.

Thompson RS, Taplin SH, McAfee TA, Mandelson MT, Smith AE. Primary and secondary prevention services in clinical practice: twenty years experience in development, implementation, and evaluation. JAMA 1995;273:1130–1135.

Woolf SH, DiGuiseppi CG, Atkins D, Kamerow DB. Developing evidence-based clinical practice guidelines: lessons learned by the U.S. Preventive Services Task Force. Annu Rev Public Health 1996;17:511–538.

REFERENCES

Aday LA. At Risk in America: The Health and Health Care Needs of Vulnerable Populations in the United States. San Francisco: Jossey-Bass; 1993:117–160.

Baker EL, Melton RJ, Stange PV, et al. Health reform and the health of the public: forging community health partnerships. JAMA 1994;272:1276–1282.

Beckles GL, Blount SB, Jiles RB. African Americans. In: CDC. Chronic Disease in Minority Populations. Atlanta: Centers for Disease Control and Prevention; 1994:2–13

Brownson RC, Reif JS, Alavanja MC, Bal DG. Cancer. In: Brownson RC, Remington PL, Davis JR, eds. Chronic Disease Epidemiology and Control. Washington, DC: American Public Health Association; 1993:137–167.

Cadman D, Chambers L, Feldman W, Sackett D. Assessing the effectiveness of community screening programs. JAMA 1984;251:1580–1585.

Casper M, Wing S, Strogatz D, et al. Antihypertensive treatment and U.S. trends in stroke mortality, 1962 to 1980. Am J Public Health 1992;82:1600–1606.

Centers for Disease Control and Prevention. Testing for antibodies to human immunodeficiency virus Type 2 in the United States. Morb Mortal Wkly Rep 1992;41(No. RR-12):1–9.

Centers for Disease Control and Prevention. Prevention and managed care:opportunities for managed care organizations, purchasers of health care, and public health agencies. Morb Mortal Wkly Rep 1995a;44(14):1–12.

Centers for Disease Control and Prevention. Update: National Breast and Cervical Cancer Early Detection Program—July 1991–September 1995. Morb Mortal Wkly Rep 1996a;45(23):484–487.

Centers for Disease Control and Prevention. Breast Cancer Incidence and Mortality—United States, 1992. Morb Mortal Wkly Rep 1996b;45:833–837.

Coffey E, Moscovice I, Finch M, Christianson JB, Lurie N. Capitated Medicaid and the process of care of elderly hypertensives and diabetics. Am J Med 1995;98:531–536.

Dasbach E, Teutsch SM. Cost-utility analysis. In: Haddix AC, Teutsch SM, Shaffer PA, Dunet DO, eds. Prevention Effectiveness: A Guide to Decision Analysis and Economic Evaluation. New York, NY:Oxford University Press; 1996:130–141.

DePue JD, Wells BL, Lasater TM, et al. Volunteers as providers of heart health programs in churches: a report on implementation. Am J Health Promot 1990;4:361–366.

Eddy DM. Clinical decision making: from theory to practice. Rationing resources while improving quality. How to get more for less. JAMA 1994;272:817–824.

Field MJ, Lohr KN, eds. Guidelines for Clinical Practice: From Development to Use. Institute of Medicine (U.S.). Committee on Clinical Practice Guidelines, Division of Health Care Services. Washington, DC: National Academy Press; 1992.

Fielding JE, Piserchia PV. Frequency of worksite health promotion activities. Am J Public Health 1989;73:538–542.

Fletcher SW, Black W, Harris R, River BE, Shapiro S. Report of the international workshop on screening for breast cancer. J Natl Cancer Inst 1993;85:1644–1656.

Gargiullo PM, Rothenberg RB. Confidence intervals, hypothesis tests, and sample sizes for the prevented fraction in cross-sectional studies. Stat Med 1995;14: 51-72.

Garraway WM, Whisnant JP. The changing pattern of hypertension and the declining incidence of stroke. JAMA 1987;258:214–217.

Gold MR, Hurley R, Lake T, Ensor T, Berenson R. A national survey of the arrangements managed-care plans make with physicians. New Engl J Med 1995;333: 1678–1683.

Grad FP. Public Health Law Manual: A Handbook on Legal Aspects of Public Health Administration and Enforcement. Washington, DC: APHA; 1990.

Green LW, Kreuter MW. Health Promotion Planning: An Educational and Environmental Approach. Second Edition. Mountain View, CA: Mayfield; 1991.

Haddix AC, Teutsch SM, Shaffer PA, Dunet DO. Prevention Effectiveness: A Guide to Decision Analysis and Economic Evaluation. New York: Oxford University Press; 1996.

Institute of Medicine. The Future of Public Health. Washington, DC: National Academy Press; 1988.

Kelsey JL, Whittemore AS, Evans AS, Thompson WD. Methods in Observational Epidemiology. Second Edition. New York: Oxford University Press; 1996.

Kinne DW. Staging and follow-up of breast cancer patients. Cancer 1991;67 (Suppl):1196–1198.

Kosary CL, Ries LAG, Miller BA, et al., eds. SEER Cancer Statistics Review, 1973–1992: Tables and Graphs. Bethesda, MD: US Department of health and Human Services, Public Health Service, National Institutes of Health, National Cancer Institute; pub. no. (NIH)96-2789; 1996.

Lantz PM, Stencil D, Lippert MT, Beversdorf S, Jaros L, Remington PL. Breast and cervical cancer screening in a low-income managed care sample: the efficacy of physician letters and phone calls. Am J Public Health 1995;85:834–836.

Lasater TM, DePue JD, Wells BL, et al. The effectiveness and feasibility of delivering nutrition education programs through religious organizations. Health Promotion Int 1990;(5):253–257.

Lasater TM, Carelton RA, Wells B. Religious organizations and large-scale health-related lifestyle change programs. J Health Educ 1991;(22):233–239.

Last JM, ed. A Dictionary of Epidemiology. Second Edition New York: Oxford University Press; 1995.

Law MR, Frost CD, Wald NJ. III. Analysis of data from trials of salt reduction. Br Med J 1991;302:819–824.

Leitch AM. Controversies in breast cancer screening. Cancer (Suppl) 1995;76(10): 2064–2069.

Levine DM, Green LW, Deeds SG, Chwalow J, Russell RP, Finlay J. Health education for hypertensive patients. JAMA 1979;241:1700–1703.

Levine DM, Becker DM, Bone LR, Hill MN, Tuggle MB, Zeger SL. Community-academic health center partnerships for underserved minority populations: one Solution to a national crisis. JAMA 1994;272:309–311.

Luce BR, Manning WG, Siegel JE, Lipscomb J. Estimating costs in cost-effectiveness analysis. In: Gold MR, Russell LB, Siegel JE, Weinstein MC, eds. Cost-Effectiveness in Health and Medicine: Report of the Panel on Cost-Effectiveness in Health and Medicine. New York: Oxford University Press;1996:176–213.

Mandel JS, Bond JH, Church TR, et al. Reducing mortality from colorectal cancer by screening for fecal occult blood. N Engl J Med 1993;328:1365–1371.

Miller BA. What is the role of early detection and screening in cancer control. J Public Health Policy 1993;Winter:403–412.

Mittelmark MB, Hunt MK, Heath GW, Schmid TL. Realistic outcomes: lessons from community-based research and demonstration programs for the prevention of cardiovascular diseases. J Public Health Policy 1993;Winter:437–452.

Morisky DM, Levine DM, Green LW, Shapiro S, Russell RP, Smith CR. Five year blood pressure control and mortality following health education for hypertensive patients. Am J Public Health 1983;73:153–162.

Morrison AS. Screening in Chronic Disease. New York: Oxford University Press; 1992.

Mullen PD, Evans D, Forster J, et al. Settings as an important dimension in health education/promotion policy, programs, and research. Health Educ Q 1995;22(3):329–345.

National Center for Health statistics (NCHS). Health United States, 1995. Hyattsville, MD: Public Health Service; 1996a.

National Committee for Quality Assurance. HEDIS 3.0: Health Plan Employer Data and Information Set. Developed under the auspices of the committee on performance measurement, July 1996 (Draft for public comment.).

National High Blood Pressure Education Program (NHBPEP). The fifth report of the Joint National Committee on Detection, Evaluation, and Treatment of High Blood Pressure. National Heart, Lung, and Blood Institute, NIH. Arch Intern Med 1993;153:154–183.

NCHS. Healthy People 2000 Review, 1995–96. Hyattsville, MD: Public Health Service; 1996b.

Petitti DB. Meta-Analysis, Decision Analysis, and Cost-Effective Analysis: Methods for Quantitative Synthesis in Medicine. New York: Oxford University Press; 1994.

Pew Health Professions Commission. Health Professions Education for the Future: Schools in Service to the Nation. Report of the Pew Health Professions Commission. Durham, NC: The Pew Health Professions Commission; 1993.

Rose G. The Strategy of Preventive Medicine. New York: Oxford University Press; 1992.

Rothenberg RB, Hahn RA. Measures of attribution. In: Haddix AC, Teutsch SM, Shaffer PA, Dunet DO, eds. Prevention Effectiveness: A Guide to Decision Analysis and Economic Evaluation. New York: Oxford University Press; 1996:193–202.

Rothman KJ. Modern Epidemiology. Boston, MA: Little Brown; 1986.

Sackett DL, Haynes RB, Guyatt GH, Tugwell P. Clinical Epidemiology: A Basic Science for Clinical Medicine. Boston: Little, Brown; 1991.

Shapiro S. Screening for secondary prevention of disease. In: Armenian H, Shapiro S, eds. Epidemiology in Health Services. New York: Oxford University Press (in press).

Shapiro S, Venet W, Strax P, Venet L. Periodic Screening for Breast Cancer: The Health Insurance Plan Project and Its Sequella, 1963–1986. Baltimore, MD: The Johns Hopkins University Press; 1988.

Smart CR, Hendrix RE, Rutledge JH, Smith R. Benefit of mammography screening in women ages 40–49. Cancer 1995;75:1619–1626.

Smith CA, Pratt M. Cardiovascular disease. In: Brownson RC, Remington PL, Davis JR, eds. Chronic Disease Epidemiology and Control. Washington, DC: American Public Health Association; 1993:83-107.

Stamler J, Rose G, Stamler R, Elliott P, Dyer A, Marmot M. Intersalt study findings: public health and medical care implications. Hypertension 1989;14:570–577.

Starfield B. Public health and primary care: a framework for proposed linkages. Am J Public Health 1996;86:1365–1369.

Stillman F, Bone L, Rand C, Levine D, Becker D. Heart, body, and soul: a church-based smoking cessation program for urban African Americans. Prev Med 1993;2:335–349.

Stokols D, Pelletier KR, Fielding JE. Integration of medical care and worksite health promotion. JAMA 1995;273:1136–1142.

Svane G, Potchen EJ, Sierra A, Azavedo E. Screening Mammography: Breast Cancer Diagnosis in Asymptomatic Women. St. Louis, MO: Mosby; 1993.

Taplin SH, Thompson RS, Schnitzner F, et al. Revisions in the risk-based breast cancer screening program at Group Health Cooperative. Cancer 1990;66:812–818.

Teutsch SM. A framework for assessing the effectiveness of disease and injury prevention. Morb Mortal Wkly Rep 1992; 41(No. RR-3):1–12.

Trehu EG, Cooper JN. Cost of screening for colorectal cancer: results of a community mass screening program and review of the literature. South Med J 1992;85:248–254.

U.S. Department of Health and Human Services (USDHHS). 1992 national survey of worksite health promotion activities: summary. Am J Health Promotion 1993;7:452–464.

U.S. Dept of Health and Human Services. Healthy People 2000: National Health Promotion and Disease Prevention Objectives. Washington, DC: U.S. Department of Health and Human Services; Publication PHS 91-50212;1991.

U.S. Preventive Services Task Force (USPSTF). Guide to Clinical Preventive Services. Second Edition. Baltimore: Williams & Wilkins; 1996.

Wilson JM, Jungner G. The Principles and Practice of Screening for Disease. W.H.O. Public Health Papers 34. Geneva: World Health organization; 1968.

Wingo PA, Tong T, Bolden S. Cancer statistics, 1995. CA Cancer J Clin 1995;45:8-30.

Woolf SH, DiGuiseppi CG, Atkins D, Kamerow DB. Developing evidence-based clinical practice guidelines: lessons learned by the US Preventive Services Task Force. Annu Rev Public Health 1996;17:511–538.

8

Epidemiologic Issues
in Outcomes Research

DIANA B. PETITTI

Outcomes are those changes, either favorable or adverse, in the actual or potential *health status* of persons, groups, or communities that can be attributed to medical care (Donabedian 1985). The Institute of Medicine has defined *outcomes research* as the study of "the end results of the structure and processes of health care on the health and well-being of patients and populations" (Feasley 1996). This definition of outcomes research is similar to that of the Foundation for Health Services Research (1994).

Outcomes research is interdisciplinary research that involves health services researchers, epidemiologists, economists, sociologists, statisticians, and ethicists. It incorporates elements of epidemiology, health services research, health economics, and psychometrics (Epstein and Sherwood 1996; Foundation for Health Services Research 1994). Although not requisite, outcomes research often involves analysis of computer-stored information collected for administrative purposes or routinely in the course of clinical care.

Until recently, much of medical research has focused on the assessment of the *efficacy* of interventions—that is, the effect of the intervention under ideal circumstances. Outcomes research seeks to measure the *effectiveness* (use under everyday practice conditions) as opposed to the efficacy (use under ideal conditions) of interventions. The outcomes movement has clarified the goals of health care in improving not only the quantity of life but the ability of individuals to fulfill their personal and social roles and to maintain the *"quality" of their lives* through the efficient delivery of high-quality care. A key feature of outcomes research is the broad range of outcomes addressed. These include economic and humanistic outcomes and patient satisfaction, as well as clinical outcomes.

This chapter gives the background for the development of outcomes research. It describes the designs used most often in outcomes research. Measurement of health status and of *preferences for health states* is introduced.

Statistical issues in outcomes research and the similarities and differences between statistical approaches in epidemiology and outcomes research are discussed. The chapter identifies some of the major limitations that arise from the uses of administrative and routinely collected clinical data for outcomes research. It can also serve as a starting point for bridging epidemiologists to a broad and diverse set of literature on outcomes research.

Framework and Historical Background

Outcomes research has its origins in the "outcomes movement" (Wennberg et al. 1980; Relman 1988; Epstein 1990). Its development is closely linked with the focus on measuring and assuring *quality* in the delivery *of health services.* The specific use of the term "outcomes research" can be traced to the efforts, beginning in the 1980s, of opinion leaders in health services research (e.g., Wennberg et al. 1980) and the Agency for Health Care Policy and Research to shift the focus of health services research from issues of the organization and processes of medical care to the outcomes of medical care. Many kinds of studies previously conducted under the rubric of clinical epidemiology, health services research, or clinical research are now called outcomes re-search. Other kinds of studies, especially the *analysis of variations* in practice, have been developed specifically under the rubric of outcomes research.

Information from outcomes research studies provides part of the information base for development of clinical practice guidelines. When definitive information from a large body of experimental research is not available, the result of outcomes research is the basis for decisions about how to manage patients in the clinical setting. Outcomes research is an element of evidence-based medicine (Naylor and Guyatt 1996) and increasingly, of continuous quality improvement and "disease management." Figure 8-1 shows how out-comes research flows into disease management and outcomes management toward the ultimate goal of improving the quality of care and patient outcomes (Epstein and Sherwood 1996).

Design of Outcomes Research Studies

Overview

Cohort studies and the analysis of variations in practice are the most common methodologic approaches in outcomes research. Because both kinds of studies are nonexperimental, the interpretation of cohort studies and the analysis of variations must consider confounding (see Chapter 2). Comorbidity and se-

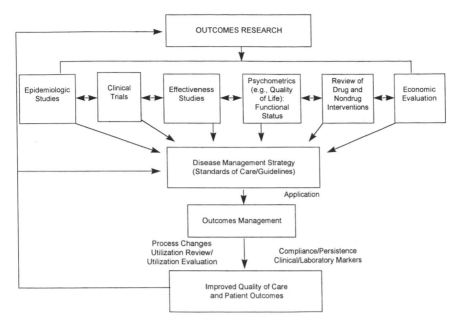

Figure 8-1. The manner in which outcomes research encompasses other kinds of research and flows into disease management with continuous improvement of the quality of health care and patient outcomes as the ultimate goal. *Source:* Epstein and Sherwood (1996)

verity of illness are particularly important potential confounders in outcomes research. Experimental designs are also used in outcomes research, but experimental outcomes research studies differ in a number of important ways from traditional randomized trials.

Cohort Studies

Many outcomes research studies are retrospective or prospective cohort studies. In outcomes research, the "exposure" studied is a medical or surgical treatment or a preventive intervention. The outcomes are varied and may include morbidity, mortality, functional status, quality of life, cost, and satisfaction with care. Table 8-1 gives some of the outcomes that are included in cohort studies to illustrate their broad range.

The goal of one kind of outcomes research that uses the cohort design is to describe what happens to patients who have an intervention. These descriptive studies are analogous to studies of the natural history of disease in traditional epidemiology. The descriptive data are used to counsel patients about what to expect following an intervention, to identify topics for further research, and as input to decision analysis or cost evaluation. The cohort study

Table 8-1. Potential Health Outcomes in Outcomes Research

Death
Length of life
Complications of disease
Complications of medical care
Physical function
Psychosocial function
Role function (e.g., return to work)
"Quality of life"
Cost of care
Service utilization (e.g., length of stay, physician visits)
Patient preferences

Source: Iezzoni (1994b).

may be retrospective or prospective. It may use administrative data collected for purposes other than research or data collected specifically for the study. Petitti and Sidney (1991) reported on short-term (30-day) and long-term (5-year) mortality in a cohort of members of a large health maintain organization who fractured their hip. This was a retrospective cohort study that used computer-stored hospital discharge data linked with computer-stored data from death certificates to assess long-term mortality. Daniel et al. (1995) reported on the functional status in a cohort of patients with anterior cruciate ligament injuries who were managed in a large orthopedic practice. This was a prospective cohort study that involved periodic reexamination of patients with anterior cruciate ligament tears who were managed by this group of orthopedists.

The goal of another kind of outcomes research that uses the cohort design is to describe *changes* in symptoms, functional status, or quality of life in patients who undergo a treatment or are the subject of a preventive intervention. These data are also used to counsel patients about what to expect following an intervention, to identify topics for research, and in decision analysis or cost evaluation. Studies of changes in symptoms, functional status, or quality of life must almost always be prospective cohort studies in which preintervention and postintervention assessments of functional status, health status, or symptoms are made and compared.

One of the most important concerns in a descriptive outcomes study has to do with the representativeness of the study population. An institution might choose to conduct a descriptive outcomes study because its outcomes are particularly good. These studies may rely on computer-stored data, limiting the range of outcomes that can be studied.

The goal of most outcomes research studies that use the cohort design is to compare alternative interventions or to compare an intervention with no intervention. Studies of this type could also be labeled clinical epidemiology. Outcomes research studies differ from traditional observational cohort studies by including a broader range of outcomes, which might include functional status, cost, and quality of life as well as (or in place of) mortality or a measure of the effect of the intervention on a specific disease-related symptom. For example, in a retrospective cohort study of outcomes in men with minimally invasive prostate cancer, symptoms of sexual and urinary dysfunction as well as mortality were compared (Litwin et al. 1995).

Analysis of Variations in Practice

A common methodologic approach in outcomes research is analysis of *variations* in practice. The units of analysis in a study of variations might be organizations (e.g., hospitals), providers (e.g., surgeons), counties, states, or even countries.

Analysis of variations generally uses administrative data, such as data from hospital discharge abstracts, insurance claims, pharmacy prescriptions, or vital records as the starting point for defining the units of analysis and the outcomes. The outcomes may also be assessed using the same administrative database or by linkage with other computer-stored information. Information may be supplemented by record review and sometimes by direct survey of patients.

Variations may be simply described. Wennberg and Gittelsohn (1975), for example, described the large variations in rates of various common surgical procedures in Maine. These descriptions focused attention on the lack of evidence about when various surgical procedures were indicated.

Analysis of variations is also often used to attempt to assess the quality of medical care. For example, New York and Pennsylvania have projects that release data on mortality following coronary bypass procedures for hospitals that perform these procedures (New York State Department of Health 1992; Pennsylvania Health Care Cost Containment Council 1991). The goal is to identify hospitals that may be delivering low-quality care and to provide information to consumers so that they can take quality of care into account in making decisions.

The analysis of variations is also used in an attempt to draw generalizable conclusions about the causes of good and bad outcome. For example, a number of authors (Hannan et al. 1991; Showstack et al. 1987; Luft et al. 1990) have used information about the variation in mortality among hospitals performing coronary artery bypass procedures to assess the relationship between surgical volume and mortality, concluding that hospitals that perform more procedures have lower mortality.

Confounding by Severity of Illness and Comorbidity

When interventions are not assigned at random, it is possible that un-measured differences between those who received the intervention and those who did not, or between those receiving alternative interventions, may account for the observed difference in outcome. Variations in outcomes between different hospitals or physicians or states might be due to underlying differences in the populations served. In both cases, confounding is a concern.

As discussed in Chapter 2, a confounding variable is a variable that is (1) causally associated with the outcome under study independently of the exposure (or intervention) of interest and (2) is associated with the exposure of interest but is (3) not a consequence of the exposure. Confounding might occur because of differences in age, gender, ethnicity, income, smoking, or the risk variables considered in traditional epidemiologic studies. In outcomes studies, confounding because of differences in severity of illness and comorbidity is a major concern. For example, the risk of death following CABG surgery is lower in men with two-vessel coronary artery disease who are otherwise healthy than in men with three-vessel disease and chronic obstructive pulmonary disease. Both the number of diseased arteries (severity of illness) and the existence of chronic obstructive pulmonary disease (comorbidity) affect the risk of mortality. In an analysis of variations among hospitals in mortality following coronary artery bypass graft surgery (CABG), the severity of coronary artery disease and the existence of illnesses other than coronary artery disease among patients in the hospitals must be taken into account in order to draw valid conclusions about the "effect" of the hospital on mortality outcome. Similarly, in a nonexperimental outcomes study examining the effectiveness of two different drugs on health status in men with coronary artery disease, disease severity and comorbidity must be taken into account to draw valid conclusions concerning the independent effect of the drug on health status.

Some methods used to measure severity of illness and comorbidity via administrative databases and clinical records in studies of variation are described later in this chapter.

Experimental Outcomes Research Studies

When an outcomes research study is experimental, it is designed to test the effectiveness (use under typical practice conditions) as opposed to the efficacy (use under ideal conditions) of an intervention. Experimental studies of the efficacy of interventions may not reflect the effectiveness of the treatments in real life because the subjects selected for traditional randomized study are rarely representative of the people for whom the treatment is used in real life. The unrepresentative nature of the study population in traditional randomized trials aimed at assessing efficacy occurs for many reasons. The study may have features such as a run-in period that makes compliance of subjects in the trial unrepresentative of compliance in real life. Only patients free of comorbidity may be eligible for the study, distorting the picture of side effects for the intervention in the real world. The study may be done in a setting that is particularly safe (e.g., a study of carotid endarterectomy is done in premier institutions with low surgical mortality). The frequency of follow-up may be dictated by the trial, making utilization and cost unrepresentative of usual care.

The Diabetes Control and Complications Trial (Diabetes Control and Complications Trial Research Group [DCCT] 1993), for example, evaluated the effect of strict control of serum glucose on the risk of nephropathy, neuropathy, and retinopathy in persons with insulin-dependent (type I) diabetes mellitus. The purpose of the study was to evaluate definitively whether strict control of serum glucose could prevent the complications of diabetes. For this reason, the subjects in the study were selected for their willingness to comply with the strict regimen imposed by study participation. Significant resources were expended to achieve strict control of serum glucose. The subjects in the study were managed in special clinics by personnel who were devoted to the study. DCCT was a study of the *efficacy* of strict control of glucose on disease outcome. The study demonstrated that strict control had the potential to lower the incidence of nephropathy, neuropathy, and retinopathy. It is uncertain whether these outcomes can be achieved in other settings and whether the cost of intervention is acceptable.

Experimental outcomes research studies are less highly controlled than experimental studies aimed at assessing efficacy. To be implemented in real-life settings, studies of the effectiveness of treatments must be less intrusive than studies of efficacy. Experimental outcomes studies recruit from a broader spectrum of patients than experimental studies of efficacy in order to enhance generalizability. Experimental outcomes research, like observational outcomes research, includes a wider variety of outcome measures than traditional experimental studies of efficacy. Measures of functional status, quality of life, and cost are typical.

Clinical trials to determine the effectiveness of strict control of glucose are now in progress. These studies attempt to enroll all patients with diabetes seen in the participating clinics. Patients are managed in regular office settings by regular personnel. The costs of the intervention and the effect of strict control on functional status and quality of life are being assessed along with the effect on achievement of strict glucose control.

Measuring Health Status Outcomes

Overview

A key feature of outcomes research is a focus on evaluating the effect of interventions on a broad range of outcomes, encompassing humanistic as well as clinical outcomes. An increasingly large amount of effort and energy in outcomes research is devoted to developing global measures of health status, health related "quality of life," and disease-specific measures of health status and "quality of life." The literature on the methods for the development of these measures is very large. There is a journal—the *Journal of Quality of Life Research*—that is devoted entirely to this topic. Equally large is the literature that compares and critiques the measures that have already been developed. There are also recent books on the topic (McDowell and Newell 1996; Spilker 1995).

The next sections of this chapter describe some of the most important methodologic considerations in the development of scales and questionnaires to measure general health status and health related quality of life. Several of the most commonly used "generic" measures of health status are described and compared. The chapter gives a brief description of methods to measure preferences for health states.

Although the chapter discusses generic measures of health status, their limitations should be recognized (Greenfield and Nelson 1992; McHorney 1996). Commonly used generic measures of health status are subject to "floor" and "ceiling" effects. That is, in people who are very ill, these instruments may not have categories that distinguish gradations of poor functional status (floor effect), and in people who are very healthy, the instruments may not distinguish gradations of good functional status (ceiling effect). Responsiveness—the ability to detect changes in function longitudinally—may also be a problem for generic measures of health status (McHorney 1996; Greenfield and Nelson 1992).

Methodologic Considerations in the Development of Measures of Health Status and Health-Related Quality of Life

Conceptual issues. To measure health, it is necessary first to be certain that we know what is meant by the term. The definition of "health," or more accurately the *conceptual* definition of health, justifies the content of an instrument to measure it and relates the measure to a broader body of theory, showing how the results obtained may be interpreted in light of that theory (McDowell and Newell 1996).

In 1948, the World Health Organization (WHO 1948) defined health as a state of "complete physical, mental, and social well-being, and not merely the absence of disease and infirmity." The WHO definition is now widely accepted. Instruments to measure health based on this definition should encompass these dimensions of health or present an alternative definition, or conceptual framework, for the measure of health.

A second main thrust of outcomes research is an attempt to incorporate measures of "quality of life" into assessment of the effect of interventions. There is a growing consensus that the effects of medical care on quality of life are critically important to measure and that medical care should strive to improve quality of life. Despite the consensus that evaluations of interventions should consider their effect on quality of life, there is no agreement on a definition of quality of life. Measures of health status are often described as measures of health-related quality of life. However, health and quality of life are distinct concepts. Quality of life encompasses, in addition to physical, mental, and social functioning, environmental quality, subjective well-being, and life satisfaction (McDowell and Newell 1996).

A number of measures used in outcome studies attempt to simultaneously assess physical, social, and emotional aspects of health. These measures are often called measures of "general health status," "generic" measures of health status, or measures of "health-related quality of life." The description of generic measures of health status as measures of "quality of life" coincides with the growing emphasis on economic analysis in the evaluation of interventions. Many economic evaluations attempt to derive measures of "quality-adjusted" life expectancy.

Many researchers believe that all measures that are called measures of "quality of life" are suitable for use in cost analysis and that all of them can be used to derive estimates of quality-adjusted life expectancy. Measures of health status can be categorized as being preference-based and nonpreference-based methods. In practice, only preference-based measures of quality of life can be used in to estimate quality-adjusted life expectancy in an economic analysis. Preference-based methods are linked with judgments about the *value* placed on a particular health state and yield a single score that is scaled from 0.0 (death) to 1.0 (complete health). Nonpreference-based measures assign scores to individual components of health and sum the components to a single score or a series of scores measuring dimensions of health (e.g., mobility, physical activity, communication/speech).

Because most measures of health status are not preference-based, this chapter will use the term "generic measures of health status" to avoid misleading the reader about the usefulness of the commonly used measures in economic evaluation.

Reliability. A measure is reliable if the same measure is observed across time, persons, or observers. Epidemiologists are generally familiar with assessments of reliability that compare the similarity of replicate measures on the same subject at the same time (intrarater reliability), the similarity of the same measurements made at different times on the same person (test–retest reliability), and the similarity of the measure made by two or more raters (interrater reliability). Each of these assessments of reliability is used to a greater or lesser extent in constructing and evaluating measures of health status.

Internal consistency (internal reliability), which is not as familiar to epidemiologists, is also important in the construction and interpretation of measures of health status and quality of life. Statistical measures of internal consistency calculate the intercorrelation between items of a scale that are meant to measure the same concept. When the internal consistency of a scale is high, it is inferred that the items that make up the scale are measuring the same thing. In theory, when internal consistency is high, test–retest reliability would also be high.

Cronbach's alpha is the most commonly used measure of internal consistency (McDowell and Newell 1996). The values of Cronbach's alpha range from 0.0 to 1.0, higher values indicating greater internal consistency. The formulas for calculating Cronbach's alpha are presented in introductory textbooks (Nunnally 1967). Widely used statistical software packages, SPSS and SAS, calculate Cronbach's alpha.

An important issue in medical research is response burden. In general, the larger the number of items in an instrument, the higher the internal consistency. However, more items increase the response burden. More items also translate to higher cost. When items in a scale are highly intercorrelated, there may be redundancy. Measures of internal consistency are also used as a tool to reduce the number of items in a scale.

Validity. A measure of health must be not only reliable but also valid. A measure is valid if it measures the phenomenon it claims to measure. A measure may be reliable but invalid. For example, a bathroom scale that is not properly zeroed will give the same wrong weight each time it is used to weigh something. It is reliable. It is not valid.

There are many ways to assess validity (Nunnally 1967). These include face validity (the extent to which an instrument "looks like" it measures what it is intended to measure), criterion validity (how the instrument compares with a "gold standard" measure), predictive validity (the ability of the instrument to predict an outcome), and convergence validity (the relationship of the instrument to other instruments that measure the same thing).

Assessing the validity of instruments to measure health involves empiric investigation. Criterion validity would involve assessment of a measure in relation to a "gold standard" measure of the phenomenon. Since there is no gold-standard measure of quality of life or of many of the other functional status measures, criterion validity is not often assessed in construction and evaluation of measures of health. Convergence validity is often assessed, and when an instrument shows convergence validity, it is considered to be a valid measure of the same phenomenon.

"Generic" Measures of Health Status

Overview

This chapter discusses in detail four generic measures of health status—the Sickness Impact Profile (SIP; Bergner et al. 1976, 1981), the 36-item Medical Outcomes Study short form (SF-36; Ware and Sherbourne 1992; Ware et al. 1993), the Quality of Well-Being Scale (QWB; Kaplan and Anderson 1988) and the EuroQol Quality of Life Scale (EuroQol Group 1990; Essink-Bot et al. 1993). These generic measures of health status are broadly applicable measures for which there is empiric data on reliability and validity. All four scales were developed to be used to evaluate the outcomes of health care, in program planning and policy formulation, and in monitoring patient progress. Documentation of how to score each of them is readily available.

McDowell and Newell (1996) describe a large number of generic and other measures of health and health status in detail and comment on the strengths and limitations of each. Spilker's book (1995) also reviews this topic in depth.

This chapter also briefly describes other methods for deriving preference-based measure of health status—i.e., utilities. Chapter 10 describes how preference-based utilities are used to estimate quality-adjusted life expectancy as an outcome. A more detailed discussion of the derivation of preference-based measures is found in Gold et al. (1996).

Sickness Impact Profile (SIP)

The SIP (Bergner et al. 1976, 1981) measures health status by assessing the way that sickness changes daily activities and behavior; 136 statements about activities and behavior (e.g., "I do not walk at all," "I sleep or nap during the day") are presented to respondents, who check the statement (or respond "yes") if it applies to them. The statements are scored in 12 separate categories of health (e.g., ambulation, sleep, and rest). Scores for some of the categories are summed to obtain additional scores for two broad dimensions of health—physical and psychosocial.

The SIP instrument can be administered by an interviewer, or it can be self-administered. It takes 20–30 minutes for an interviewer to administer and about the same amount of time to self-administer.

Test–retest reliability and internal consistency of the SIP are both high—greater than 0.80 (Bergner et al. 1981). Correlations of SIP category scales with other instruments used to measure health status are summarized in McDowell and Newell (1996). A limitation of SIP is its insensitivity to small changes in a patient's daily situation (DeBruin et al. 1992). Table 8-2 describes some of the most important features of the SIP.

36-Item Short Form Questionnaire (SF-36)

The SF-36 (Ware and Sherbourne 1992; Ware et al. 1993) assesses health status by asking respondents to answer 36 questions about their view of their overall health, about how well they feel, and about how well they are able to perform their usual activities. Thirty-four of the 36 questions are used to calculate scores, scaled from 0 to 100, that assess eight dimensions of health (Table 8-3). Two items are used to measure change in health status.

The SF-36 can be self-administered or administered in telephone or face-to-face interviews. It takes about 15 minutes for an interviewer to administer and about 10 minutes to self-administer, although the time that it takes to self-administer is dependent on reading skills and on age (McHorney 1996). Machine-readable (bubble format) forms are available, and there is software that automates processing of the SF-36 forms.

Internal reliability of the SF-36 scales has been studied extensively and is

Table 8-2. Important Features of the Sickness Impact Profile (SIP)

Major Category	Description
Domains assessed	Independent categories of function: sleep and rest, eating, work, home management, recreation Physical function: ambulation, mobility, body care and movement Psychosocial function: social interaction, alertness behavior, emotional behavior, communication
Time to administer	20–30 minutes: interviewer 20–30 minutes: self-administered
Reliability	Well studied: 0.81 to 0.97
Preference-based	No

Table 8-3. Important Features of the 36-Item Short Form Health Survey (SF-36)

Major Category	Description
Domains assessed	Physical functioning
	Role limitation due to physical health problems
	Bodily pain
	Social functioning
	General mental health
	Role limitation due to emotional problems
	Vitality, energy, fatigue
	General health perceptions
Time to adminster	1–10 minutes: telephone interview[a]
	5 minutes: self-administered
Reliability	Well-studied: 0.90
Preference-based	No

[a]Elderly may require 15 minutes.

high—greater than 0.80—for all eight scales. Test–retest reliability is also high for all scales. Correlations of the SF-36 with other functional status measures are summarized by Ware et al. (1993). The main advantage of the SF-36 is the ease of administration and the extensiveness of the documentation of its validity and reliability. Table 8-3 describes some of the most important features of the SF-36.

Quality of Well-Being Scale (QWB)

The QWB (Kaplan and Anderson 1988) assesses health status by asking about symptoms and level of function in three areas—mobility, physical activity, and social activity. These ratings are linked with weights that were derived from a general population sample to yield a single index, scaled from 0.0 to 1.0, that represents a judgment about the social undesirability of the overall problem. Unlike the SIP and the SF-36, the scaled QWB values can used in economic analysis to estimate quality-adjusted life expectancy.

The QWB is an interviewer-administered instrument, although a self-administered version is being developed. The amount of time it takes for an interviewer to administer varies according to the respondent's health, ranging from 7 to 20 minutes.

The reliability of the preference weights has been shown to be 0.90 (Kaplan and Bush 1982). Information on the sensitivity of the QWB to changes in health and correlations with other measures of functional status are summarized by McDowell and Newell (1996).

The QWB has been criticized mainly for its focus on the physical dimensions of health status and function. The methods for deriving the weights used to score the data so that they can be scaled from 0.0 to 1.0 are also criticized. Table 8-4 describes some of the most important features of the QWB.

EuroQol Quality of Life Scale (EuroQol)

The EuroQol (EuroQol Group 1990; Essink-Bot et al. 1993) was developed beginning in the late 1980s by a multinational group. The goal of the group was development of a simple measure of general health that would provide a single index value of health status. The 1993 version of the EuroQol covers five dimensions of health: mobility, self-care, usual activities, pain/discomfort, and anxiety/depression. Respondents rate themselves in each one of three mutually exclusive categories (no problem, some problem, major problem) for each dimension, leading to 243 distinct health states. Two states for death and unconsciousness are added. The ratings are scored to yield a single index of health status, scaled from 0.0 to 1.0. The scoring algorithm is based on values assigned to each of the 245 health states derived from interviews of a large and representative national sample of adults in Great Britain. The instrument was designed so that it can be self-administered. It takes only 2–3 minutes to complete. Test–retest reliability has been reported to be 0.85–0.90 (Van Agt et al. 1994).

Measuring Preferences for Health States

Preference-based measures of health status are necessary to estimate quality-adjusted life expectancy. The methods that are used most often to measure preferences for health states are the standard gamble, the time trade-off, and direct scaling methods.

The standard gamble involves having raters choose between two alternatives. One alternative has a certain outcome and one alternative involves a

Table 8-4. Important Features of the Quality of Well-Being Scale (QWB)

Major Category	Description
Domains assessed	Mobility
	Physical activity
	Social activity
	Symptoms
Time to administer	20 minutes
Reliability	Preference weights: 0.90–0.95
Preference-based	Yes, using weights derived from population-based sample

gamble. The certain outcome is the health state to be rated. The gamble has two possible outcomes—the best health state (usually complete health), which is described as occurring with a probability, p; or an alternative state, the worst state (usually death), which is described as occurring with a probability of $1 - p$. The probability, p, is varied until the rater is indifferent between the indifferent between the alternative that is certain and the gamble that might bring the better health state. The gamble is repeated for all of the health states that are to be rated. The points of indifference associated with each health state are the values used in the scale of health preferences. Values from 0.0 to 1.0 are assigned to each health status, and these values are used to estimate quality-adjusted life expectancy.

The time trade-off method was developed as an alternative to the standard gamble by Torrance et al. (1972). The time trade-off also presents the rater with a choice. The choice is between two alternatives that both have a certain outcome. Raters are asked to value a choice of being in a less desirable health state for a longer time followed by death compared with being in a more desirable state for shorter period of time followed by death. The time in the less desirable state is decreased to the point of indifference between a longer period of time in the less desirable state and the shorter period of time in the more desirable state.

Both the standard gamble and the time trade-off methods are difficult to apply. For this reason, direct scaling methods are used commonly to derive preferences. The most used direct scaling methods are interval scaling, category rating, and magnitude estimation (Froberg and Kane 1989). Interval scaling starts by depicting the scale as a line on a page with clearly defined end-points called anchors. The rater identifies the best and worst health states and places these at the anchor points. The rater then rates the preference for each health state by placing each state at a point on the line between the anchors. In category rating, raters sort the health states into a specified number of categories, and equal changes in preference between adjacent categories are assumed to exist. In magnitude estimation, the rater is given a "standard" health state and asked to indicate, with a number or a ratio, how much better or worse each health state is compared with the standard.

Statistical Issues in Outcomes Research: Risk Adjustment and Predictive Modeling

Most outcomes research studies are nonexperimental. Although these studies take advantage of "natural experiments," the possibility that differences in outcomes might be due to differences in patients' characteristics or factors other than the intervention or unit of care cannot be dismissed. Risk adjustment aims to take confounding into account. When outcomes research involves the comparison of the effectiveness of an intervention in one or more groups of patients, risk adjustment is directly analogous to adjustment for confounders in traditional risk factor epidemiology. In this case, the approaches to identification of confounders are the same as in traditional epidemiologic studies. The models used to control for confounders and the software packages used to operationalize the statistical approach are identical in outcomes research and in traditional epidemiology. Logistic regression, proportional hazards models, linear and categorical regression are all applicable in outcomes research that compares the effectiveness of interventions.

The goals of risk adjustment when comparing outcomes among institutions or other units of observation are the same as the goals when adjusting for confounders in traditional epidemiology—to take into account differences in the characteristics of patients treated at different institutions or by different providers. The risk adjustment methodologies used in comparisons of outcome among hospitals often involve "predictive modeling." This is directly analogous to indirect standardization of rates. A detailed technical explanation of predictive modeling as it is applied to compare hospitals and physicians is beyond the scope of this chapter. The interested reader is referred to Iezzoni (1994a,b) and Blumberg (1986).

In predictive modeling, models aimed at predicting outcome based on patient characteristics are developed based on large databases of historical data. Modeling approaches familiar to epidemiologists, such as logistic regression, are often used at this stage. The model results are then applied to data from an institution or another unit of analysis (e.g., surgeon) to calculate the expected outcome for individual patients seen at each institution (or managed by each surgeon) based on adjustment for the characteristics of patients. The number of outcome events predicted by the model based on patient characteristics are summed across all patients for the given unit of analysis. The ratio of the observed to expected number of events is computed. This yields a ratio (O/E) of observed to expected events that is the same as an indirectly standardized mortality ratio. Since the number of outcome events is often small for any single unit of observation, the comparison of the number of observed to the number of expected outcomes is usually "corrected" for small sample size. This step is not taken in analysis of SMRs in traditional epidemiology because the number of events in most studies that use SMRs is large.

The SMR for each unit of observation can be multiplied by the rate in the whole study population to yield an indirectly standardized rate. More often further analysis on the calculated ratios is carried. The results of the application of the predictive model are also used to rank hospitals or other units of analysis by the deviation of their expected from observed outcomes, taking into account sample size.

The results of the analysis after risk adjustment are used in many ways. Ranks based on the model may be used to identify outliers, which then become the target for quality improvement efforts. The characteristics of "outlier" hospitals may be described to try to identify commonalities among them. Factors associated with the standardized rate or the rank, such as surgical volume (e.g., Hannan et al. 1991; Showstack et al. 1987; Luft et al. 1990), might be explored. Decisions about how to allocate resources or which hospitals to award contracts are often made based on these kinds of analyses. The risk-adjusted ranks have also been used as a "report card" comparing institutions or providers (New York State Department of Health 1992; Pennsylvania Health Care Cost Containment Council 1991).

More than a dozen tools that use information from hospital discharge abstracts and/or medical records to measure severity of illness and comorbidity in hospitalized patients in order to adjust for risk have been developed. These tools include MedisGroups (Steen et al. 1993), Disease Staging (Gonella et al. 1984; Markson et al. 1991; Naessens et al. 1992), and the All Patient Refined Diagnosis Related Groups (3M 1993). The tools are mostly proprietary, and they are marketed widely to hospitals, payers, and governments.

Problems that arise in adjustment for confounding and in model building in traditional epidemiology apply equally to risk adjustment and predictive modeling as they are used in outcomes research. These problems include limitations due to missing and inaccurate data on measured confounders, failure to identify confounders, small sample size, and model misspecification. Steen (1994) describes the particular challenges of predictive modeling in outcomes research. Iezzoni et al. (1995) show that four different widely used methods for estimating the probability of death in hospitalized patients (MedisGroups, APACHE III, APR-DRGs, and Disease Staging) are poorly correlated with each other. The risk adjusted measures of expected mortality also differed in their ability to predict observed mortality, illustrating the challenges of risk adjustment in outcomes research.

Data Sources in Outcomes Research

Administrative Data

Outcomes research often uses administrative or billing data or other routinely collected clinical data. Using administrative data that has already been collected is attractive to outcomes researchers because there are no costs associated with collecting the data, because the number of people or events included in administrate databases is often large, and because the data are often "population-based." The Medicare claims data, for example, represent essentially the entire US population older than 65.

Administrative data were not, however, collected for the purposes of research. Quality control of coding and data entry rarely achieve the levels achieved in data collection efforts done specifically for research. The completeness and accuracy of data elements in administrative databases are almost never as good as in planned research. The sheer volume of data collected routinely in health care settings makes assurance of the completeness and accuracy of each element difficult.

Administrative data may contain errors that are familiar to epidemiologists because these errors are common concerns in data collected specifically for research (e.g., missing values, miscodes, out-of-range values). In addition, nuances of coding and data collection that are not under control of the outcomes researcher and that may not be documented have the potential to seriously distort analyses based on administrative data. A 1988 editorial in the *New England Journal of Medicine* (Caper 1988) drew attention to a threefold difference in the rate of coronary artery bypass surgery between La Jolla, California, and Palo Alto, California, that had been found in an analysis of practice variation based on administrative data on hospitalizations. The difference in CABG rates was used to illustrate the irrationality of allocation of health resources. In a subsequent letter to the editor, Cherry et al. (1988) pointed out that the billing office of the large hospital carrying out CABG procedures in La Jolla assigned all members of the Kaiser Permanente Medical Care Program undergoing surgery to the La Jolla residential zip code regardless of their true residence. When data were recoded to their true address, the difference in CABG rates between La Jolla and Palo Alto disappeared.

Billing data and other administrative data used to reimburse hospitals and physicians are subject to a problem that is not familiar to epidemiologists, called "upcoding"—in which codes for conditions that do not exist or for a more serious form of the illness (e.g., myocardial infarction for ischemia) are recorded. "Upcoding" is a concern when hospitals or physicians are paid more for more complex cases or where there are other financial incentives to overstate the severity of the patient's illness. For example, the DRG payment is higher for a hospital admission for a patient with acute myocardial who has hypertension, diabetes, and congestive heart failure than for an admission for myocardial infarction in a patient with no comorbidities. This may tempt the coder (who is paid by the hospital) to include a code for diabetes in a patient who may have only glucose intolerance. When some hospitals are more likely to upcode than others, risk adjustment based on hospital discharge codes as indicators of comorbidity is treacherous.

As the outcomes research movement has matured, the serious limitations of administrative data have become increasingly apparent. Marklan et al. (1994) describe the waning of the initial enthusiasm of researchers involved in the Agency for Health Care Policy and Research's initial PORT (Patient Outcomes Research Team) project concerning use of Medicare claims data for outcomes research. Problems identified included a limited range of information about the patient's condition at the time of treatment, failure to code the side of bilateral anatomic structures (e.g., hips, eyes, knees), inability to identify patients whose illness was untreated (e.g., patients with symptoms of gallbladder disease not treated with surgery), and failure to record information on services not covered by Medicare (e.g., use of outpatient drugs).

Experience using administrative data for outcomes research shows that this kind of research is not done by "pushing a button." It is much more difficult to make sense of data of uncertain completeness and accuracy than it is to make sense of "research quality" data.

Data Collected Routinely During Clinical Care

The problems of incomplete or inaccurate data in administrative databases can be ameliorated by supplementing the information collected routinely during clinical care with information recorded in charts. Chart review is, however, expensive and time-consuming. Some information critical to proper interpretation of a comparison between patients cared for in hospitals (e.g., income, ethnicity, smoking) may not be recorded in charts. Finally, there is no protocol for the recording of information in medical records. Providers may differ in their threshold for recording whether the patient had a comorbid condition or may use different criteria to make a diagnosis.

Data Quality and the Results of Outcomes Research Studies

Evaluations of the agreement between administrative data and chart data have been done. Hartz and Kuhn (1994) showed that only 59% of major complications recorded in clinical charts were recorded in the administrative data from hospital discharge records. When hospital ranks based on risk adjustment using administrative data were compared with hospital ranks based on chart review, the coefficients of correlation between hospital rank and mortality, major complications, and any complication were not statistically significant (Table 8-5). In the case of any complication, the correlation coefficient was negative (Table 8-5).

Table 8-5. For Three Outcomes, Hospital Ranks Based on Risk Adjustment Using Administrative Data Compared with Chart Review

Hospital	Mortality		Major Complication		Any Complication	
	Administrative Data Rank	Chart Review Rank	Administrative Data Rank	Chart Review Rank	Administrative Data Rank	Chart Review Rank
A	1	2	2	1	5	10
B	2	4	1	2	1	4
C	3	3	10	3	9	2
D	7	7	5	7	2	7
E	4	10	3	8	4	9
F	6	6	6	6	3	1
G	10	8	7	9	6	8
H	9	9	8	10	8	3
I	5	5	4	4	7	5
J	8	1	9	5	10	6
Rank correlation	0.48		0.21		−0.14	
p	>0.05		>0.05		>0.05	

Source: Hartz and Kuhn (1994).

Summary

Outcomes research uses observational study designs that are the same as the observational designs used in traditional epidemiology. Outcomes research studies often require primary data collection that entails designing chart review forms and survey instruments, determining appropriate sample size, deciding on a sampling frame, and supervising data collection. These are all components of traditional epidemiologic research.

When outcomes research does not involve primary data collection, it usually involves analysis of computer-stored data collected for other purposes. These analyses often use the same software packages and statistical models as those used in traditional risk factor epidemiology. Finally, an understanding of confounding and of statistical approaches to control for confounding are critical to outcomes research just as they are essential in traditional epidemiology.

Outcomes research is closely related to the measurement of quality. The line between outcomes research and performance measurement is not a sharp one. In this book, performance measurement is used to refer to activities designed to compare health plans, hospitals, and communities in terms of indicators of the quality of health care. Outcomes research is used to refer to attempts to contribute to generalizable knowledge about the effectiveness of interventions. Because economic outcomes are often assessed in outcomes research studies, there is also direct overlap between outcomes research and cost analysis.

CASE STUDIES

Initial Antidepressant Choice in Primary Care

Background

Antidepressants that selectively inhibit serotonin reuptake (SRIs; e.g., Prozac) have captured popular attention (Kramer 1993), although randomized trials comparing SRIs with other classes of antidepressants do not show greater efficacy (i.e., relief of depression) for SRIs compared with tricyclic antidepressants (Song et al. 1993; Workman and Short 1993). SRIs have fewer adverse effects than tricyclic antidepressants (Stokes 1993), and treatment adherence may be higher (Song et al. 1993). However, SRIs are more expensive than tricyclic antidepressants. Thus, their advantages need to be weighed against their higher cost.

Simon et al. (1996) undertook a randomized trial comparing fluoxetine (Prozac) with imipramine and desipramine in primary care clinics of the Group Health Cooperative of Puget Sound, Washington, a group-model health maintenance organization. Depressed patients identified in primary care settings were screened to identify absolute contraindications to use of either fluoxetine or imipramine. They were then randomly assigned to initial treatment with one of the three drugs. All subsequent decisions regarding antidepressant management (initial dose, dosage changes, treatment discontinuation, specialty referral) were made by patients and the primary care physician. Outcomes assessed in the trial included relief of depression, health-related "quality-of-life" using the SF-36, side effects, and cost.

There were no differences in relief of depression between the three treatment groups. Patients on fluoxetine had significantly fewer adverse effects. There were no differences between the three groups for any of the eight subscales of the SF-36. The cost of fluoxetine was $100 higher than for the other two antidepressants but the fluoxetine group had lower visit costs, resulting in equal outpatient costs.

Key Questions

1. Was this randomized trial designed to evaluate the efficacy or the effectiveness of fluoxetine?

This study was a study of the *effectiveness* of fluoxetine. Studies of efficacy assess outcomes in ideal circumstances. They seek to determine whether the intervention works at all. Studies of effectiveness evaluate outcome in conditions of usual care. They are designed to determine whether the intervention works in real life.

2. What features of this trial distinguish it from an efficacy trial?

The first feature of this trial that distinguishes it from an efficacy trial is the nonrestrictive entry criteria. In the trial, only patients with absolute contraindications were excluded. Second, after randomization, all aspects management were relegated to the primary care physician. Finally, the study focused on a broad range of outcomes, including cost and quality of life, not just clinical outcomes (i.e., relief of depression and side effects of the drugs).

3. What is the cost per quality-adjusted life-year for fluoxetine treatment?

The SF-36 is a nonpreference-based measure of health status. It cannot be used to estimate quality-adjusted life expectancy.

4. Which antidepressant is best as a starting therapy for depressed patients in primary care?

A conclusion about which treatment is "best" depends on which outcome is considered to be the most important one. If relief of depression is the only outcome of interest, the three drugs are equivalent. If the SF-36 measure of "quality of life" is the outcome of interest, there is also no difference. The three treatments are equal in their net cost, although the cost of fluoxetine was higher. In settings where the cost of the drug is born by the patient and the savings accrue to the system, patients might prefer the drugs other than fluoxetine, whereas the system is neutral.

Fluoxetine had fewer side effects. Preference for initial starting therapy would depend on the value that the patient and the physician place on the lower side-effect profile. The fact that the lower rate of side effects from fluoxetine is not reflected by differences in scores on the SF-36 instrument is noteworthy. Generic measures of health status may be insensitive to changes in minor symptoms even though the symptoms might be bothersome to the patient.

Implications for Practice.

Randomized trials of the effectiveness of treatments can be useful guides to clinical policy by highlighting the trade-offs between various outcomes. Measures of general health status cannot be relied on exclusively to assess the effects of interventions on outcome. The SF-36 cannot be used to estimate quality-adjusted life expectancy because it is not a preference-based measure.

Regionalization and Outcome of Cardiac Surgery

Background

In some states (e.g., New York) and countries (e.g., Canada), because of a variety of public policies, cardiac surgery services have become regionalized. A number of studies have shown a relationship between higher volumes of coronary artery bypass surgery and lower mortality after taking clinical factors into account (Showstack et al. 1987; Hannan et al. 1991). Regionalization results in the delivery of cardiac surgery being done in a fewer number of high-volume facilities. The effect of such regionalization on access to care and on outcomes is of interest.

Grumbach et al. (1996) used computerized hospital discharge abstracts submitted to state agencies in New York and California and provincial health plans in Ontario, British Columbia, and Manitoba to ascertain all CABG procedures performed form 1987 through 1989. They linked information on patients' zip code or postal code to ascertain distance that patients lived from the hospital of surgery. Mortality was determined from the hospital discharge records. Information from the discharge records, including discharge codes, were used to risk-adjust mortality rates.

In New York and Canada, 60% of all CABGs were performed in hospitals performing 500 or more operations per year. In California, only 26% of CABGs were performed in hospitals performing this number of operations per year. In New York, California, and Canada, risk-adjusted mortality outcomes were lower in hospitals performing 500 or more procedures per year. In Canada, where the distance between hospitals performing CABGs was large, there was no difference in the population rate of CABG procedures. In California and New York, CABG rates were lower for populations living 100 miles or more from the nearest CABG hospital.

Key Questions

1. What is the design of this study?

This is a study of variations in practice. It seeks to draw generalizable conclusions about the organization of the delivery of health services and the outcomes of care. It is representative of studies of variations in practice in that it is based solely on computer-stored administrative data. It is also representative of this kind of study in that it used risk adjustment to try to take into account differences between patients managed at different hospitals.

2. What are the major limitations of this study?

The study ascertains only in-patient mortality. If discharge practices differ between hospitals of different sizes or between Canada and the United States, in-patient mortality may be biased. For example, if smaller hospitals are less likely to discharge patients early, in-patient mortality may be biased upward compared with hospitals with shorter lengths of stay.

Differences in risk that have not been measured could confound the relationship between hospital and mortality. Although the data were adjusted for measured differences, conclusions are dependent on the correctness of the adjustment model and the completeness of measurement of confounders.

The data on distance from residence to the hospital were based on ZIP code or postal code as recorded on the discharge record. This chapter gave an example where use of ZIP code recorded on routine records to assign a patient's residence can lead to erroneous conclusions (Cherry et al. 1988).

The study is based solely on computer-stored administrative data. The reliability and validity of important data elements used in the analysis, including the designation of person as having died in the hospital, are not established.

3. What are the advantages of using computer-stored administrative data in this analysis?

Analysis of computer-stored data is cheap because the data already exist. The administrative data are population based, covering virtually all CABG procedures in three large geographic areas. Because of the size of the administrative database, the number of fatal events is large.

4. What other outcomes should be studied to evaluate regionalization?

Patient satisfaction with care is a relevant outcome. The willingness of patients to trade higher mortality for shorter travel time and convenience could also be measured. The total cost of care taking into account the cost of travel and lost work time for family members is another outcome of interest (see Chapter 9).

Implications for Practice

Regionalization of some procedures may have beneficial effects on some outcomes. Computer-stored administrative records provide an important source of outcome data for evaluations of policies like regionalization.

SUGGESTED READINGS

Epstein RS, Sherwood LM. From outcomes research to disease management: a guide for the perplexed. Ann Intern Med 1996;124:832–837.

Iezzoni LI. Using risk-adjusted outcomes to assess clinical practice: an overview of issues pertaining to risk adjustment. Ann Thorac Surg 1994;58:1822–1826.

Marklan CW, Greene R, Cummings MA. Methodologic challenges and innovations in patient outcomes research. Med Care 1994;32:S13–21.

McDowell I, Newell C. Measuring Health. A guide to Rating Scales and Questionnaires. Second Edition. New York: Oxford University Press; 1996.

Naylor CD, Guyatt GH, for the Evidence-based Medicine Working Group. Users' guides to the medical literature. X. How to use an article reporting variations in the outcomes of health services. JAMA 1996;275:554–558.

Steen PM. Approaches to predictive modeling. Ann Thorac Surg 1994:58:1836–1840.

REFERENCES

All Patient Refined Diagnosis Related Groups. Definition Manual. Wallingford, CT: 3M Information Systems; 1993.

Bergner M, Bobbitt RA, Kressel S, Pollard WE, Gilson BS, Morris JR. The Sickness Impact Profile: conceptual formulation and methodology for the development of a health status measure. Int J Health Serv 1976;6:393–415.

Bergner M, Bobbitt RA, Carter WB, Gilson BS. The Sickness Impact Profile: development and final revision of a health status measure. Med Care 1981;19:787–805.

Blumberg MS. Risk adjusting health care outcomes: a methodologic review. Med Care Rev 1986;43:351–393.

Caper P. Solving the medical care dilema. N Engl J Med 1988;318:1535–1536.

Cherry JK, Carmichael DB, Shean FC, Ritt DJ. Inaccurate data in "Solving the health care dilemma." N Engl J Med 1988;319:800.

Daniel DM, Stone ML, Dobson BE, Fithian DC, Rossman DJ, Kaufman K. Fate of the ACL injured patient: a prospective outcome study. Am J Sports Med 1995;22:632–644.

De Bruin AF, De Witte LP, Stevens F, Diedericks JP. Sickness Impact Profile: the state of the art of a generic functional status measure. Soc Sci Med 1992;35:1003–1014.

Diabetes Control and Complications Trial Research Group. The effect of intensive diabetes treatment on the development and progression of long-term complications in diabetes mellitus: the Diabetes Control and Complications Trial. N Engl J Med 1993;329:977–986.

Donabedian A. The Methods and Findings of Quality Assessment and Monitoring: An Illustrated Analysis, Volume 3. Ann Arbor, MI: Health Administration Press; 1985; 286.

Epstein A. The outcomes movement—will it get us where we want to go? N Engl J Med 1990;323:266–269.

Epstein RS, Sherwood LM. From outcomes research to disease management: a guide for the perplexed. Ann Intern Med 1996;124:832–837.

Essink-Bot ML, Stouthard ME, Bonsel GJ. Generalizabiity of valuations on health states collected with the EuroQol questionniare. Heath Econ 1993;2:237–246.

EuroQol Group. EuroQol: a new facility for measurement of health-related quality of life. Health Policy 1990;16:199–208.

Feasley JC, ed. Health Outcomes for Older People: Questions for the Coming Decade. Washington, DC: Institute of Medicine, National Academy Press; 1996.

Foundation for Health Services Resarch. Health Outcomes Research: A Primer. Washington, DC: Foundation for Health Services Research; 1994.

Froberg DG, Kane RL. Methodology for measuring health-state preferences. II: scaling methods. J Clin Epidemiol 1989;42:459–471.

Gold MR, Siegel JE, Russell LB, Weinstein MC. Cost-Effectiveness in Health and Medicine. New York:Oxford University Press; 1996.

Gonnella JS, Hornbrook MC, Louis DZ. Staging of disease. A case-mix measure. JAMA 1984;251:637–644.

Greenfield S, Nelson EC. Recent developments and future issues in the use of health status assessment measures in clinical settings. Med Care 1992;30(Suppl):MS23–MS41.

Grumbach K, Anderson GM, Luft HS, Roos LL, Brook R. Regionalization of cardiac surgery in the United States and Canada: geographic access, choice, and outcomes. JAMA 1996;274:1282–1288.

Hannan EL, Kilburn H Jr, Bernard H, O'Donnell JE, Lukccik G, Shields EP. Coronary artery bypass surgery: the relationship between inhospital mortality rate and surgical volume after controlling for clinical risk factors. Med Care 1991;29:1094–1107.

Hartz AJ, Kuhn EM. Comparing hospitals that perform coronary artery bypass surgery: the effect of outcome measures and data sources. Am J Public Health 1994;84:1609–1614.

Hunt SM, McEwen J, McKenna SP. Measuring health status: a new tool for clinicians and epidemiologists. J R Coll Gen Pract 1985;35:185–188.

Iezzoni LI. Using risk-adjusted outcomes to assess clinical practice: an overview of issues pertaining to risk adjustment. Ann Thorac Surg 1994a;58:1822–1826.

Iezzoni LI. Risk Adjustment for Measuring Health Care Outcomes. Ann Arbor, MI: Health Administration Press; 1994b.

Iezzoni LI, Ash AS, Shwartz M, Daley J, Hughes JS, Mackiernan YD. Predicting who dies depends on how severity is measured: implications for predicting patient outcomes. Ann Intern Med 1995;123:763–770.

Kaplan RM, Anderson JP. A general health policy model: update and applications. Health Serv Res 1988;23:203–205.

Kaplan RM, Bush JW. Health-related quality of life measurement for evaluation research and policy analysis. Health Psychol 1982;1:61-80.

Kramer P. Listening to Prozac. New York, NY: Viking; 1993.

Litwin MS, Hays RD, Fink A, et al. Quality of life outcomes in men treated for localized prostate cancer. JAMA 1995;273:129–135.

Luft HS, Garnick DW, Mark DH, et al. Hospital Volume, Physician Volume, and Patient Outcomes: Assessing the Evidence. Ann Arbor, MI: Health Administration Press; 1990.

Marklan CW, Greene R, Cummings MA. Methodologic challenges and innovations in patient outcomes research. Med Care 1994;32:S13–21.

Markson LE, Nash DB, Louis DZ, Gonnella JS. Clinical outcomes management and disease staging. Evaluation Health Professions 1991;14:201–227.

McDowell I, Newell C. Measuring Health. A Guide to Rating Scales and Questionnaires. Second Edition. New York: Oxford University Press; 1996.

McHorney CA. Measuring and monitoring health status in elderly persons: practical and methodological issues in using the SF-36 Health Survey. Gerontologist 1996;36:571–593.

Naessens JM, Leibson CL, Krishan I, Ballard DJ. Contribution of a measure of disease complexity (COMPLEX) in prediction of outcome and charges among hospitalized patients. Mayo Clin Proc 1992;67:1140–1149.

Naylor CD, Guyatt GH, for the Evidence-based Medicine Working Group. Users' guides to the medical literature. X. How to use an article reporting variations in the outcomes of health services. JAMA 1996;275:554–558.

New York State Department of Health. Coronary Artery Bypass Grafting Surgery in New York State, 1989–1991. Albany: New York State Department of Health; 1992.

Nunnally JC. Psychometric Theory. New York: McGraw-Hill Book; 1967: 194–198.

Parkerson GR, Gehlbach SH, Wagner EH, James SA, Clapp NE, Muhlbaier LH. The Duke-UNC Health Profile: an adult health status instrument for primary care. Med Care 1981;19:806–828.

Pennsylvania Health Care Cost Containment Council. A Consumer Guide to Coronary Artery Bypass Graft Surgery. Harrisburg, PA: Health Care Cost Containment Council; 1991.

Petitti DB, Sidney S. Hip fracture in women: incidence, in-hospital mortality, and five-year survival probabilities in members of prepaid health plan. Clin Orthopaedics 1989;246:150–155.

Relman AS. Assessment and accountability: the third revolution in medical care. N Engl J Med 1988;319:1220–1222.

Showstack JA, Rosenfeld KE, Garnick DW, Luft HS, Schaffarzick RW, Fowles J.

Association of volume with outcome of coronary artery bypass graft surgery: scheduled vs. nonscheduled operations. JAMA 1987;257:785–789.

Simon GE, VonKorff M, Heiligstein JH, et al. Initial antidepressant choice in primary care. JAMA 1996;275:1897–1892.

Song F, Freemantle N, Sheldon T, et al. Selective serotonin reuptake inhibitors: meta-analysis of efficacy and acceptability. BMJ 1993;306:683–687.

Spilker B, ed. Quality of Life and Pharmacoeconomic Clinical Trials. Philadelphia, PA: Lippincott-Raven; 1995.

Steen PM. Approaches to predictive modeling. Ann Thorac Surg 1994;58:1836–1840.

Steen PM, Brewster AC, Bradbury RC, Estabrook E, Young JA. Predicted probabilities of hospital death as a measure of admission severity of illness. Inquiry 1993;30:128–141.

Stokes PE. Fluoxetine: a five-year review. Clin Ther 1993;15:216–243.

Torrance GW, Thomas WH, Sackett DL. A utility maximization model for evaluation of health care programs. Health Serv Res 1972;7:118-133.

Van Agt HM, Essink-Bot ML, Krabbe PF, Bonsel GJ. Test-retest reliability of health state evaluations collected with the EuroQol questionnaire. Soc Sci Med 1994;39:1537–1544.

Ware JE, Sherbourne CD. The MOS 36-item Short-Form Health Survey (SF-36). I. Conceptual framework and item selection. Med Care 1992;30:473–483.

Ware JE Jr, Snow KK, Kosinski M, et al. SF-36 Health Survey: Manual and Interpretation guide. Boston, MA: The Health Institute, New England Medical Center; 1993.

Wennberg JE, Gittlesohn A. Health care delivery in Maine. I. Patterns of use of common medical procedures. J Maine Med Assoc 1975;66:123–130.

Wennberg JE, Bunker JP, Barnes B. The need for assessing the outcome of common medical procedures. Annu Rev Public Health 1980;1:277–295

Workman EA, Short DD. Atypical antidepressants versus imipramine in the treatment of major depression: a meta-analysis. J Clin Psychiatr 1993;54:5–12.

World Health Organization. Constitution of the World Health Organization. Basic Documents. Geneva, Switzerland: WHO; 1948.

9

Economic Evaluation

DIANA B. PETITTI

Economic evaluation of health care has become an increasingly important tool to guide decision-making in applied settings. Employers are demanding greater accountability for expenditures for health care on behalf of their employees. The federal government is struggling to contain health care expenditures to balance the federal budget and maintain the solvency of the Medicare trust fund. Local and state policy-makers, both in public health and health care settings, are operating within fixed budgets that make it impossible to offer everything that modern health care can deliver.

Economic evaluation requires skills in decision analysis and in economics as well as an understanding of study design. Some kinds of economic evaluation require skills in psychometrics. Interpretation of the results of economic evaluations often raises complex moral and ethical issues. It is impossible to cover the topic of economic evaluation of health care comprehensively in one chapter. There are several excellent textbooks (Warner and Luce 1982; Drummond et al. 1987; Haddix et al. 1996; Gold et al. 1996) devoted solely to the technical details of economic evaluation of health programs. The book by Gold et al. (1996), based on the deliberations of an expert panel on cost-effectiveness analysis appointed by the US Public Health Service, presents an explicit set of guidelines for the conduct of cost-effectiveness analysis for health and medicine. It is particularly recommended. A short summary of these recommendations is also useful (Weinstein et al. 1996).

This chapter presents an introduction to economic evaluation of health interventions that allows the reader to distinguish the basic types of economic evaluation. It presents the most detail on cost-effectiveness analysis, because cost-effectiveness analysis is done most often to assess health care interventions. Estimation of cost, which is central to economic analysis, is also described. The incorporation of preference-based measures of health status to estimate quality-adjusted life expectancy for use in cost-utility analysis is described. Finally, some of the limitations of economic evaluation are discussed especially as they apply to decision-making in public health agencies.

Definitions

Types of Economic Evaluation

Most authors (O'Brien 1995; Epstein and Sherwood 1996) describe four main types of economic valuation—cost-minimization analysis, cost-benefit analysis, cost-effectiveness analysis, and cost-utility analysis. The assumption and questions addressed in these four kinds of economic evaluation are summarized briefly in Table 9-1.

There is substantial overlap between the types of studies shown in Table 9-1. Cost-minimization analysis, cost-benefit analysis, and cost-effectiveness analysis all compare the cost of alternative interventions. In cost-minimization analysis, the effectiveness of the interventions is assumed or has been shown to be the same, and only the cost difference in the interventions is determined. A cost-minimization analysis asks the question, "Which intervention is least expensive given that they are equally effective?" Both cost-effectiveness analysis and cost-benefit analysis compare decision options in terms of their monetary cost, assuming that the interventions differ in their nonmonetary outcomes.

In cost-benefit analysis, all of the consequences of the decision options are valued in monetary terms. Cost-benefit analysis addresses the question, "What is the overall economic trade-off between the interventions?" In cost-effectiveness analysis, at least some of the consequences of the decision options are valued in nonmonetary terms, such as lives saved, years of life saved, or disability avoided. Cost-effectiveness analysis asks the question, "What is the comparative cost of the two interventions per outcome?" Studies of the cost of interventions per year of quality-adjusted life expectancy are cost-

Table 9-1. Types of Health Economic Evaluations

Type of Analysis	*Assumption/Question Addressed*
Cost-minimization	The effectiveness (or outcome) of two or more interventions is the same. Which intervention is the least costly?
Cost-benefit	The effectiveness (or outcome) of two or more interventions differs. What is the economic trade-off between interventions when all of the costs and benefits of the intervention and its outcome are measured in monetary terms?
Cost-effectiveness	The effectiveness of two or more interventions differs. What is the comparative cost per unit of outcome for the intervention?
Cost-utility	The question is the same as for cost-effectiveness analysis. The outcome is a preference measure that reflects the value patients or society places on the outcome

Source: Epstein and Sherwood (1996).

utility analyses. Cost-effectiveness and cost-utility analysis are identical except that the effectiveness measure used in a cost-utility analysis is one that reflects societal or individual preferences for the outcomes.

There is also overlap between these types of economic evaluation studies and outcomes research. Economic outcomes are often included as a component of an outcomes research study. A cost-effectiveness or cost-utility analysis can be an explicit component of a health outcomes research study. Information that is used in cost-utility analysis is often collected as a part of an outcomes research study.

Cost-of-illness studies are sometimes identified as a fifth type of economic evaluation study. The goal of a cost-of-illness study is to estimate the total societal costs of caring for persons with an illness compared with persons without the illness without reference to a specific alternative intervention. A cost-of-illness study asks the question, "What is the economic cost of caring for persons with this illness compared with persons free of the illness?"

Cost-Benefit Analysis Versus Other Types of Economic Evaluation

In cost-benefit analysis all of the consequences of interventions are valued in monetary terms. For example, in a cost-benefit analysis of renal dialysis, a dollar value is assigned to a life saved by providing this treatment. In a cost-benefit analysis of a worksite injury reduction program, a dollar value is placed on the pain and suffering prevented by the program.

Assigning a monetary value to human life or to pain and suffering is a difficult task. There are several ways it can be done. These methods can be classified into two groups—human capital approaches and willingness-to-pay approaches. When human capital approaches assign a monetary value to life, the monetary value of the life of a person who is economically productive, such as a working man, is higher than the monetary value of the life of a person who is not economically productive, such as a child, a retiree, or the disabled. Willingness-to-pay approaches do not have this problem.

Cost-benefit analysis has the advantage of allowing comparisons of disparate programs, such as programs to vaccinate children and building highways. These kinds of decisions are very important in making public policy decisions.

Cost-benefit analysis is, however, rarely used to address health issues for a number of reasons. Placing monetary values on many of the outcomes of health care is considered immoral by some even though it is based on rational methods. Analysts in health care are rarely deciding whether to vaccinate children or build highways. Rather, they are trying to find ways to maximize health given a fixed number of health care dollars. Because cost-benefit analysis is seldom used in public health and health care settings, it will not be discussed further in this chapter. The interested reader should consult Sugden and Williams (1990) and Warner and Luce (1982) for details on the conduct of cost-benefit analysis.

Cost-effectiveness and cost-utility analysis are used with increasing frequency in public health and health care settings. Most of the important methods and concepts applicable to cost-effectiveness studies are also applicable to cost of illness, cost-minimization, and cost-utility studies. When economic outcomes are a component of an outcomes research project, the analysis usually includes cost-effectiveness analysis and/or cost-utility analysis. Because of the importance of cost-effectiveness analysis and the broadness of the application of the principles of economic analysis illustrated by cost-effectiveness analysis, the remainder of this chapter will mainly address cost-effectiveness and cost-utility analysis.

When Is an Intervention "Cost-Effective?"

The term "cost-effective" is often misused (Doubilet, et al. 1986). An intervention is sometimes called cost-effective in the absence of data on both cost and effectiveness. The term is misused as a synonym for effectiveness in the absence of information on cost. The term is sometimes restricted to situations where the intervention is cost saving relative to its alternatives. None of these uses of the term cost-effective is correct.

In health applications, the term cost-effective should be used when an intervention *provides a benefit at an acceptable cost* (Doubilet, et al. 1986). An intervention is deemed cost-effective if it meets at least one of three criteria (Doubilet, Weinstein, and McNeil 1986). First, an intervention is cost-effective when is less costly and at least as effective as its alternative. Second, an intervention is cost-effective when is more effective and more costly, but the added benefit is "worth" the added cost. Third, an intervention is cost-effective when it is less effective and less costly, and the added benefit of the alternative is not "worth" the added cost. Interventions that are cost saving are cost-effective (Warner and Luce 1982).

Average Versus Incremental Cost-Effectiveness

Cost-effectiveness is measured as a ratio of cost to effectiveness. An *average* cost-effectiveness ratio and an *incremental* or *marginal* cost-effectiveness ratio should be distinguished (Detsky and Naglie 1990). An average cost-effectiveness ratio is estimated by dividing the cost of the intervention by a measure of effectiveness without regard to its alternatives. An incremental or marginal cost-effectiveness ratio is an estimate of the cost per unit of effectiveness of switching from one intervention to another, or the cost of using one intervention in preference to another.

In estimating an incremental or marginal cost-effectiveness ratio, both the numerator and denominator of the ratio represent differences between the alternative interventions (Weinstein and Stason 1977):

$$\text{Difference in cost} \ / \ \text{Difference in effectiveness}$$

where

$$\text{Difference in cost} = \text{Cost of the intervention} - \text{Cost of the alternative}$$

and

$$\text{Difference in effectiveness} = \text{Effectiveness of the intervention} \\ - \text{Effectiveness of the alternative}$$

Cost-effectiveness analysis should almost always estimate an incremental or marginal cost-effectiveness ratio. Estimating an average cost-effectiveness ratio is not generally useful (Detsky and Naglie 1990). The unspecified implicit alternative to an intervention is usually doing nothing. But doing nothing has costs and effects that should be taken into account in the analysis (Detsky and Naglie 1990). Furthermore, explicit declaration of "doing nothing" as the alternative intervention helps to frame discussions of the desirability of the intervention.

Perspective

It is important to define perspective in a cost-effectiveness analysis. Costs are seen differently from different perspectives. For example, the cost of vaccinating children against chickenpox from the perspective of a health department or health care organization is the cost of providing the service (which includes the price paid to purchase the vaccine and the labor costs to give the vaccine), the costs of the building in which the services are provided, and other overhead costs. In contrast, the cost of vaccination from the perspective of the family whose child receives the vaccine is the amount they pay out of pocket for the vaccine, the cost of travel to location where the vaccine is given, the cost of parking, and the cost of lost wages because of missed work. The cost of vaccination from the perspective of the child is the cost of pain from receiving the injection and the cost of missed daycare or school. The societal perspective encompasses all of these costs.

The perspective of a cost-effectiveness analysis should be stated explicitly, because the perspective determines which costs should be included in the analysis and what economic outcomes are considered as benefits. The usual perspectives in cost-effectiveness analysis are the societal perspective and the program perspective. An analysis that takes the societal perspective seeks to determine the total costs of the intervention to all payers for all persons. Analyses that take a program perspective are more heterogeneous in their aims. An analysis that takes the program perspective might, for example, address the question of the immediate cost of an intervention and its outcome in order to compare it with other interventions and outcomes for the same condition. It might seek to determine whether coverage for the intervention would save money for the program in the long run. An intervention might save money for the program but not, in the long run, for society. For example, deciding *not* to provide a costly preventive service for young persons who are insured by a company might save money for the program if the consequence of failing to provide the service is an event that occurs when the person is old and covered by another kind of health insurance.

It is generally agreed that cost-effectiveness studies done by public health agencies to evaluate programs done to affect the health of populations should take the societal perspective (Gold et al. 1996; Haddix et al. 1996).

Contributors to Cost

Overview

The economic concept of opportunity cost is central to cost-effectiveness analysis. The opportunity cost of a resource is its total value in another use. When a public health agency spends money to provide health care, this money is not available for housing, education, highway construction, space programs, or as a reduction in income taxes. When a health care organization spends money for bone marrow transplantation, this money is not available for mammography outreach, enhanced prenatal care, or as a reduction in the premium charged to employers or individuals for health care. When an elderly man spends time being vaccinated for influenza, this time is not available to play golf. An overall goal conceptual goal in cost-effectiveness analysis is comprehensive identification of all of the costs of the intervention and its alternative, including all of the opportunity costs.

Definitions

The terms used to describe the contributors to cost (e.g., direct cost, production cost, indirect cost, opportunity cost) are used in different ways in different textbooks and in published cost-effectiveness analyses. The use of these terms is confusing and contradictory, and one term may be used for different concepts by different authors. The term "indirect" cost is especially trouble-some because it has a common meaning as an accounting term which is very different from its use by those who conduct cost-effectiveness analysis. Table 9-2 gives the definitions of key cost terms in cost-effectiveness analysis as they are used in this chapter. Others use different terms for the same concepts. An understanding of the concepts underlying each term is more important than the choice of terms.

Total Direct Cost

Total direct cost includes the cost of all the goods, services, and other re-sources that are consumed in the provision of an intervention or in dealing with the side effects of the intervention or other current or future conse-quences of the intervention (Gold et al. 1996). Identification of the contribu-tors to total direct cost should be exhaustive. This is one of the most impor-tant challenges in a cost-effectiveness analysis. Only when all of the contributors to total direct cost have been enumerated can reasoned decisions about which costs to include in the analysis be made and justified.

There are several categories of cost that should be considered as possible contributors to total direct cost. These are described in Table 9-3. The first category of total direct cost is direct health care cost. There are a number of possible contributors to direct health care costs. These include tests, drugs, supplies, personnel, and equipment. Rent and depreciation, space prepara-tion and maintenance, utilities, other support services, and administrative support services needed to produce the intervention are also counted as a direct health care cost. Induced costs should be included. Induced costs include costs due to added (or averted) treatments or tests attributable to the intervention. For example, the cost of visits to the emergency department to care for children who have fever as a result of being vaccinated for chickenpox are induced costs of a vaccination program.

The second category of total direct cost is direct non–health care cost. These costs include, for example, the cost to patients to partake of the inter-

Table 9-2. Definition of Terms Used to Describe Various Components of Cost in this Chapter

Term	Definition
Opportunity cost	Total value of a resource in another use
Total direct cost	The cost of all goods, services, and other resources that are consumed in the provision of an intervention or in dealing with the side effects of the intervention or other current or future consequences of the intervention
Indirect cost	Monetary value of lost wages and productivity due to morbidity and death

Table 9-3. Categories of Cost That Contribute to Total Direct Cost

Category	What Is Included
Direct health care costs	Tests, drugs, supplies, personnel, equipment Rent, depreciation, utilities maintenance Support services Costs (savings) due to added (averted) treatments attributable to intervention[a]
Direct non-health care costs	Costs to partake of the intervention
Informal caregiver costs	Monetary value of time of family members or volunteers to provide home care
Cost of patient time	Lost wages to partake of intervention Monetary value of time spent to partake of intervention

[a]Induced costs

vention (e.g., transportation, child care). In the example of a chickenpox vaccination program, the cost of a babysitter is a direct non–health care cost that should be included as a contributor to total direct cost.

The third category of total direct cost is the cost of informal caregiver time. This is the monetary value of the time of family members or volunteers who provide home care. The fourth category of total direct costs is the cost of the use of patient time.

Indirect Costs

Indirect costs are also called productivity costs (Gold et al. 1996). These costs include the monetary value of lost wages and productivity due to morbidity and death. Gold et al. (1996) provide cogent arguments that these costs are encompassed as health effects of the intervention and that they should not be valued monetarily. They state that a comprehensive measurement of effectiveness (quality-adjusted life-years) includes the ability to be productive. Exclusion of lost productivity from the numerator of cost will have a large impact on cost-effectiveness ratios for highly disabling and lethal conditions. In practice, cost-effectiveness analyses have rarely included the costs of lost productivity as direct costs in the numerator.

Measuring Cost

After the contributors to cost have been identified, they must be valued. Determining the correct monetary value for each contributors to cost can be difficult and time-consuming, especially if micro-costing methodologies are used (Gold et al. 1996; Haddix et al. 1996). Micro-costing involves the direct enumeration and costing out of every input consumed in the intervention. Micro-costing methodologies are described in detail by Gold et al. (1996) and, for prevention programs, by Haddix et al. (1996). They will not be discussed further in this chapter.

In practice, in evaluations of health interventions, gross-costing approaches are used most often. These approaches use estimates of cost that are large relative to the intervention (e.g., the average cost of a hospital day, the average cost of a physician visit). Fee schedules or data on average charges or payments for various services are often the source of these estimates. For example, the Medicare fee schedule is used to estimate cost for laboratory tests and outpatient services. The DRG payment for various conditions is used to estimate the cost of care for various hospitalized conditions. The average payment based on insurance outpatient records is used to estimate the cost of procedures.

Using charge or payment is usually correct when the perspective of the analysis is a program perspective, since payments and charges are true costs from the point of view of the program. For example, Medicare would likely save the amount projected in a cost analysis based on Medicare payment data. Elimination of coverage for a specified procedure would save an insurance company the amount projected from a cost analysis of that procedure based on the amount paid for that procedure.

Medicare reimbursement for various services is based on attempts to relate the procedures to a standardized scale of input to produce the service—a relative value unit. Furthermore, information on the cost-to-charge ratio is available for hospitalizations, and this can be used to adjust data on charges when conducting a cost analysis from the society perspective.

When the perspective of the cost-effectiveness analysis is not the societal perspective, using fee schedules and data on payment or charge as a substitute for cost can lead to unwarranted conclusions (Finkler 1982). Savings projected by using an inappropriate source of cost data may fail to materialize when the costs used in the analysis are not the true costs of the intervention or its consequence in that setting.

Discounting

Costs

Most people would prefer to receive $1 today rather than $1 a year from today because a dollar received today can be invested (or put in a savings bank) and will be worth more in a year than it is today. The preference for a dollar today is called the *time preference for money*. In economic analysis, the time preference for money necessitates *discounting* future costs. The necessity for discounting is particularly important in the economic evaluation of health programs because in most situations involving health not all of the costs of an intervention are incurred at a single point in time, and many of the monetary benefits of an intervention are reaped in the future. Discounting cost adjusts future costs and expresses all costs and monetary benefits of an intervention in terms of their present value.

The formula for discounting is as follows:

$$c_{present} = c_0 + c_1 / (1 + r)^1 + c_2 / (1 + r)^2 + \ldots c_n / (1 + r)^n$$

where $c_{present}$ is the cost in current dollars, r is the discount rate, and c_0, $c_1, \ldots c_n$ are costs in future years. Spreadsheet programs and business calculators will do discounting automatically.

The process of discounting at a positive rate gives greater weight to costs and monetary benefits the earlier they occur. High positive discount rates favor alternatives with costs that occur late.

Benefits

When discounting costs, most authors believe that nonmonetary health benefits (e.g., lives, years of life saved) should be discounted at the same rate, because the nonmonetary benefits are being valued relative to dollars (Weinstein and Fineberg 1980; Drummond et al. 1987; Keeler and Cretin 1983; Gold et al. 1996; Haddix et al. 1996). When costs are discounted and benefits are not discounted, for any program begun now, a delayed program that should be funded first can always be defined. Therefore, among an infinite set of programs of equal cost, no program with a finite starting date can be selected (Keeler and Cretin 1983). It is thus impossible to make a decision to begin a program based on its cost-effectiveness.

Choice of the Discount Rate

Although it is generally agreed that costs and benefits should be discounted and that costs and benefits should be discounted at the same rate, there is less agreement about the discount rate that should be used. The discount rate reflects the rate of return on investment, or, alternatively the rate of growth of the economy. There is, however, not a single rate of return on investment, and this rate, as well as the rate of growth of the economy, may vary over time. More important, the use of the private sector return for public sector program costs, such as the costs of a public health program, may not be correct (Sugden and Williams 1990).

An approach based on the "shadow price of capital" has gained support more recently. The expert panel commissioned by the US Public Health Service to make recommendations about the conduct of cost-effectiveness analysis in the evaluation of health care (Gold et al. 1996) based their recommendation on this approach, and they present a set of careful arguments for using this approach. The use of the shadow-price-of-capital approach led this group to recommend using a discount rate of 3% for economic evaluations involving public investment in health programs. However, most published cost effectiveness analyses use a discount rate of 5% in the "base case" or "reference case" analysis. In recognition of the use of discount rates of 5% in most published cost-effectiveness analyses, the panel also recommended an analysis using a discount rates of 5% in the base-case or reference-case analysis.

Quality-Adjusted Life-Years—an Outcome Measure in Cost-Effectiveness Analysis

Quality-adjusted life-years attempt to combine, in a single metric, expected increments in the quantity of life from an intervention with the effects on quality of life (LaPuma and Lawlor 1990). An analysis that uses quality-adjusted life-years seeks to evaluate the trade-off between mortality, morbidity, the preferences of patients and society for various types of morbidity, and the willingness of patients and society to accept a shortening of life to avoid certain morbidities. The incorporation of measures of quality of life into decision-making about allocation of resources is a cornerstone of the outcomes movement. The concept of the quality-adjusted life-year is explicit recognition that there are states of health for which people are willing to take a measurable risk of a bad outcome (usually death) to avoid.

Calculation of quality-adjusted life expectancy involves, first, the estimation of life expectancy and the amount of life spent in various health states. Second, it is necessary to measure the value that individuals or society place on the time spent in each health state. These two pieces of information are used to estimate quality-adjusted life-years by multiplying the amount of time spent in each health state by the measure of value for time spent in that health state.

Measuring Life Expectancy

Life expectancy is defined by actuaries as the average future lifetime of a person. It is usually estimated for persons of a specific age, sex, and race. Actuarial methods to estimate life expectancy are based on specialized statistical lifetable functions that rely on data on mortality rates specific for age, sex, and race. The age-, sex-, and race-specific mortality rates are based on death certificate data and census data.

In very rare cases, life expectancy for interventions has been compared directly in a randomized trial or in a follow-up study. In these rare cases, the empirically measured information on life expectancy from the relevant studies can be used directly.

More often, available information on life expectancy in persons with a disease is in the form of overall mortality rates, 5-year survival rates, or median survival. The available information on interventions consists of a measure of the relative risk or the odds of mortality in those who have the intervention compared with those who do not. These two pieces of information do not translate directly into information about life expectancy. For example, an intervention that halves the relative risk of death in a 5-year follow-up interval does not double life expectancy. The effect on life expectancy of a disease that increases 5-year survival is dependent on the age, sex, and race of the person, since life expectancy in the absence of the intervention is also dependent on these factors.

The estimation of life expectancy from information on overall mortality, 5-year survival, median survival, and the relative risk of death in a given interval can be done with actuarial methods using information on age-, sex-, and race-specific mortality. These actuarial methods are complex calculations, and they will not be described.

Beck et al. (1982a,b) described a simpler method for estimating life expectancy that requires only information on the age-, sex-, and race-specific life expectancy from a table of vital statistics and an estimate of the effect of the disease, treatment, or intervention on mortality. The method, called the declining exponential approximation of life expectancy (DEALE), has been shown to closely approximate estimates of life expectancy based on actuarial methods (Beck et al. 1982a).

Use of the DEALE assumes that survival follows a declining exponential curve. If this assumption is true, then life expectancy for a person of a given age, sex, and race can be estimated as the reciprocal of the mortality rate:

$$\text{Life expectancy} = 1 \,/\, \text{mortality}$$

For a person of a specific age, sex, and race, this relationship can be used to estimate mortality from published lifetables:

$$m_{asr} = 1 \,/\, le_{asr}$$

where m_{asr} is the average mortality rate of a person of a given age, sex, and rate and le_{asr} is the life expectancy of a person of a given age, sex, and race as described in published life tables.

If an intervention decreases mortality by an amount, m_i, then life expectancy for the person who has the intervention, le_i, is estimated as:

$$le_i = 1 \,/\, (m_{asr} - m_i)$$

When the goal of the analysis is to estimate the effect of a disease on life expectancy, the same method can be used. In this case, excess mortality from the disease, m_e, is added to the mortality rate specific for age, and race.

Excess mortality from various diseases and the effects of interventions on mortality per year are sometimes measured directly, and these equations are then directly applicable. More often, available information consists of overall mortality rate, life expectancy, 5-year survival, or median survival in persons with the disease or in those who had the intervention. These measures are all compound measures of mortality. They consist of baseline mortality—the mortality expected in the general population—plus either the excess mortality due to the disease or lower mortality due to the intervention. Before applying the DEALE, measures of compound mortality must be decomposed into baseline mortality and excess mortality (for diseases) or baseline mortality and saved mortality (for interventions). Methods to decompose different kinds of compound measures of mortality so that they can be used to estimate life expectancy using the DEALE are described in detail by Beck et al. (1982b), and they will not be described here.

Adjusting the Measure of Life Expectancy

The measurement of preferences for health states was discussed in Chapter 8. Application of these techniques results in assignment of a value to time spent in each health state. This value is often called Q. The Q factor for each health state is to adjust the life expectancy for each health state by multiplying the amount of time spent in each health state by the Q factor for that health state.

In the simplest case, the disease causes a consistent reduction in quality of life over all remaining years of life expectancy and the intervention returns quality of life to what it would have been in the absence of disease. Quality-adjusted life expectancy for those with the disease is calculated by multiplying life expectancy for those with the disease by Q. Quality-adjusted life expectancy for those with the intervention is calculated by multiplying life expectancy in the absence of the disease by 1.0. The difference between the two estimates is used as the denominator in the cost-effectiveness ratio.

Sensitivity Analysis

Sensitivity analysis evaluates the stability of the conclusions of an analysis relative to assumptions made in the analysis. It is a way of estimating the uncertainty in the analysis. When a conclusion is shown to be invariate to the assumptions, confidence in the validity of the conclusions of the analysis is enhanced. Sensitivity analysis also helps identify the most critical assumptions of the analysis.

In one-way sensitivity analysis, the assumed values of each variable in the analysis are varied, one at a time, while the values of the other variables in the analysis remain fixed. In one-way sensitivity analysis of a cost-effectiveness analysis, one-way sensitivity analysis should include varying the discount rate for costs and benefits while keeping the values of the other variables in the analysis fixed.

Threshold analysis is an extension of one-way analysis. In threshold analysis, the value of one variable is varied until the alternative interventions are found to have equal outcomes, and there is no benefit of one alternative over the other in terms of estimated outcome. The point at which there are equal outcomes is called the "break-even" point. Estimating the break-even cost can be used to decide how much should be paid for an intervention to make total expenditures for an intervention neutral.

In two-way sensitivity analysis, the expected outcome is determined for every possible combination of reasonable estimates of two variables, while the values of all of the other variables in the analysis are held constant at baseline. In three-way sensitivity analysis, the expected outcome is determined for combination of reasonable estimates of three variables, while the values of all of the other variables in the analysis are held constant at baseline. In *n*-way sensitivity analysis, the expected outcome is determined for every possible combination of every reasonable value of every variable. *N*-way sensitivity analysis is analogous to *n*-way regression.

A sensitivity analysis varying the discount rate should always be done. Most experts recommend a range that starts at zero and goes to 7% (Gold et al. 1996) or 8% (Haddix et al. 1996). Most other variables should be subjected to one-way sensitivity analysis. The most influential variables in the one-way sensitivity analysis should be subjected to two-way and three-way sensitivity analysis, although this is seldom done in practice.

Limitations of Cost-Effectiveness Analysis in Public Health and Health Care Settings

Cost Data

True measures of cost for particular settings are difficult to obtain. The use of charge data as a substitute for cost in such analyses can lead to unwarranted conclusions about efficiency (Finkler 1982). Thus, estimated "savings" may not materialize if the costs are overestimated.

Estimating true cost is especially difficult in public health settings. The cost of delivering services in these settings may be different from costs estimated from large national data sources. Most public health agencies have high fixed costs (e.g., buildings) and little flexibility in changing the labor pool. The cost of interventions may be higher when they are delivered in a public health settings, making the results of cost-effectiveness analysis done based on national estimates of cost invalid in practice. Cost savings estimated from elimination of a program may not materialize because of high fixed costs. In public health settings, the failure of projected savings to materialize may have serious political consequences because it may lead to a decision to not provide a service or to end a service that ultimately has no counterbalancing social good.

Problems With Life Expectancy and Quality-Adjusted Life Expectancy as Measures Used to Set Health Policy

Life expectancy in the absence of an intervention is a function of current age and sex and, in most populations, of race. When life expectancy is used as the measure of effectiveness, an intervention that prolongs life will have the smallest effect on the estimated gain in life expectancy in the group with the shortest life expectancy. Thus, the cost per year of life gained will be greatest in the group with the shortest life expectancy in the absence of the intervention. When cost-effectiveness evaluates a choice between alternative therapies—for example, a choice between two different types of pneumococcal vaccine in the elderly, this theoretical problem does not pertain. When, however, cost-effectiveness analysis is used to guide choices between an intervention for a person with a short life expectancy and similar interventions for persons with a longer life expectancy, use of life expectancy as an outcome will "discriminate" against the group whose life expectancy is shortest (Harris 1987). For example, a public health agency might be faced with a choice between funding a program to prevent falls in the elderly and a program to prevent auto crashes in adolescents. Even if the net costs of the programs (compared with doing nothing) are the same and the effectiveness of the programs is identical in terms of the number of lives saved, the program for adolescents will be more cost-effective in terms of years of life saved because the number of years of life available to be saved is greater for adolescents than for the elderly.

Quality-adjusted life-years can also be used in two ways—to choose between two interventions for the same group or in the same person, or to choose which intervention to use for different groups or which conditions to prioritize in the allocation of health resources. The use of quality-adjusted life-years to help guide choices between alternative interventions for a single patient and investments of society in one invention in preference to another intervention for the same condition is generally held to be useful (Smith 1987; Harris 1987). The use of estimates of quality-adjusted life-years to make decisions about interventions and about how to determine which patients to target for treatment is controversial. It has been called "positively dangerous and morally indefensible" by one author (Harris 1987) and based on "false premises, faulty reasoning, and unjust principles" by another (Rawles 1989).

Concerns about the justness and the morality of the use of quality-adjusted life-years to determine whom to treat are mostly concerns made in the context of their use in cost-utility analysis. Drummond (1987) points out that investing in the interventions that have the lowest cost per quality-adjusted life-year ignores the principle of equity (Drummond 1987). The use of quality-adjusted life-years to decide who to treat or what to pay for ignores what might be the choices of individuals, denying the ethical principle of autonomy, which is generally most important for individual patients, in favor of the principle of justice or fairness, which is generally most important for a community (LaPuma and Lawlor 1990). Since quality-adjusted life-years depend on life expectancy, using them discriminates against the aged and the disabled, because they have less life years to gain from an intervention (Harris 1987).

Value Judgments

Cost-effectiveness and cost-utility analysis do not resolve the ethical dilemmas of allocating scarce resources. Except when an intervention is cost saving, demonstration that it is "cost-effective" does not avoid difficult value judgments. There is no criterion that can be used to say, based on a cost-effectiveness analysis, that an intervention should be recommended. A decision to do something because it is "worth the added cost" is an ethical and moral, not an economic, judgment. Opinions about whether something is "worth" a certain amount of money are subject to variations in the perspective and the values of those making the judgment of worth. Judgments about whether added cost is "worth it" are subject to political forces.

The political problems that occur when cost-effectiveness analysis is used as the sole basis for allocating scarce resources are illustrated by the state of Oregon's Medicaid reform effort. In 1990–1991, Oregon attempted to set priorities for the allocation of Medicaid resources for its low income population based on cost-effectiveness analysis. The Oregon Health Services Commission generated a list of condition-treatment pairs ordered by their cost-effectiveness and then attempted to make funding decisions based on this ordering. The sole use of these cost-effectiveness ratios for resource allocation was ultimately rejected by the state of Oregon based on many criticisms (e.g., Hadorn 1991; Office of Technology Assessment [OTA] 1992). In the end, cost-effectiveness analysis was only one of 13 factors used to prioritize funding of services for the poor.

Tengs et al. (1995) compiled information from analyses that assessed the cost-effectiveness of life-saving interventions. Table 9-4 shows the estimated cost per year of life saved for some commonly accepted medical and public health interventions. There are large variations in the amount of money ex-

Table 9-4. Estimate Cost per Year of Life Saved for Life-Saving Interventions

Category	Description	Cost/Life Saved
Safety	Mandatory seat-belt use and child restraint laws	$ 98
	Smoke detectors in airplane lavatories	$ 30,000
	Flashing lights at rail-highway crossings	$ 42,000
Toxin control	Banning asbestos in roofing felt	$ 550,000
	South Coast of California ozone control program	$ 610,000
	Radionuclide emission control at Department of Energy facilities	$ 730,000
Medicine	Mammography every 3 years for women 60–65	$ 2,700
	Lovastatin for men 45–54 with no heart disease and cholesterol ≥300 mg ldl	$ 34,000
	Prophylactic AZT following needlestick injuries in health care workers	$ 41,000
	Misoprostol to prevent drug-induced gastrointestinal bleed	$ 210,000
	Intensive care for seriously ill patients with multiple trauma	$ 460,000
	Lovastatin for women 45–54 with no heart disease and cholesterol ≥300 mg ldl	$1,200,000

Source: Tengs et al. (1995).

pended per life saved for these accepted interventions. Thus, in practice, society makes decisions to allocate resources in ways that do not reflect their cost-effectiveness.

Ubel et al. (1996) did an empirical study in which prospective jurors, medical ethicists, and experts in medical decision analysis choose between two screening tests for a population at low risk of colon cancer. One test cost $200 per life saved; the other cost $181 per life saved. The second test was, therefore, more cost-effective because it saves more lives for the number of dollars spent. In the example, it would cost $200,000 to offer the first test to everyone—saving 1,000 lives. It would cost $400,000 to offer the second test to everyone—saving 2,200 lives. The subjects were posed with a hypothetical situation in which they could spend only $200,000 for screening. Within this budget, it would be possible to screen all of the population with the first test or half of the population with the second test. Using the first test in everyone would save 1,000 lives. Using the second test in half the population would save 1,100 lives. Fifty-six percent of the jurors, 53% of the ethicists, and 41% of the experts in medical decision analysis recommended offering the less effective screening test to everyone, in spite of the fact that this strategy was less cost-effective and saved 100 fewer lives. The authors concluded that their study illustrated people's discomfort with policies based on cost-effectiveness analysis, in keeping with the Oregon experience.

The counterarguments to the use of quality-adjusted life-years to decide who to treat and how to allocate resources focus on the seriousness of the dilemma of allocating resources and the lack of rational alternatives to cost-effectiveness analysis (Danford 1990; Kaplan and Ganiats 1990). "Rationing" is occurring already, it is argued, and cost-effectiveness analysis simply makes explicit the basis for decisions about how to allocate resources.

Russell et al. (1996), writing for the US Public Health Service Panel on Cost-Effectiveness in Health and Medicine (Russell et al. 1996), concluded that "no method of making decisions about health care resources allocation provides a complete procedure for resolving ethical issues." Cost-effectiveness analysis is, therefore, one of many inputs to decisions about resource allocation and clinical policy.

Summary

Cost-effectiveness and cost-utility analysis are closely related methods to evaluate cost as one outcome of medical care. These kinds of analysis are increasingly important tool to guide decision-making in applied settings in spite of their limitations and the technical difficulties of doing them in a way that assures their credibility. Cost evaluation is one of many inputs into decisions about resource allocation and clinical policy. A better understanding of the strengths and limitations of different kinds of cost evaluation, especially cost-effectiveness and cost-utility analysis, will enhance their usefulness.

CASE STUDY

Cost-Effectiveness of Incorporating Inactivated Poliovirus Vaccine Into the Routine Childhood Immunization Schedule

Background

Both inactivated poliovirus vaccine (IPV) and oral attenuated poliovirus vaccine (OPV) are highly effective. Use of polio vaccine has led to a dramatic decrease in poliomyelitis incidence in the United States. The advantages of OPV are ease of administration and, because there are no combination vaccines containing IPV, avoidance of pain from an additional injection. OPV is less costly than IPV and it confers greater immunity to indigenous wild-type virus. OPV causes vaccine-associated paralytic poliomyelitis (VAPP), which is sometimes fatal and often disabling. About 10 cases per year of VAPP occur in the United States.

Until 1995, the Advisory Committee on Immunization Practices (ACIP) of the US

Public Health Service recommended three doses of OPV at 2, 4, and 6 months of age and 6 to 18 months (primary series), with a supplemental dose of OPV at school entry. This recommendation was based on the ease of administration of OPV and continued concern about wild-type poliomyelitis.

In 1991, wild-type poliomyelitis was eradicated from the Western Hemisphere (deQuadros and Henderson 1993). The hemisphere was certified as polio free by an international commission in 1994 (Pan American Health Organization 1994). In addition, in the last decade, substantial progress has been made toward global eradication of poliomyelitis eradication. Because the importation of wild-type poliomyelitis is now considered low, one of the main advantages of OPV over IPV for childhood vaccination has been essentially eliminated.

The eradication of wild-type poliovirus and concern about VAPP cases led to reconsideration of the childhood immunization schedule. In 1995, the ACIP recommended a change in the poliomyelitis vaccination policy from four recommended doses of OPV to a sequential schedule using two doses of IPV followed by two doses of OPV. In 1996, Miller et al. (1996) published the results of a cost-effectiveness analysis comparing the old and new ACIP recommended poliomyelitis immunization schedules.

Key Questions

1. What is the appropriate perspective for a cost-effectiveness analysis comparing the old and the new immunization schedule?

Miller et al. (1996) took the societal perspective in their analysis. This is the appropriate perspective for an analysis that informs national policy aimed a maximizing the health and welfare of the total population. An analysis from the perspective of a health care organization might yield a different estimate of the cost-effectiveness of the new compared with old schedule because the price paid by the organization for vaccine and vaccine delivery might differ from the average societal cost and because the health care organization does not bear some of the costs of the program (e.g., travel costs).

2. In comparing the old and the new immunization schedules, what assumption should be made about the risk of wild-type poliovirus for the old and new poliomyelitis immunization schedules? How would one assess the importance of this assumption in the cost-effectiveness analysis?

Miller et al. (1996) assumed that the risks of wild-type virus are the same for the new and old vaccination schedules. A major argument for the old (4 OPV) schedule is protection against wild type virus. If the new (2 IPV, 2 OPV) schedule carries a risk of polio cases due to imported wild-type virus, the benefits of the new schedule are diminished. This is, therefore, a very important assumption and should be tested in a sensitivity analysis. Miller et al. (1996) did not test this assumption in their analysis. However, they point out that in the absence of known wild poliovirus transmission in the United States the OPV schedule is difficult to justify politically.

3. What are the direct costs of a OPV and IPV program? Identify contributors to direct health care cost, direct non–health care costs, informal caregiver cost, and the costs of time spent to partake of the intervention.

Miller et al. (1996) included vaccine administration costs, clinic travel costs, and vaccine cost as contributors to direct health care cost. Excess visits might be generated by the new (2 IPV, 2 OPV) schedule. These were considered as direct health care costs. Lost wages for the parent to partake of the program were identified as direct non–health care costs. There were no caregiver costs for the program. The cost of pain and suffering for the child who undergoes multiple vaccines was not monetarized directly. Rather, it was assumed that multiple injections would lead parents to elect additional visits, which would add to the cost of the program.

4. What number of dollars per case of VAPP prevented would justify a change to the new vaccine schedule?

Miller et al. (1996) estimated that the new (2 IPV, 2 OPV) schedule would prevent about five of 10 VAPP cases. VAPP cases are currently compensated, on average, $1,200,000. Miller et al. found that it would cost about $3,100,000 more per VAPP case prevented to implement the new (2 IPV, 2 OPV) schedule. The cost of this program was higher than those of other public health prevention programs.

5. How does the mandatory nature of the program affect the recommendation based on the cost-effectiveness analysis?

Individuals offered a voluntary choice between an "extra" injection for their child and a one out a million chance of VAPP for which they would be compensated might make a decision that is different from the public policy decision. The ACIP voted to recommend the new (2 IPV, 2 OPV) schedule notwithstanding its high cost compared with other programs, reasoning that public concern about the adverse events from a government-mandated program in a country with no wild type virus outweighed considerations of cost.

Implications for Practice

The cost-effectiveness analysis of the poliomyelitis vaccine schedule was careful and "state of the art." Only about half of all VAPP cases would be prevented by the new recommended (2 IPV, 2 OPV) schedule. The cost for the new (2 IPV, 2 OPV schedule) for the number of cases of VAPP prevented ($3.1 million) is higher than most public health programs. In spite of the carefulness of this cost-effectiveness analysis and the demonstration that the new (2 IPV, 2 OPV) schedule was not "cost-effective" using conventional benchmarks, the new (2 IPV, 2 OPV) schedule was recommended.

SUGGESTED READINGS

Danford DA. QALYs: their ethical implications. JAMA 1990;264:2503.

Doubilet P, Weinstein MC, McNeil BJ. Use and misuse of the term "cost effective" in medicine. N Engl J Med 1986;314:253–256.

Gold MR, Siegel JE, Russell LB, Weinstein MC. Cost-Effectiveness in Health and Medicine. New York: Oxford University Press; 1996.

Haddix AC, Teutsch SM, Shaffer PA, Dunet DO. Prevention Effectiveness. A Guide to Decision Analysis and Economic Evaluation. New York: Oxford University Press; 1996.

Russell LB, Gold MR, Siegel JE, Daniels N, Weinstein MC, The role of cost-effectiveness analysis in health and medicine. Panel on Cost-Effectiveness in Health and Medicine. JAMA 1996;276:1172–1177.

Weinstein MC, Stason WB. Foundations of cost-effectiveness analysis for health and medical practices. N Engl J Med 1977;296:716–721.

REFERENCES

Beck JR, Kassirer JP, Pauker SG. A convenient approximation of life expectancy (the "DEALE"). I. Validation of the method. Am J Med 1982a;73:883–888.

Beck JR, Pauker SG, Gottlieb JE, Klein K, Kassirer JP. A convenient approximation of life expectancy (the "DEALE"). II. Use in medical decision-making. Am J Med 1982b;73:889–897.

Danford DA. QALYs: their ethical implications. JAMA 1990;264:2503.

de Quadros CA, Henderson DA. Disease eradication and control in the Americas. Biologicals 1993;21:335–343.

Detsky AS, Naglie IG. A clinician's guide to cost-effectiveness analysis. Ann Intern Med 1990;113:147–154.

Doubilet P, Weinstein MC, McNeil BJ. Use and misuse of the term "cost effective" in medicine. N Engl J Med 1986;314:253–256.

Drummond MF. Resource allocation decisions in health care. a role for quality of life assessments? J Chron Dis 1987;40:605–616.

Drummond M, Stoddart G, Torrance G. Methods of Economic Evaluation of Health Care Programmes. Oxford: Oxford University Press; Oxford, 1987.

Epstein RS, Sherwood LM, from outcomes research to disease management. A guide for the perplexed. Ann Intern Med 1996;124:832–837.

Finkler SA. The distinction between cost and charges. Ann Intern Med 1982;96:102–109.

Gold MR, Siegel JE, Russell LB, Weinstein MC. Cost-Effectiveness in Health and Medicine. New York: Oxford University Press; 1996.

Haddix AC, Teutsch SM, Shaffer PA, Dunet DO. Prevention Effectiveness. A Guide to Decision Analysis and Economic Evaluation. New York: Oxford University Press; 1996.

Hadorn DC. The role of public values in setting health care priorities. Soc Sci Med 1991;32:773–782.

Harris J. QALYfying the value of life. J Med Ethics 1987;13:117–123.

Kaplan RM, Ganiats TG. QALYs: their ethical implications. JAMA 1990;264:2503.

Keeler EB, Cretin S. Discounting of life-saving and other non-monetary benefits. Management 1983;29:300–306.

LaPuma J, Lawlor EF. Quality-adjusted life-years. ethical implications for physicians and policymakers. JAMA 1990;263:2917–2921.

Miller MA, Sutter RW, Strebel PM, Hadler SC. Cost-effectiveness of incorporating inactivated poliovirus vaccine into the routine childhood immunization schedule. JAMA 1996;276:967–971.

O'Brien B. Principles of economic evaluation for health care. J Rheumatol 1995;22:1399–1402.

Office of Technology Assessment (OTA). U.S. Congress. Evaluation of the Oregon Medicaid proposal. OTA-H-531. Washington, DC: U.S. Government Printing Office; 1992.

Pan American Health Organization. The certification of wild poliovirus eradication from the Western Hemisphere. Epidemiol Bull 1994;15:1-3.

Rawles J. Castigating QALYs. J Med Ethics 1989;15:143–147.

Russell LB, Gold MR, Siegel JE, Daniels N, Weinstein MC, The role of cost-effectiveness analysis in health and medicine. Panel on Cost-Effectiveness in Health and Medicine. JAMA 1996;276:1172–1177.

Smith A. Qualms about QALYs. Lancet 1987;i:1134–1136.

Sugden R, Williams A. The Principles of Practical Cost-Benefit Analysis. Oxford: Oxford University Press; 1990.

Tengs TO, Adama ME, Pliskin JS, et al. Five-hundred life-saving interventions and their cost-effectiveness. Risk Anal 1995;15:369–390.

Ubel PA, Dekay ML, Baron J, Asch DA. Cost-effectiveness analysis in a setting of budget constraints: is it equitable. N Engl J Med 1996;334:1174–1177.

Warner KE, Luce BR. Cost-Benefit and Cost-Effectiveness Analysis in Health Care. Principles, Practice, and Potential. Ann Arbor: Health Administration Press; 1982.

Weinstein MC, Stason WB. Foundations of cost-effectiveness analysis for health and medical practices. N Engl J Med 1977;296:716–721.

Weinstein MC, Fineberg HV. Clinical Decision Analysis. Philadelphia:WB Saunders; 1980.

Weinstein MC, Siegel JE, Gold MR, Kamlet MS, Russell LB. Recommendations of the Panel on Cost-Effectiveness in Health and Medicine. JAMA 1996;276;1253–1258.

10

Measuring the Quality of Health Care

DIANA B. PETITTI
ANDY AMSTER

The measurement and improvement of quality of care have been a part of health care for decades. Recently, attempts to measure and monitor quality have become more intense as a response to demands for accountability in the delivery of services (Relman 1988) and as an outgrowth of the quality and outcomes "movement." The development of systems to measure the performance of organizations that deliver health care is a part of the attempt to assure accountability. It is also a response to consumer concern—about how new ways of organizing and financing medical care effect quality.

This chapter discusses definitions of the of health care quality. Approaches to measuring the quality of care are recounted. Several systems designed to measure the performance of organizations are described. Important statistical and ethical issues in performance measurement are delineated.

Defining Quality

Experts have struggled for decades to formulate a single concise, meaningful, and generally applicable definition of the quality of health care (Blumenthal 1996). In arriving at its definition of quality of care published in 1990, the Institute of Medicine collected over 100 definitions from the literature (Lohr 1990).

Three definitions of quality in health care are commonly cited. These definitions came from Donabedian (1980), the American Medical Association (1986), and the Institute of Medicine (Lohr 1990) and are reproduced in Table 10-1. These three definitions are conceptually similar. They differ in their emphasis on quality of life, the delivery of services, and processes of care as components of quality. Donabedian (1988) has suggested that there is more

Table 10-1. Three Commonly Cited Definitions of Quality of Health Care

Source	Definition
Donabedian (1980)	"That kind of care which is expected to maximize an inclusive measure of patient welfare, after one has taken account of expected gains and losses that attend the process of care"
American Medical Association (1986)	"Care that consistently contributes to the improvement or maintenance of quality and/or duration of life"
Institute of Medicine (Lohr 1990)	"The degree to which health services for individuals or populations increase the likelihood of desired health outcomes and are consistent with current professional knowledge"

than one legitimate formulation of quality depending on the system of care and the nature and extent of responsibilities.

Blumenthal (1996) goes further to clarify the relationship between different perspectives and the definition of quality of care. He describes four main perspectives on quality—the health care professional perspective, the patient perspective, the perspective of health care plans and organizations, and the purchaser perspective. These different perspectives lead to different definitions of quality. Health care providers tend to define quality in terms of the attributes of care and the results of care. This leads to definitions of quality that have an emphasis on technical excellence and the characteristics of patient/professional interaction (Palmer 1995; Donabedian 1988). The patient perspective leads to definitions of quality that take into account the preferences and values of patients and their opinions about their care. This leads to definitions of quality that encompass satisfaction with care, as well as outcomes such as morbidity, mortality, and functional status. Health care plans and organizations tend to place greater emphasis on the general health of the enrolled population and on the function of the organization (Leape 1994). This perspective leads to a definition of quality that takes into account the ability of the plan to meet the needs of enrollees; it encompasses decisions to limit some care to assure essential services for all and acknowledges the reality of fixed resources. Purchasers, like health care organizations, tend to be concerned about population-based measures of quality and organizational performance (Blumenthal 1996). The purchaser perspective leads to a definition of quality that is similar to that of health care organizations. However, purchasers are very concerned about the "value" of care, and this concern incorporates the price of care and the efficiency of the delivery of care.

Blumenthal (1996) and others (Brook et al. 1996; Donabedian 1988) recognize that different perspectives and definitions of quality call for different measurement approaches. Thus, it is important that the definition of quality and the perspective be specified so that the measure of quality is appropriate to the definition and the perspective.

Measuring Quality: Structure, Process, Outcome

Quality of care can be measured based on structure, process, or outcome (Donabedian 1980, 1982, 1985). Structural measures are the characteristics of the resources in the health system. For providers, these variables include professional characteristics (e.g., specialty, board certification). For institutions, they include size, location, ownership, and licensure status, as well as physical attributes (e.g., number of beds, ownership) and other organizational factors (e.g., staff-to-patient ratios).

Processes embody what is done to and for the patient (e.g., ordering of a immunization, prescription of a medication). Process measures of quality can be made for individual practitioners, groups of practitioners, or for entire systems of care. Much of the current emphasis in measuring quality focuses on the quality of care of delivered by systems that are defined according to the structure of their financing (e.g., managed care).

Outcomes are the end results of care or the effect of the care process on the health and well-being of patients and populations. Elinson (1987) describes the relevant health care outcomes as "the five Ds"—death, disease, disability, discomfort, and dissatisfaction. More positively, Lohr (1988) frames relevant health care outcomes as survival, states of physiologic, physical and emotional health, and satisfaction.

Early attempts to measure quality centered on the measurement of the structural aspects of care. For example, many structural measures are made in decisions about accreditation of hospitals. Implicit in the use of structural measures of care to measure quality is the assumption that structure affects outcome. It is assumed that if a hospital has a certain number of nurses for each patient or a certain number of square feet of space in each room, the hospital is delivering high-quality care. In fact, the link between measures of structure and measures of outcome is difficult to demonstrate directly. Notwithstanding this limitation, quality assurance programs and organizations, such as the Joint Commission on the Accreditation of Health Care Organizations (JCAHO) and the National Committee on Quality Assurance (NCQA), that accredit institutions, rely on structural measures to infer quality and confer accreditation on this basis. It is probably true that compliance with a certain minimum standard of structure is necessary to assure quality of some kinds of care. For example, brain surgery done by a general practitioner is certainly low-quality care and a dirty operating room virtually assures poor outcomes. Assuring that structures are in place is not sufficient to assure quality, and demonstration that structure meets certain criteria does not assure that processes are appropriate or that outcomes are good.

Much of the current debate about quality measurement centers on the use of process versus outcome measures of quality. Most authors agree that both process and outcome measures can provide valid information about the quality of health care (Donabedian 1980; Lohr 1990; Brook et al. 1996a,b). The advantages and disadvantages and the arguments for and against process and outcome measures are important to understand.

Process measures have several advantages (Lohr 1990). They are appealing to providers because they are directly related to what providers do. It is relatively easy to explain process measures because the links with outcomes may be very direct. Process measurement can often point directly to areas where care needs to be improved. For example, the percentage of a pediatrician's patients who are fully immunized is directly relevant to the pediatrician. A measure of the percentage of children fully immunized against polio is easy to justify as a measure of quality because the link between the process (immunization) and the desired outcome (prevention of disease) is clear. If the percentage of children who are fully immunized is low, the points of intervention to increase rates are easy to identify.

Process criteria are more sensitive measures of quality than outcome measures when a deficiency in process invariably leads to a poor outcome. Outcome measures may not be sensitive to deficiencies in quality because a poor outcome does not occur each time there is a deficiency in the quality of care (Brook et al. 1996a,b). For example, failure to give thrombolytic therapy within 8 hours to patients who present in the emergency department with acute chest pain does not result in a death from myocardial infarction each time the failure to provide prompt thrombolysis occurs. Failure to immunize a child against polio rarely (if ever) results in a case of poliomyelitis. However, as a practical matter, there are few incontrovertibly proven direct links between process and outcome for most clinical conditions.

Process measures may be essential to the measurement of the quality of care for chronic conditions. In these cases, the goal of care is often prevention of complications of the condition. The time between performance of key processes of care and a favorable outcome of that care is long. For example, the effect of providing adjuvant chemotherapy following a diagnosis of breast cancer on mortality from breast cancer may not be evident for a decade. Using mortality rates from breast cancer to assess the quality of care in women with breast cancer will not be a sensitive measure of quality of care in the short term. Using prescription of appropriate adjuvant chemotherapy, a process measure, is the better measure of the quality of care.

The advantages of measures of outcome mirror those of process measures (Lohr 1990). Most (e.g., mortality, reduction in pain) are easy to explain and interpret. The reliability and validity (see Chapter 8) of some of them have been established. They, too, can be used to target quality improvement efforts. Outcomes such as functional status and satisfaction with care reflect the patient perspective.

There are several arguments against process measures as measures of quality of care. Processes are not necessarily important predictors of outcome. Directing resources at processes that do not affect outcomes may increase health care cost without producing any improvement in health (Ellwood 1988). The resources necessary to collect process data may be high compared with the resources necessary to collect outcomes data. Readily accessible data sources may be poor. Finally, it may not be possible to achieve consensus on the correct process for many clinical problems.

Outcome measures are criticized because, it is argued, many differences in outcome are not under the control of providers, and conclusions about the quality of care based on outcome measures may be invalid. For example, mental health status is affected by personal and economic factors (e.g., divorce, unemployment) that are not subject to control of the health care provider. Providers have a limited influence on the smoking behavior of their patients, whose decisions to smoke are subject to peers, personality, the media, and economic forces (e.g., the amount of tobacco tax). Lohr (1990) also points that it may be difficult to assign responsibility for outcomes to a single provider or a system of care when there are no clear points of entry or exit to the health care system. For example, a case of hepatitis B in an adult member of a health care organization might occur because of the failure of the pediatrician in another organization to vaccinate appropriately during infancy. Renal failure in a person with diabetes who is insured by one health care plan may be due to failure of another plan to have provided adequate screening and treatment for microalbuminuria during the early stages of the condition.

Many outcomes (e.g., mortality) are rare. Comparisons of quality based on rare outcomes are often of low statistical power (Brook et al. 1996a). Poor outcomes care may be hidden by low statistical power. The problem of statistical power is especially acute when using outcome measures to assess the quality of care of individual providers, since the number of expected outcome events for any single provider is low. For example, the average mortality rate following coronary artery bypass surgery is about 5%. The expected number of deaths for a thoracic surgeon who performs 200 coronary artery bypass procedures a year is only 10. If this surgeon has 15 deaths per year, it is still within the limits of sampling variation.

Outcomes such as functional status and "quality of life" are multidimensional, and a complete assessment of the effect of care on these outcomes requires the measurement of general, physiologic, mental, physical, and social health (Brook et al. 1996a). Satisfaction with care is another important multidimensional component of quality. Assessments of these multidimensional outcomes may be costly when attempts are made to measure them on large and representative populations.

Using patient satisfaction to measure quality may hide deficiencies in the technical quality of care. Patients may be very satisfied with care that is inappropriate. They may be very dissatisfied with care that is appropriate. For example, patients with uncomplicated viral upper respiratory infections may be satisfied with an encounter in which they received broad-spectrum antibiotics and dissatisfied if they receive only advice to rest and drink lots of fluids. Prescribing broad-spectrum antibiotics for viral upper respiratory infections is poor quality care. A patient may be dissatisfied with the care of an orthopedist because the orthopedist states that the patient is physically able to return to work before the patient wishes to return. Saying that injured persons are unready for work when they are physically healed is poor quality care.

Methods for Quality Assessment

Brook and Appel (1973) and Brook et al. (1996b) delineate five methods of quality assessment. The first three methods are "implicit." That is, there are no prior standards or agreements about what constitutes quality of care. A health professional reviews data and, based on this review, answers one of three global questions—"Was the process of care adequate?" "Could better care have improved the outcome?" or "Was the overall quality of care acceptable?" None of these three methods for measuring the quality of care bears a strong relationship to epidemiology. For this reason, implicit measures of quality will not be discussed further in this chapter.

The fourth method for quality measurement evaluates care using explicit process criteria. The process criteria should ideally be based on review of the scientific literature and data that shows that the process affects outcome causally. For example, an explicit process measure for the care of patients with type I (insulin-dependent) diabetes would be control of serum glucose. A measure of control would be performance of glycosylated hemoglobin and a result consistently less than 8%. This process measure is justified based on the observations in the Diabetes Control and Complications Trial showing that strict control of serum glucose reduced the likelihood of nephropathy, neuropathy, and retinopathy in type I diabetics (Diabetes Control and Complications Trial Research Group 1993).

The fifth method also uses explicit criteria. Here it is determined whether the observed results of care are consistent with the outcome predicted by a model that has been validated using scientific evidence or clinical judgment.

For example, mortality in patients who received one type of treatment is compared with mortality in patients who received another type of care. The chapter on outcomes research discusses the conceptual basis for this method in more detail.

Performance Indicators and Performance Indicator Systems

Overview

A performance indicator system is an "interrelated set of process and/or outcome measures that facilitate internal and external comparisons of an organization's performance over time" (Loeb and Buck 1996). Performance indicator systems attempt to assess the quality of care delivered by an organization through collection of a variety of structural, process, and outcome measures. Within each performance indicator system, each of the individual performance indicators is ideally a measure of the quality of care.

At least 140 performance indicator systems for evaluation and comparison of hospital care have been developed (Loeb and Buck 1996). There has been tremendous growth in the development of other performance indicator systems as well. Both Medicare and Medicaid are in the process of developing performance indicator systems to assess the quality of care provided to beneficiaries by managed-care organizations. The Health Plan Employer Data and Information Set (HEDIS) is a performance indicator system (Corrigan and Nielsen 1993) developed by the National Committee on Quality Assurance (NCQA) to compare the quality of care of Health Maintenance Organizations (HMOs). The Foundation for Accountability (FACCT) has developed another performance indicator system to compare organizations in terms of the quality of the health care they deliver (Graham 1997). The project to Develop and Evaluate Methods to Promote Ambulatory Care Quality (DEM-PAQ) is an indicator system for measuring the quality of ambulatory care (Lawthers et al. 1993). A set of performance indicators to be used in public health settings is also being developed (Institute of Medicine 1996).

Information from performance indicator systems is used in a variety of ways. Most prominently, it is used to make "report cards" that purchasers and consumers of health care are supposed to be able to use to assess the quality and the "value" of different providers of health care. Performance indicators are also used to monitor the quality of care over time. In these cases, performance indicator systems are directly analogous to public health surveillance. Finally, performance indicator systems are used within organizations to identify where the quality of care needs to be improved. Thus, performance indicators are a key component of approaches to continuous quality improvement that has the following components: (1) agreement about how to measure quality of performance, (2) measurement of performance, (3) identification of targets for improvement based on the measurements, (4) intervention, and (5) remeasurement of performance to assess the effect of the intervention (Palmer and Peterson 1995).

Development of Performance Indicator Systems

There are a multiplicity of groups involved in the development of performance indicator systems. For example, HEDIS was developed by a group made up of representatives of the perceived main users of the system (purchasers of health care), the health plans that were being asked to provide the measures, and experts in quality measurement. DEMPAQ was developed by a coalition of health providers and academic health services researchers with funding from the Health Care Financing Administration (Palmer and Peterson 1995). FACCT is a coalition of major purchasers and consumer organizations such as American Express, the Health Care Financing Administration, the Oregon Health Plan, and the American Association of Retired Persons. Federal grants are also supporting the development and testing of some performance indicators and performance indicators systems. Many systems of hospital performance indicators have been developed by firms that either started as for-profit firms or became for-profit firms when the large sums of money to be made in performance measurement became apparent. More recently, publicly traded for-profit consulting corporations have become involved in providing advice to employer groups and corporations about performance indicators. State governments are also developing performance indicator systems.

Deciding to use a particular system to monitor quality and for performance measurement may affect decisions about resource allocation and the focus of quality improvement activities. There may be substantial financial gains for commercial firms whose performance indicator system is chosen to guide decisions about hospital accreditation. There is prestige involved in having a performance indicator system chosen for use by a variety of organizations. The high-stakes nature of the development and adoption of performance indicators and the large potential for profit and influence have led to competition among these systems and indicators.

Approaches to choosing among different performance indicator systems are being developed. This process is most advanced for performance indicator systems for hospital care. Thus, the Joint Commission on the Accreditation of Healthcare Organizations approved a plan to evaluate the more than 140 different performance indicator systems using a specified set of attributes and to allow hospitals to use any of the systems that were in conformance with these guidelines and met the specified criteria. Table 10-2 shows the attributes of an acceptable performance indicator system that were defined by this commission (Loeb and Buck 1996).

It is uncertain how choices will be made among performance indicator systems to compare the quality of care among managed-care organizations such as HEDIS and FACCT. Some influential commentators (Brook et al. 1996a) have made a strong recommendation for the use of indicator systems that rely on process (versus outcome) to assess quality. These recommendations are directly in conflict with FACCT, which has strongly advocated outcome measures. In the absence of a consensus of what measures should be used, purchasers, consumers, and government will likely demand information from several different systems. If this happens, the amount of required measurement is likely to overwhelm health care organizations. Ultimately, the information may also overwhelm consumers and purchasers. The cost of acquiring data to measure performance is an issue, especially as the number of different performance indicators systems and the number of indicators within each system increase. The expenditure of resources for measurement may divert resources from changes in systems and processes that directly improve the quality of care. Measurement unlinked with an action plan based on the measurement is not worthwhile.

Choosing Quality-of-Care Indicators

The specific quality indicators within a performance indicator system can be measures of structure, process, or outcome. To be credible, it must be demonstrated that changes in the processes that are used as measures of quality lead to differences in outcome and that measures of outcome that are used as measures of quality are ones that can be altered by health professionals (Brook et al. 1996a). For example, unless it has been demonstrated that use of an acetyl cholinesterase inhibitor in unselected hypertensive diabetics leads to better outcomes in type II diabetes, the percentage of diabetics patients on an ACE inhibitor is not a credible measure of quality of care. Unless it can be demonstrated that mental health measured using the SF-36, which is a mea-

Table 10-2. Joint Commission on Accreditation of Health Care Organizations: Attitudes of Acceptable Performance Measurement Systems

---

- Includes appropriate performance measures, focusing on processes and/or outcomes related to patient care, including measures at the individual level
- Has automated database permitting trend analysis and intrasystem comparison
- Ensures data quality through audits of accuracy and completeness
- Utilizes risk adjustment and stratification
- Makes feedback available to participating organizations at least annually
- Is relevant to the accreditation process

---

sure of functional outcome (see Chapter 8), can be altered by health care, these scores are not a credible measure of quality of care.

Measures used to compare institutions or providers should reflect differences in the quality of care among the units of analysis (e.g., hospital, health plan, community) and not differences in demographic characteristics or underlying risk factors among patients managed in each setting. For example, if it is concluded that mortality after coronary artery bypass surgery (CABG) at hospital A is greater than at hospital B because of differences in the quality of care, it is essential that differences in ethnicity, age, and comorbidities be ruled out as explanations for the difference. The difficulties of risk adjustment have hampered attempts to compare mortality outcomes between hospitals as a way of assessing quality of care. The challenges of risk adjustment were discussed in detail in Chapter 8. Epidemiologists will be very familiar with these challenges, which are identical to the challenges in controlling for confounding in traditional case-control and cohort studies.

Although the desirable theoretical features of a measure of quality are easily specified, in practice, finding specific indicators for the consensus that they measure is difficult. Some of the successful examples of developing indicator measures of quality are reviewed by Brook and colleagues (1996a). The most successful and useful quality indicator measures are evidence based. For example, the US Preventive Health Task Force's evidence-based guidelines for mammography and Pap smear screening were, in part, the basis for the decision by HEDIS to include mammography and Pap screening as clinical quality indicator measures (Lee and McGinnis 1995). American Diabetes Association guidelines influenced the decision by HEDIS to include retinopathy screening as a clinical quality indicator.

Standardization of Indicators

When comparing organizations or providers, it is essential that the information on quality indicators be collected in a standardized way so that comparisons between indicators are not due to differences in measurement methodology. Standardization is meant to assure comparability between units so that differences can be correctly attributed to differences in the quality of care and not to differences in methodology. Initially, it was believed that standardization would also allow for monitoring trends in quality. However, as measurement methods and data quality improve, they become incomparable over time. That is, the price of better data is inability to compare over time.

Standardization is often achieved by providing specific rules for data collection and reporting and by developing protocols for collecting data for the measures. The next section provides a detailed example of how HEDIS has attempted to standardize its measures of quality.

Health Plan Employer Data and Information Set (HEDIS)

The Health Employer Data and Information Set (HEDIS) is a well-known system of performance indicators that is being used by the Health Care Financing System and by the private sector to compare the quality of care delivered by HMO's. HEDIS was developed by the National Committee for Quality Assurance (NCQA). It was introduced in 1993 and was revised in 1995 and again for 1997. The HEDIS system has been influential and is the model for many other performance measurement efforts. Medicaid and Medicare HEDIS and HEDIS-like systems for evaluating indemnity insurance providers, PPOs and IPAs are all being developed.

The HEDIS performance indicator system was designed to evaluate a number of aspects of health plan performance including clinical quality of care, access to care, satisfaction with care, utilization of services, and the financial performance of the health care organization. Selection of initial measures was based on three criteria (Corrigan and Nielsen 1993): (1) relevance and value to the employer community, (2) reasonable ability of health plans to develop and provide the data, and (3) potential impact on improving patient care and reducing morbidity and mortality.

The specific measures of the quality of clinical care included in HEDIS version 3.0 are shown in Table 10-3. The clinical quality-of-care indicators were chosen to address aspects of the medical care process for which there was strong evidence in the literature to support the relationship between medical care process and desired outcomes.

For each HEDIS measure, exact specifications are provided. These specifications were designed to enable accurate trending of performance and to assure valid comparisons of units of care. Table 10-4 gives the HEDIS specifi-

---

Table 10-3. Health and Employer Data and Information Set (HEDIS)[a] Effectiveness of Care Performance Measurement Indicators

- Childhood immunization status
- Adolescent immunization status
- Advising smokers to quit
- Flu shots for older adults
- Breast cancer screening
- Cervical cancer screening
- Prenatal care in the first trimester
- Low birth-weight babies
- Check-ups after delivery
- Treating children's ear infections
- Beta-blocker treatment after a heart attack
- Eye exams for people with diabetes
- The health of seniors
- Follow-up after hospitalization for mental illness

[a] Version 3.0.

Table 10-4. Health and Employer Data and Information Set (HEDIS)[a]
Specifications for Mammography Screening as a Performance Measure

Description

The percentage of Medicaid, commercial, and Medicare risk women age 52–69 years, who were continuously enrolled during the reporting year and the preceding year, and who have had no more than one break in enrollment of up to 45 days per year should be included in this measurement

Administrative data specification

Calculation

This specification uses membership data to identify women age 52–69 years and claims/encounter data to identify those women who received one or more mammograms during the reporting year or the year before the reporting year. Separate calculations are required for the Medicaid, commercial, and Medicare risk populations

Denominator

Three separate denominators, one for each of the three required calculations, are derived using all enrolled women age 52–69 as of December 31 of the reporting year, who were members of the plan as of December 31 of the reporting year, and who were continuously enrolled during the reporting year and the preceding year. Members who have had no more than one break in enrollment of up to 45 days per year should be included in this measure

Numerator

The number of members in the denominator for each of the three populations (Medicaid, commercial, and Medicare risk) who have had one (or more) mammogram(s) during the reporting year or the year before the reporting year. A woman is considered to have had a mammogram if a submitted claim/encounter meets any of the following criteria:

CPT-4 code: 76090 or 76091 or 76092
OR
Revenue code: 401 or 403
OR
ICD-9-CM procedure code: 87.37 or 87.36
OR

(*continued*)

cations for mammography to exemplify how data sources and indicators are standardized for HEDIS.

The first versions of HEDIS were developed by an expert group comprised of representatives of health care organizations, employers, and academic experts. In developing HEDIS 3.0, there was a broad-based public "call for measures." Individuals and organizations were asked to nominate indicator measures to be included in HEDIS 3.0, based on delineation by HEDIS of the desirable attributes of measures. HEDIS specified criteria that they stated would be used to evaluate candidate quality indicator measures. The desirable attributes of indicator measures and the criteria for selection of performance indicators for HEDIS 3.0 are shown in Table 10-5.

Table 10-4. (*continued*)

Revenue code: 320 or 400 in conjunction with the following breast-related ICD-9-CM diagnosis codes: 174.xx, 198.81, 217, 233.0, 611.72, 793.8, V10.3, V76.1.

Hybrid method specification

Calculation

This specification uses membership data to identify women age 52–69 years. Claims/encounter data and/or medical record review is used to identify those women who received one or more mammograms during the reporting year or the year before the reporting year. Separate calculations are required for the Medicaid, commercial, and Medicare risk populations

Denominator

Three separate denominators, one each for the three required calculations, are derived using random samples of 411 Medicaid members, 411 commercial members, and 411 Medicare risk members from the plan's eligible populations. Eligible members include Medicaid enrolled women or commercially enrolled women or Medicare risk enrolled women age 52–69 as of December 31 of the reporting year, who were members of the plan as of December 31 of the reporting year, and who were continuously enrolled during the reporting year and the preceding year. Members who have had no more than one break in enrollment of up to 45 days per year should be included in this measure

Numerator

The number of enrolled women in the denominator for each of the three populations (Medicaid, commercial, and Medicare risk) who have had one (or more) mammogram(s) during the reporting year or the year before the reporting year) as documented through either administrative data or medical record review. Documentation in the medical record must include, at a minimum, an author-identified note indicating the date the mammogram was performed and the result or finding.

*a*Aversion 3.0.

Data Sources for Quality Measurement

Once the specific quality indicators have been chosen, appropriate sources of data must be specified. Data sources available for measurement include computer-stored administrative data (e.g., claims data, encounter data) and clinical data (e.g., prescriptions databases, ambulatory diagnosis databases), paper medical records, patient reports, and direct observation of an encounter.

Direct observation of encounters can provide an objective record of what occurred. It is costly to conduct direct observations. In practice, direct observation is rarely used to measure quality of care, and it will not be discussed further.

Table 10-5. Desirable Attributes of Performance Measures and Criteria Used to Select Measures for HEDIS 3.0

Relevance
- Meaningful: The measurement should be meaningful to at least one of the audiences for HEDIS
  - Health importance: The measure should capture as much of the plan's activities relating to quality as possible
  - Financial importance: The measure should be related to activities that have high financial costs to health plans, or purchasers or consumers of health care
  - Cost-effectiveness: The measure should encourage the use of cost-effective activities and/or discourage the use of activities that have low cost-effectiveness
  - Strategically important: The measure should encourage activities that deserve high priority in terms of using resources most efficiently to maximize the health of their members
  - Controllability: There should be actions that health plans can take to improve their performance on a measure
  - Variance between plans: If the primary purpose of the measure is to differentiate among plans, then there should be potentially wide variations across plans with respect to the measure
  - Potential for improvement: If the primary purpose of the measure is to support negotiations between plans and purchasers, or to stimulate self-improvement by plans, there should be substantial room for plans to improve their performance with respect to the measure

Feasibility
- Precisely specified: The measure should have clear operational definitions, specifications for data sources, and methods for data collection and reporting
- Reasonable cost: The measure should not impose an inappropriate burden on health plans
- Confidential: The collection of data for the measures should not violate any accepted standards of member confidentiality
- Logistically feasible: The data required for the measure should be available during the time period allowed for collection

Scientific validity
- Reproducible: The measure should produce the same results when repeated in the same population and setting
- Valid: The measure should make sense logically, clinically, and if it focuses on a financially important aspect of care, financially (face validity), and should correlate well with other measures of the same aspect of care (construct validity)
- Accurate: The measure should accurately measure what is actually happening
- Risk adjustable: Either the measure should not be appreciably affected by any variables that are beyond the plan's control ("covariates"), or any extraneous factors should be known, they should be measurable, and there should be validated models for calculating an adjusted result that corrects for the effects of covariates
- Comparability of data sources: The accuracy, reproducibility, risk adjustability, and validity of the measure should not be affected if different plans have to use different data sources for the measure

It is widely recognized that measures of quality and performance measures are limited by the quality of the data used to construct them. Chapter 8 discussed the problems of data quality as these problems affect outcomes research. They apply equally to the use of the same data sources for measuring quality. The reader should review the material on data quality in Chapter 8.

In measuring quality, the appropriateness of the source of data depends on the purpose of gathering the information (Siu et al. 1991; Palmer and Peterson 1995; Brook et al. 1996a). Thus, it is not possible to say that there is one "best" source of information for all kinds of quality measures. The sources of data clearly are not interchangeable (Gerbert and Hargreaves 1986). For example, data on immunization recorded in a computer database is a function of not only the provision of immunization, but also the completeness of recording. Self-reported immunization captures not only immunizations given in the traditional health care setting but immunizations given in shopping malls and senior centers. Each data source has advantages and disadvantages for measuring quality. Table 10-6 shows one assessment of the suitability of administrative data, medical records, and patient report for several categories of quality measures (Siu et al. 1991).

Computer-stored administrative and clinical records are easily accessible. They do not contain much clinical detail. As discussed in Chapter 8, the reliability of some of the data is uncertain because of the circumstances under which the data are collected. The data may be incomplete because some of the care obtained by a patient is not recorded. For example, influenza shots given at a community clinic will not be recorded in a health plan's immunization database. Prescriptions filled in the local drugstore will not be recorded in the prescription database. It is rare that it is possible to obtain a meaningful measure of quality using solely administrative data (Brook et al. 1996a).

Paper charts contain clinical detail. As discussed in Chapter 8, it is costly to retrieve charts. We estimate that it costs $2.50 in labor to pull and refile a chart. A trained record abstraction service costs $50.00 per hour. When a patient has charts at several locations, it may be difficult to identify all of them. Charts are not good sources of data on mortality outcomes, functional status, or patient satisfaction. Clinical charts may not themselves be complete even for delivered services. Laboratory data, for example, may not be recorded consistently in the paper chart if computer-stored data are also available.

A patient's report is theoretically an ideal source of information on processes. It is the only source of data on satisfaction with care and most measures of functional status. Obtaining patient reports to assess quality requires surveys, which are costly. All surveys have nonrespondents, and bias can arise from nonresponse. Finally, patients do not always accurately report their receipt of services. For example, for preventive services, there is a

Table 10-6. Data Sources for Obtaining Quality-of-Care Information

Information Needed	Computer-Stored Administrative and Clinical Records	Paper Medical Records	Patient Report
Access to care	Time-to-appointment, number of visits, use of specialty care	Number of visits	May be best source of information
Use of services	May be best source of information, if available	Adequate, but data may need to be obtained from several charts	Lacks detail, "telescoping" a problem, not reliable
Symptoms	Not useful	Limited data	May be best source of information
Interpersonal aspects of care	Not useful	Not useful	May be best source of information
Technical aspects of of care	Linkage of multiple sources may allow use for limited purposes	Data available on most important processes	Unknown accuracy
Diagnostic tests	May be best source of information, if available	Good for abnormal results; hospital records miss outpatient tests and vice versa	Lacks detail, uncertain accuracy
Medications	Good source for prescription, if available	Good source for important drugs	Fair source for current medication
Patient education	Not useful	Not necessarily documented	Unknown accuracy
Mortality	May be best source	Incomplete	Not useful
Functional status	Not useful	Not useful	Best source of information
Satisfaction with care	Not useful	Not useful	Sole source of accurate information

Source: Siu et al. (1991).

tendency to "telescope," reporting receipt of services more recently than they were actually performed. Surprisingly, many individuals simply do not know what kinds of tests and procedures they have received. For example, a person may know that they had a "shot" but not know whether the shot was for influenza or pneumococcal pneumonia. Finally, the questions asked in surveys may use words to describe procedures that are not understandable to the respondent, leading to inaccurate reporting. For example, a person may not know that they had a "sigmoidoscopy" although they might remember that they had "an uncomfortable procedure in which a tube was inserted into the rectum."

Ethical Concerns in Performance Measurement

The enhanced ability to collect and handle data electronically has greatly expanded the potential for the use of these data to make improvements in the quality of care. The use of such databases, however, raises "a spectre of misuse that could harm patients, health care providers, and the public at large" (Donaldson 1994). Disclosure of inaccurate data about quality of care has the potential to cause direct economic harm to providers and health care organizations, and it may mislead the public. Disclosure of information about medical conditions in the course of measuring quality has the potential to embarrass, distress, or directly harm individuals. For example, disclosure of treatment for HIV, mental illness, or pelvic inflammatory disease; a diagnosis of epilepsy or impotence; and the performance of an abortion or an examination for rape all have the potential to stigmatize an individual. Disclosure of the existence of a genetic disease may make a person as well as his/her offspring uninsurable.

The Department of Health and Human Services has established rigorous regulations governing access by researchers to information about health and illness that would allow individuals to be identified. When doing research based on these regulations, the importance of protecting these data from harm due to breaches of confidentiality and invasions of privacy is emphasized. The ethical principle of autonomy, upon which the regulations are based, encompasses the right of the individual to decide when and under what circumstances to disclose to others the existence of illness and medical treatments.

Data gathered for quality assessment and improvement, performance measurement, and outcomes management is often considered to be exempt from the regulations governing access to individually identifiable data collected for research and from the ethical principles that underlie the federal regulations governing research. Many contracts between health care organizations and purchasers of care (usually employers) state that data and information related to quality of care may be reviewed without the explicit prior authorization of the patient or the review of a body charged with assuring protection of confidentiality and privacy (i.e., institutional review boards). Groups involved in performance measurement, quality assessment, and outcomes monitoring sometimes request information that reveals the diagnoses and the treatments of identifiable individuals without specifying how privacy and confidentiality will be protected and without acknowledging the potential risk of breaches of privacy and confidentiality. There appear to be two standards for access to health data—the research standard and the quality-of-care measurement standard.

The tension between protection of privacy and demands for access will continue until there are structures and processes that allow the potential of data to measure and improve quality to be exploited while protecting the individual from harm due to breaches of privacy and confidentiality. When Clinton's health care reform package was being discussed, anticipating the availability of, and need for, large amounts of data about health, the Institute of Medicine (1994) sponsored a conference to explore these issues in depth. The suggestions made at this conference are a useful starting point for the discussion of privacy, confidentiality, and access in the postreform era.

Summary

Performance measures relate to a defined population (e.g., the members of a health plan, persons hospitalized in a certain hospital, residents of a community). The link with the epidemiologic concept of "population-based" is strong. Measures of quality and performance measures are quantitative measures—rates, proportions, populations means, etc. The skills of the epidemiologist in interpreting measures in the face of sampling variation are directly relevant. Obtaining specific measures of quality and performance often requires primary data collection, which may entail designing chart review forms and questionnaires, determining the appropriate sample size, deciding on a sampling frame, and supervising data collection. These are all components of traditional risk-factor epidemiology. Explicit methods to measure quality of care have particularly close linkages with epidemiology. They use data collection methods and statistical approaches that are the same as in traditional risk-factor epidemiology. Finally, just as in outcomes research, an understanding of confounding and of statistical approaches to control for confounding (i.e., risk adjustment) is critical to the interpretation of measures of quality and performance.

Figure 10-1 shows a schematic of the relationships of quality (as a construct) and the measurement of quality, outcomes research, and cost evalua-

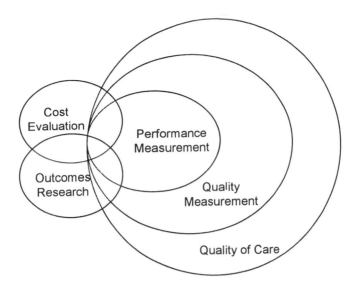

Figure 10-1. The overlap of economic evaluation, outcomes research, performance measurment, quality measurement, and quality

tion. Outcomes research is often, but not always, aimed at measuring quality of care. It overlaps and is in many, but not all cases, indistinguishable from performance measurement or methods for quality measurement. As described in Chapter 8, cost evaluation is often a component of outcomes research. It is also a component of the measurement of quality and performance measurement. Finally, operationally, just as outcomes research flows into outcomes management (see Figure 8-1), performance measurement flows into performance monitoring and then into intervention.

Performance measurement and surveillance have many features in common. Both involve ongoing measurement. Both seek to develop standardized measures. Both use information from measurement to decide on interventions and evaluate the effects of the interventions by monitoring the same measures over time.

The measurement of quality provides employment opportunities for epidemiologists with an interest in the delivery of health services as a vehicle to improve health. Many managed care organizations have a population perspective that is closely aligned with the goals of public health epidemiologists. Finally, the field of quality measurement is in need of technical experts with the skills that most epidemiologists possess.

CASE STUDIES

Selecting Quality Indicators for the Health Plan Employer Data and Information Set (HEDIS): Diabetes

Background

The Health Plan Employer Data and Information Set (HEDIS) is a performance indicator system that was developed by the National Committee on Quality Assurance (NCQA) to compare the quality of care of Health Maintenance Organizations (HMOs) (Corrigan and Nielsen 1993). The desirable attributes of performance measures and the criteria for selection of performance measure for HEDIS 3.0 were presented in Tables 10-5. Imagine that you are on the committee charged with selecting clinical quality of care indicators for HEDIS.

Key Questions

1. A candidate quality indicator measure for diabetics for HEDIS 3.0 was the percentage of diabetics who have had a hemoglobin (Hgb) A1C measurement in the past year. Is this a process indicator or an outcome indicator?

The percentage of diabetics who have a HgbA1C is a process indicator. It is a reflection of what is done to and for the patient.

2. How would you rate the validity of HgbA1C as a clinical quality of care indicator?

The Diabetes Complications and Control Trial was a randomized controlled trial (Diabetes Control and Complications Trail Research Group 1993). It showed that strict control of serum glucose in type I (insulin-dependent) diabetes prevents nephropathy, neuropathy, and retinopathy. Hemoglobin A1C is a valid and reproducible measure of control of serum glucose over a period of 2–3 months. Measurement of HgbA1C and attempts to keep it below 8.0% are supported by data from this well-conducted clinical trial.

Randomized trials of strict glucose control in type II (non–insulin dependent) diabetes have not been completed. Many believe that the mechanisms for development of the microvascular complications of type I and type II diabetes are the same and that extrapolation from findings in type I diabetes is justified. However, there is concern that tight control of serum glucose might lead to serious episodes of hypoglycemia in elderly patients and patients with comorbidities, who comprise a large proportion of patients with type II diabetes. Thus, while there is a growing consensus that HgbA1C should be measured and monitored for type II diabetics, there is no evidence from randomized trials that it affects outcome favorable. Those who would hold clinical quality-of-care process indicators to the standard of proof in randomized trials would not accept this measure as a valid quality-of-care indicator for type II diabetes.

Implications for Practice

It is difficult to identify clinical quality-of-care indicators for which there is universal agreement. Even when data from clinical trials supports the efficacy of an intervention, it may be difficult to define a quality-of-care indicator based on the data that is feasible and is unequivocally a measure of high quality care.

Quality of Care Measures for Post-MI Patients

Background

There is substantial evidence from randomized trials that patients with acute myocardial infarction (MI) who are treated with thrombolytic therapy within 8 hours of symptom onset have better outcomes (Yusuf et al. 1985a). Randomized trials also establish that post-MI patients treated with aspirin (Antiplatelet Trialists' Collaboration 1988) and beta-blockers (Yusuf et al. 1985b) have been better outcomes. Measures of the percentage of patients with acute MI treated with thrombolytic therapy within 8 hours of symptom onset, of the percentage treated with aspirin, and of the percentage treated with beta-blockers are all scientifically valid clinical quality-of-care process indicators.

Key Questions

1. Which of these three measures is likely to be most feasible using administrative or medical records data?

Aspirin does not require a prescription and a physician recommendation to use it would not be recorded in computer-stored prescription databases. A recommendation to use aspirin also might not be recorded in the medical record, because it is not a prescription medication. Even if a physician recorded a recommendation to use aspirin in the medical record, actual use by the patient could be assessed only by surveying the patient. Since adherence is part of the quality-of-care picture, use of aspirin, and not just a recommendation to use it, is the best measure of quality of care. Collecting data by surveys is costly. In addition, the reliability and validity of self-reported use of aspirin are uncertain. Response bias is always a concern in surveys.

Thrombolytics are given acutely in the emergency department. The completeness of recording of provision of thrombolytic therapy in computer-stored prescription databases would vary depending on the degree of integration of emergency department drug data into the computer-stored data system. The fact that a thrombolytic was given would probably be recorded in the emergency department and/or hospital record, but the time between symptom onset and the provision of the medication might not be recorded routinely in these records.

Beta-blockers are prescription drugs. For persons with a drug coverage benefit, filled prescriptions would be recorded in computer-stored prescription databases. Filled prescription data do not reflect physician recommendations or patient adherence with use. However, if restricted to persons with a drug benefit, computer-stored prescription data are a reasonably good source of data on beta-blocker use post-MI. The medical record would contain information on whether a beta-blocker was prescribed for all post-MI patients regardless of drug benefit coverage and the filling of the prescription. Obtaining data from medical records is costly.

2. What are some other reasons to be concerned about the use of the percentage of post-MI patients treated with a beta-blocker as a clinical quality-of-care indicator?

There are several contraindications to use of a beta-blocker even in post-MI patients (e.g., asthma). If the percentage of post-MI patients using beta-blockers were 100%, there should be concern that persons with contraindications to beta-blocker use were not identified, which is low quality care. It is not certain what percentage of persons have contraindications. The optimal percentage of post-MI patients on a beta-blocker might vary from population to population depending on the prevalence of contraindications. Contraindications to use of beta-blockers would not be recorded in administrative databases. Contraindications would be recorded in medical records. Obtaining data on the percentage of post-MI patients on a beta-blocker with reference to the existence of specific contraindications would make the information costly to obtain because it would require review of medical records.

Implications for Practice

Even when there is strong evidence that a given intervention constitutes high quality care, it may be difficult, or even impossible, to obtain a valid and reliable measure of the extent to which the intervention is applied in practice. The choice of measures of quality is determined as much by the feasibility and cost of obtaining data as it is by the accuracy of the data.

SUGGESTED READINGS

Blumenthal D. Quality of care: what is it? N Engl J Med 1996;335:891–894.

Brook RH, McGlynn EA, Cleary PD. Measuring quality of care. N Engl J Med 1996;335:966–970.

Donabedian A. The quality of care: how can it be assessed? JAMA 1988;260:1743–1748.

Lohr KN, Yordy KD, Thier SO. Current issues in quality of care. Health Affairs 1988;7:5–18.

Palmer RH, Peterson LE. Development and testing of performance measures for quality improvement in clinical preventive services. Am J Prev Med 1995;11:402–406.

REFERENCES

American Medical Association, Council of Medical Service. Quality of care. JAMA 1986;256:1032–1034.

Antiplatelet Trialists' Collaboration: Secondary prevention of vascular disease by prolonged antiplatelet treatment. Br Med J 1988;296:320–332.

Blumenthal D. Quality of care: what is it? N Engl J Med 1996;335:891–894.

Brook RH, Appel FA. Quality-of-care assessment: choosing a method for peer review. N Engl J Med 1973;288:1323–1329.

Brook RH, McGlynn EA, Cleary PD. Measuring quality of care. N Engl J Med 1996a;335:966–970.

Brook RH, Kamberg CJ, McGlynn EA. Health system reform and quality. JAMA 1996b;276:476–480.

Corrigan JM, Nielsen DM. Toward the development of uniform reporting standards for managed care organizations: the Health Plan Employer Data and Information Set (Version 2.0). J Quality Improvement 1993;19:566–575.

Diabetes Control and Complications Trial Research Group. The effect of intensive diabetes treatment on the development and progression of long-term complications in diabetes mellitus: the Diabetes Control and Complications Trial. N Engl J Med 1993;329:977–986.

Donabedian A. Explorations in Quality Assessment and Monitoring, Volume 1. The Definition of Quality and Approaches to its Assessment. Ann Arbor, MI: Health Administration Press; 1980.

Donabedian A. Explorations in Quality Assessment and Monitoring, Volume 2. The Criteria and Standards of Quality. Ann Arbor, MI: Health Administration Press; 1982.

Donabedian A. Explorations in Quality Assessment and Monitoring, Volume 3. The Methods and Findings of Quality Assessment and Monitoring: an Illustrated Analysis. Ann Arbor, MI: Health Administration Press; 1985.

Donabedian A. The quality of care: how can it be assessed? JAMA 1988;260:1743–1748.

Donaldson MS. Gearing up for health data in the information age. J Quality Improvement 1994;20:202–207.

Elinson J. Advances in health assessment discussion panel. J Chronic Dis 1987:40(Suppl 1):83S-91S.

Ellwood PM. Outcomes management: a technology of patient experience. N Engl J Med 1988;318:1549–1556.

Gerbert B, Hargreaves WA. Measuring physician behavior. Med Care 1986;24:838–847.

Graham J. Foundation for Accountability (FACCT): A Major New Voice in the Quality Debate. Medical Outcomes & Guidelines Sourcebook; 1997: 4–9.

Institute of Medicine, Donaldson MS, Lohr KN, ed. Health Data in the Information Age: Use, Disclosure, and Privacy. Washington, DC: National Academy Press; 1994.

Institute of Medicine, Committee on Using Performance Measurement to Improve Community Health. Using Performance Measurement to Improve Community Health: Exploring the Issues. Washington, DC: National Academy Press; 1996.

Lawthers AG, Palmer RH, Edwards JE, Fowles J, Garnick DW, Weiner JP. Developing and evaluating measures of ambulatory care quality: a preliminary report of the DEMPAQ Project. J Quality Improvement 1993;19:552–565.

Leape LL. Error in medicine. JAMA 1994;272:1851–1857.

Lee PR, McGinnis JM. Quality improvement issues: how they affect clinical preventive services. Am J Prev Med 1995;11:381–382.

Loeb JM, Buck AS. Framework for selection of performance measurement systems: attributes for conformance. JAMA 1996;275:509.

Lohr KN, ed. Medicare: A Strategy for Quality Assurance. Washington, DC: National Academy Press; 1990.

Lohr KN, Yordy KD, Thier SO. Current issues in quality of care. Health Affairs 1988;7:5–18.

Palmer RH, Peterson LE. Development and testing of performance measures for quality improvement in clinical preventive services. Am J Prev Med 1995;11:402–406.

Relman AS. Assessment and accountability: the third revolution in medical care. N Engl J Med 1988;319:1220–1222.

Siu AL, McGlynn EA, Morgenstern H, Brook RH. A fair approach to comparing quality of care. Health Affairs 1991;10:62–75.

Yusuf S, Collins R, Peto R, Furberg C, Stampfer MJ, Goldhaber SZ, Hennekens CH. Intravenous and intracoronary fibrinolytic therapy in acute myocardial infarction: overview of results on mortality, reinfarction and side-effects from 33 randomized controlled trials. Eur Heart J 1985a;6:556–585.

Yusuf S, Peto R, Lewis J, Collins R, Sleight P. Beta blockade during and after myocardial infarction: an overview of the randomized trials. Prog Cardiovasc Dis 1985b;27:335–371.

11

Communicating Epidemiologic Information

PATRICK L. REMINGTON

"The data speak for themselves"—Unknown

Although epidemiologic research has profound public health and policy implications, its meaning must be communicated effectively to a wide variety of technical and nontechnical audiences. Epidemiology courses and texts teach important research skills, but few provide the practical skills needed to communicate to a diverse public. The data may speak for themselves, but epidemiologists can translate what they say for practitioners of public health and clinical medicine.

Reaching the diverse consumers of health information is no easy task. Epidemiologic information is complex and technical, and often inconclusive or contradictory. Scientists and health care providers are overwhelmed by the information reported every day in scientific journals. The mass media and the general public seem to have an insatiable appetite for this information, with little regard for its accuracy or relevance. Policy-makers and public officials are often left to develop health policies without input from epidemiologic research. Recognizing the increasing importance and complexity of health communication, the CDC recently created a separate health communication unit to give focused attention to this field (Roper 1993).

Strategies for communicating epidemiologic information range from presentations given in a continuing education course to the development of a complex, multimillion-dollar national health education campaign. This chapter will not attempt to provide an exhaustive review of the many health communications strategies (Cwikel 1994; Maibach and Holtgrave 1995). The interested reader is encouraged to explore the excellent references listed at the end of this chapter. Rather, several communication strategies that an epidemiologist may encounter in his or her practice will be described:

- *Written communication:* the preparation of a report or manuscript describing the purpose, methods, results, and implications of a study

- *Oral communication:* the presentation of information to a group of individuals.
- *Health-related media stories:* the reporting of epidemiologic information in newspapers, television, or other news media
- *Public health surveillance:* strategies used by public health agencies to improve the dissemination of surveillance information, primarily intended for health professionals and policy-makers
- *Risk communication:* strategies to communicate risk information to the public, to assure appropriate public health policies
- *Social marketing:* social change strategies that communicate epidemiologic information by understanding the needs of the target audience
- *Media advocacy:* strategies to promote specific health policies through media coverage of health issues

Written Communication

Writing is fundamental to communicating epidemiologic information. These skills can be developed informally by reading and carefully analyzing current literature (Riegelman and Hirsch 1996) or by writing papers and submitting them for peer review and critique. In addition, writing skills can be enhanced through formal study. Many institutions offer scientific writing courses and several texts have been written for those interested in improving their writing skills (Gregg 1996). The following provides a brief overview of the steps used to write a scientific paper.

Most scientific writing is divided into distinct sections, with a title, abstract, introduction, methods, results, discussion, acknowledgments, references, and tables and figures.

Title

The title is a critically important part of a report. Like the headline of a newspaper article, it is the 'hook' that grabs the reader's attention. Titles should be brief yet provide enough information about the purpose or findings of the study. Many authors use the title to summarize the major finding of the report. Consider the subtle difference between a title such as "The Effects of Estrogen Use on Breast Cancer Risk," and "Estrogen Use Increases Risk of Breast Cancer." The former describes what the study is about, the latter provides a concise summary of the main conclusion of the article.

Abstract

The abstract provides the reader with a brief (150–200 words) yet complete overview of the paper. Each section of the paper is summarized in a sentence or two, beginning with the background or purpose of the study, the principal methods used, the key results, and the conclusions. Recently, several journals have started using structured abstracts, with specific headings (Haynes et al. 1990). For example, the *Journal of American Medical Association* recommends using the structured headings of objective, design, setting, patients or other participants, intervention, main outcome measure(s), results, and conclusions (American Medical Association 1997). The *New England Journal of Medicine* states that abstracts should consist of four paragraphs: background, methods, results, and conclusions (*New England Journal of Medicine* 1996).

Introduction

The introduction is usually brief and sets the stage for the reader. The first part describes the problem that the research is addressing. It is followed by a brief statement of other work that has been done by others. Although some writers use the introduction to present a detailed review of the literature, in most clinical and epidemiologic reports the literature review is either very brief or placed in the discussion section. Finally, the introduction should conclude with a statement regarding the specific purpose of the research, especially if an a priori hypothesis was tested. Examples of such statements include, "We hypothesize that women who consumed alcohol are at greater risk of developing breast cancer" or "The purpose of this paper is to describe the trends in breast cancer mortality in the United States for white and black women."

Methods

The methods section describes how the study was conducted. Enough information should be presented so that the reader could replicate the study in a different setting. The study design should be described, such as a cross-sectional survey, case-control study, cohort study, or randomized control trial. Subheadings are helpful for organizing the components of the study design, and include:

- Study setting and time period
- Patients or participants, with clear inclusion and exclusion criteria
- Data collection, including the main outcome measure
- Intervention or assignment methods
- Quality control measures
- Data analysis and statistical techniques

Results

The results section presents the findings of the research. The first part often describes the characteristics of the study population. Information is presented in tables or figures and referred to in the text. Only results of the study should be presented. Methods should not be described in the results section and any comment or reference to other literature should be saved for the discussion. The adage, "A picture is worth a thousand words" applies to epidemiologic reports. Tables and figures can help communicate complex numerical information presented in a table (Tufte 1987).

Discussion

Although rarely divided into subsections, the discussion should describe the major conclusion of the paper, how these findings relate to the past research, the limitations of the study, and the implications of this research for health care providers or policy-makers. The first sentence of the discussion is often a single statement of the major finding of the paper. An example would be, "In this study, we demonstrated that women who consume more than two drinks per day are at increased risk of developing breast cancer." These findings are then compared and contrasted with other research conducted in the past. Finally, the implications of the research are often described for health care providers or policy-makers.

Before the report is submitted for publication, the author should carefully review the journal for the exact writing style and format. Reviewing previously published articles, which represent the "successes," provides the best guide for how a paper should be written. Some journals tend to publish papers with more detailed introductions. Others may avoid discussion of policy implications and instead focus only on research findings. For example, the journal *Epidemiology* states that "opinions or recommendations about public health policy should be reserved for editorials, letters, or commentaries, and not presented as the conclusions of scientific research" (Epidemiology 1997). A paper that is written to conform to the journal's style and content will have a greater likelihood of being accepted for publication.

The last step before submitting a manuscript for publication is to read the entire report aloud. This single step is one of the best ways to uncover problems in the text, such as confusing or complex sentences, errors in grammar, or missing words or text. These are rarely uncovered by automated spell- or grammar-check programs.

Oral Communication

Epidemiologists are frequently called upon to present information to a variety of professional and public audiences in diverse settings, ranging from scientific conferences to town hall meetings. Effective oral presentations can impart important information to key individuals and groups (Levy 1997). One needs to prepare well in advance and understand the science base of the research or surveillance findings. It is important to listen to the audience and capture their attention with real-life examples. Many communities throughout the United States are conducting formal health and community needs assessments (Institute of Medicine 1988), and epidemiologists are called upon to help interpret community-level data for the planners and community at large.

Although there are no absolute rules for oral presentations, the following guidelines may be useful to the practicing epidemiologist:

- *Understand your audience and the purpose of the presentation:* Why have you been asked to speak? Is it to provide information on a general topic or to respond to a specific community concern? One must understand the background and expectations of the audience. A presentation at the Society for Epidemiologic Research annual scientific session will obviously differ from a presentation to a community group. Slides or overheads might be appropriate for a health audience but not for the general public.
- *Determine the time allowed for your presentation:* An otherwise excellent presentation can be ruined if the presenter talks beyond allotted time. Some scientific meetings provide very strict time allowances, such as 10 or 15 minutes. On other occasions, one might be allowed to talk for 20 minutes to an hour. Regardless of the time available, it is important to plan to use less time than scheduled and to leave more time for unanticipated questions and discussion. A general rule is to allow at least one-third of the time for discussion (e.g., 5 minutes for a 10 minute talk, 20 minutes for a 40 minute talk). A question and answer period provides an opportunity for intelligent discussion and gives the audience and the presenter greater insight on the work. Always use a timer and stop talking when the time is up.
- *Prepare audiovisuals:* Good audiovisuals make the difference between a good talk and a great talk. There are many excellent software programs available to facilitate such presentations. Despite such technical advances, a few basic rules must be followed. Use the 1-minute/one-slide rule—, e.g. no more than 20 slides should be presented in a 20-minute talk. Tables and graphs may require more than a minute, and a slide with a short list of "bulleted" statements less than a minute. Never say, "This is a busy slide." Never say, "I want you to ignore all of this and just look here." Instead, display *only* the information that you want the audience to see. If all of the information is important on a busy slide, it should be distributed among two or more separate slides.
- *Practice your presentation:* Few people can deliver a well-organized presentation "off the cuff." A presentation is always easier to give and understand the second or third time. A practice run will enable you to see how long the talk takes. Later, compare the "practice time" with the time that it actually takes to give the talk. Take any differences into account the next time. Finally, practicing a presentation provides you with a chance to present the information to colleagues. This not only lets them know more about your work but provides an opportunity to get their insight and constructive criticism.
- *Walk the viewer's eyes through the slide:* Follow the written text using a laser or

other type of pointer. Take extra time for figures. For a graph, slowly read the title and then y- and x-axis legends. Then point out the major finding of the slide. Similarly for a table, read the title and column headings and then point out the major finding. For text, point to each phrase and read it exactly as it is written. If you find yourself saying something that is different from the written text, change the slide. Short "bullet" statements can be used to make a point, and then you can elaborate further.

- *Be clear and concise:* Someone once said that a good talk has a clear introduction, concise conclusions, and, above all else, nothing in between. A different rule of thumb divides a talk into three parts: Tell them what you're going to say, say it, and then tell them what you said. It is often preferable to communicate one or two things effectively than to present all of the "interesting" findings. One will never be criticized for giving a talk that is too clear and well organized.
- *Record and review:* Finally, one way to improve the quality of your presentation skills is to evaluate your performance yourself. This can be accomplished by asking the audience to complete an evaluation form or by asking selected individuals in the audience for feedback. Presentations can be recorded on video, or, more simply, by using a hand-held tape recorder. This type of self-assessment is extremely helpful and often points out problems that are easy to remedy.

Reporting Epidemiologic Research by the News Media

Most of the information that Americans receive about science and technology comes from television news programs and newspapers (Nelkin 1987). The news media has become increasingly interested in reporting the results of research as they are published in journals or presented at scientific conferences. Science and health writers scour the hundreds of studies published each week. Their selection of which published research will be played in a lead story shapes the public image of the critical health issues of the day. Many health professionals first learn about the results of an important study by reading it in the morning paper or hearing it on the six o'clock news.

The role of the media in reporting on scientific studies was recently assessed (Wilkes and Kravitz 1992). Two journals in the United States—the *New England Journal of Medicine* and the *Journal of the American Medical Association*—account for many of the national and local stories that present health information to the public. Wilkes and Kravitz (1992) reviewed reports published in these two journals during a 10-month period in 1989, and found 414 original scientific articles. The most common type of study published during this time dealt with epidemiology or health services research (42%), compared with basic science (21%), clinical trials (26%), and other topics (11%).

The first authors of these reports stated that their research was often discussed in the lay press; coverage included print and electronic media at the local and national level (Table 11-1). In this study, most first authors were contacted by the media and most authors made special efforts to make themselves available. Many were aided by press releases issued by their institutions or the journal, or by press conferences. Thus, the dissemination of this information is a result of efforts by both media and researchers.

The media's interest in reporting health information is a result of the public interest and demand for such information. Reporters are looking for new information, startling results, or studies that contradict the status quo. Preliminary findings or seemingly trivial results are often reported boldly as "important new information" or "a study with startling findings." At times it may seem more important to sell newspapers and advertising space than to present a concise and effective health message.

Authors may conclude their work with a cautionary statement and caveat such as, "These data are preliminary and should be interpreted with caution." However, once in the press, these caveats are useless (Taubes 1995). In response to this, professional journals have published guidelines on how to deal with reporters. These guidelines serve as defensive tactics, warning epidemiologists to be aware of the reporter's motives. The *New England Journal of Medicine* warns, "Never even whisper to a reporter anything you would not care to see in screaming headlines." Potential problems can be identified if authors do a dry run with public relations staff in their agency.

At the other end of the spectrum from overly aggressive reporters is the promotion of research findings by scientists themselves. A presentation of "major research findings" at a press conference may promote the researcher's—or institution's—stature in the community. Many institutions

Table 11-1. Types of Media Coverage of Reports Published in the *New England Journal of Medicine* and the *Journal of the American Medical Association*, 1989

	Number	*Percent*
Report received media attention	239	65%
Newspaper coverage		
Local	158	43%
National	84	23%
Electronic media coverage		
Local	132	36%
National	125	34%
Trade journals	147	40%
All reports	367	100%

Source: Wilkes and Kravitz (1992).

employ a media or public relations professional to increase coverage. These professionals serve as an important link between the media and scientists, helping to package complex material in a manageable form (Nelkin 1987).

Epidemiologic research takes an incremental approach in determining the causes of disease and effectiveness of preventive interventions. Many of the major risk factors for diseases were identified decades ago. Wynder recalls that in his early study of smoking and lung cancer, "the relative risks were so large that, in fact, our paper published in 1950 included no statistical testing. For similar reasons, other studies such as those on alcohol and cancer of the upper alimentary tract, sexual habits and cervical cancer, radiation and leukemia were also easy targets to explore by even the inexperienced epidemiologist" (Wynder 1996).

Occasionally, causal relationships have been established following a few studies. For example, aspirin was determined to cause Reye syndrome, an often fatal disease of young children, as a result of a few studies published in the early 1980s (Starko et al. 1980; Waldman et al. 1982; Halpin et al. 1982). The media attention given to these studies caused a dramatic decline in aspirin use and an associated decline in the number of Reye syndrome cases (Remington et al. 1986).

Despite these occasional important health discoveries, most of the understanding about disease causation accumulates over years, and even decades, often requiring dozens of different studies using a variety of epidemiologic methods. Much of today's epidemiologic research focuses on risk factors that

Table 11-2. Media Highlights of Controversies in Epidemiology

Risk Factor	Headline or Implication	Contradiction
Coffee	Causes pancreatic cancer (McMahon et al. 1981)	Does not cause pancreatic cancer (Feinstein et al. 1981)
Type A personality	Causes heart disease (Barefoot et al. 1983)	Does not cause heart disease (Shekelle et al. 1987)
Margarine	Is good for the heart	Is bad for the heart (Willett and Asherio 1994)
Pesticides	Cause breast cancer (Falck et al. 1992)	Do not cause breast cancer (Krieger et al. 1994)
Estrogen replacement therapy	Does not cause breast cancer (Kaufman et al. 1984)	Causes breast cancer (Steinberg et al. 1991)
Beta carotene	Prevents cancer	Causes cancer (Omenn et al. 1996)
Oral contraceptives	Do not cause breast cancer (Cancer and Steroid Hormone Study Group 1986)	Cause breast cancer (Miller DR et al. 1989).

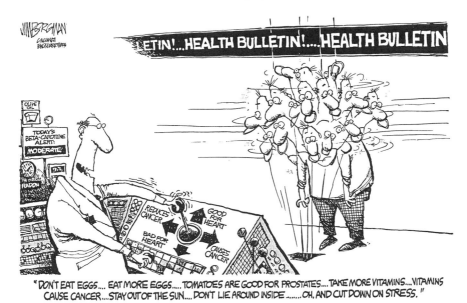

"DON'T EAT EGGS.... EAT MORE EGGS..... TOMATOES ARE GOOD FOR PROSTATES.... TAKE MORE VITAMINS.... VITAMINS CAUSE CANCER.... STAY OUT OF THE SUN.... DON'T LIE AROUND INSIDE........ OH, AND CUT DOWN ON STRESS. "

Figure 11-1. Conflicting health messages received by the public (Reprinted with special permission of King Features Syndicate)

are prevalent in society, such as alcohol consumption or exposure to environmental tobacco smoke or pesticides. Even with a small relative risk of disease among those exposed (e.g., a relative risk of 1.3), the widespread exposure to these factors creates a potentially large public health problem. Despite the potential importance of the issue, however, many of the studies that examine these risks are plagued by biases, errors in measurement, and methodologic weaknesses. Thus, some have stated that we now approach the "limits of epidemiology" (Taubes 1995). When results from studies appear to conflict, the media highlights the controversy (Taubes 1995; Angell and Kassirer 1994). Examples of this abound in the literature (Table 11-2 and Figure 11-1).

In conclusion, communicating epidemiologic information through media coverage of published research often leaves the public confused, bewildered, and in a state of "information overload." As a result, the public may begin to doubt all the information, or select only the information that conforms with their desires and existing beliefs. More organized strategies are needed to improve the public's understanding about these issues.

Public Health Surveillance

A goal of peer-reviewed research is to advance the science knowledge base. In contrast, the goal of public health surveillance is to report on the health of the population so that the information may be used to improve public health. Surveillance is considered by the Institute of Medicine to be one of the core functions of public health (Institute of Medicine 1988). As noted in Chapter 4, contemporary public health surveillance is "the ongoing systematic collection, analysis, and interpretation of outcome-specific data essential to the planning, implementation, and evaluation of public health programs, closely integrated with the timely dissemination of these data to those responsible for prevention and control" (Thacker 1988). A surveillance system must include not only the capacity for data collection and analysis but also the capacity to effectively communicate this information to a broad array of audiences (Goodman and Remington 1993). This final link in the surveillance chain is the application of surveillance findings for disease prevention and health promotion. A surveillance "system" includes a functional capacity for data collection, analysis, and dissemination linked to public health programs as illustrated in the surveillance "loop" (Figure 11-2).

Surveillance systems have evolved continuously over the past several decades, as the major health problems have evolved from infectious diseases to chronic diseases and as advances in technology have permitted the use of diverse data systems, such as hospital discharge data, random-digit-dialed telephone survey data, or cancer registries. Recently, the principles of surveillance have been used by state and national agencies to monitor the quality of health care (Chassin et al. 1996). For example, tools such as HEDIS (Health Plan Employer Data Information System) are currently being used to monitor the quality of care delivered by managed-care organizations (Iglehart 1996).

This increasing amount of surveillance data provides a wealth of information to public health agencies. However, too often these agencies simply analyze the data and report the results in agency reports, or occasionally in state or national publications. These reports are often long and contain technical jargon. In addition, the information is seldom linked to program priorities, and the reports are seldom used to promote public health practice or as a vehicle for setting priorities for action.

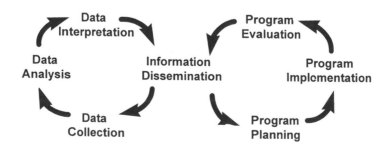

Figure 11-2. Surveillance loop (Remington and Goodman 1993)

Epidemiologists working in public health agencies are frequently asked to disseminate the results of a surveillance report, often by publishing the information in a health department report. To increase application of surveillance findings to disease prevention and health promotion programs, a basic framework for communicating surveillance information has been developed (see Table 11-3) (Remington and Goodman 1993).

Conduct the Analysis

Most surveillance reports use epidemiology to assess the time, person, and place characteristics of a disease or risk factor. A "trend" report might show an increase in the rate of a disease over time, such as an increase in the death rate due to lung cancer among women (Remington and Fiore 1989). A "person" report might show that a certain population subgroup is at increased risk of developing a disease, such as an increasing breast cancer death rate among black women, compared to a declining rate among white women (Palmersheim and Remington 1996). Finally, a "place" report might show a higher rate of a certain disease in a region, such as a higher death rate from cardiovascular disease in a rural part of a state.

Establish the Message

This is perhaps the most important step in disseminating health and surveillance information. Like businesses, public health agencies have a product (i.e., information) that they need to sell (i.e., communicate). An epidemiologist must convince the audience that it is worth their time to read, understand, and act on the information. An important adage in marketing the message is that "less is more."

Many reports produced by public health agencies are long, technical, and full of information. These reports might be mailed to the media, policy makers, or health care providers who, in turn, rarely take the time read through the report to find the important information. In order to capture their

Table 11-3. Steps in Communicating Public Health Surveillance Information

Step	Question	Action
1	What do the data show?	Conduct the analysis
2	What should be said?	Establish the message
3	What is the communication objective?	Set an objective
4	To whom should the message be directed?	Define the audience
5	What communications medium should be used?	Select the channel
6	Was the communication objective achieved?	Evaluate the impact

attention, the main point of the report must be obvious and simple to under-stand.

Set a Communication Objective

Why is the information being reported? Public health agencies often report information without any specific goal, but simply "because it is there." At other times, the purpose is to educate the general public about a health issue. This is a worthy but challenging goal given the complexity of the message and the inability to shape the message for the intended audience.

Occasionally, surveillance findings point to needed public health action. For example, recent findings of increasing smoking rates among youth em-phasize the need for effective youth smoking–prevention initiatives. There-fore, the intent of releasing this information might be to support a public health initiative, such as the FDA youth smoking rules.

Define the Audience

Once the objective for communicating the information has been established, one can define the appropriate target audience. Local health departments and health care providers have been the long-standing audience for communicable disease surveillance information since these professionals have been responsi-ble for implementing disease control strategies. In addition, physicians have been the source of these reports, and reporting back to them has shown the usefulness of the system and supported their continued reporting.

The audience for public health surveillance information is much broader today. It includes policy-makers, voluntary health organizations, professional organizations, and the general public. A report that lung cancer death rates are increasing in a state could be communicated to the general public or to young women specifically. This would increase awareness of the health conse-quences of smoking. It might also be targeted to policy-makers—such as legislators considering increasing the tax on cigarettes to fund a comprehen-sive statewide smoking prevention and control program. Finally, the report could be given to an advocacy organization, such as a state-wide women's health council to use in their efforts to advocate for women's health.

Select a Channel

A "channel" can be considered the medium through which messages must travel to reach the intended audience. Examples of channels include profes-sional journals, direct mail, television, radio, and newspapers. Public health agencies traditionally report surveillance information in newsletters or statistical bulletins. These reports are routinely mailed to local public health agencies, physicians, health care institutions, the media, and other interested individuals in the community or the state. A press release is occasionally used to increase the media interest in the story.

Careful selection of a proper communication channel increases the likelihood that the information will reach the target audience. This requires a thorough understanding, based on market research, of how those individuals get their information. For example, children and teachers might best be reached through the school system newsletter. Policy-makers might be reached through a direct mailing to their offices or via a constituent organization. Doctors might be reached through a state medical society journal.

In an effort to bring public health surveillance information to Wisconsin's doctors, the Wisconsin Division of Health established a "public health column" in the *Wisconsin Medical Journal,* the monthly journal of the state's medical society. Each month, one or more brief articles are published that present a wide variety of surveillance information. These articles are often cited in the media and are widely quoted by the journal's readership. This series represents one of the channels that a state division of health can use to bring information to the medical and health care community.

In addition, creative presentation of information can increase the media coverage of a health issues. An oft-cited example involves reporting the health impact from cigarette smoking in the United States. The government reports that over 400,000 persons die each year from smoking-related diseases. This health burden can be equated with the lives lost if two fully-loaded 747s crashed every day for a year. In Wisconsin, the health burden from tobacco was described in terms of the death of an entire city's population (Moss et al. 1990).

Evaluate the Impact

The final step in a communication plan is to evaluate how widely the information was disseminated and whether the information led to the intended outcome. The dissemination can be measured by determining the number of reports distributed, or the readership of a journal, or by assessing the coverage in the media. Newspaper clipping services will search for all articles in a defined geographic area and provide copies of each article with the selected "key words." These articles can be reviewed by the program staff to assess the geographic distribution and extent of the media coverage. In addition, the content of the clippings can be reviewed to assess both the accuracy and appropriateness of the messages.

Determining the impact of the communication effort on public health action requires an evaluation of the changes in outcomes—changes in things such as knowledge, behaviors, and disease rates. This type of evaluation often requires surveys of the target population before and after the surveillance information has been disseminated to detect these changes. These evaluations are often expensive, time-consuming, and difficult to interpret.

Risk Perception and Risk Communication

Risk communication is a specialized communication strategy used by epidemiologists who work in health agencies or industries to improve the use of risk assessments in decision-making. Many of the strategies described elsewhere in this chapter *promote* public awareness of health issues, especially public concern regarding the health aspects of behaviors such as tobacco use, diet, and exercise. In contrast, risk communication can be considered a strategy to *decrease* the public's concern about certain health risks, most often those related to environmental exposures.

Twenty years ago, few scientists were involved in the field of risk perception and communication. Today, the literature contains hundreds of articles on this topic (Fishhoff et al. 1993). This increased interest has resulted from a number of factors (Covello 1995). First, the public has become increasingly concerned about environmental health issues, such as those related to nuclear power and electromagnetic fields. Second, laws have been enacted mandating that environmental risk information be communicated to the public, media, and special interest groups. Finally, the public increasingly does not believe in government and other institutions as sources of information.

The research today focuses in two broad areas: how the public perceives the risk and how health professionals communicate with the public.

Risk Perception

The perception—and misperception—of risk creates the demand for risk communication strategies. Scientists define risk precisely as "the rate of disease among those exposed, compared to those not exposed." Epidemiologic measures, such as relative risk, absolute risk, and risk differences provide a variety of measures of the potential impact of the "actual risk" on individuals and in populations. However, the risks from many environmental exposures, such as chemical toxins, pesticides, or electromagnetic fields, are often difficult to determine in scientific studies.

In response to these uncertainties, government agencies such as the Environmental Protection Agency, the Food and Drug Administration, and the Occupational Safety and Health Administration estimate risk using the best available data and then extrapolate this risk estimate it to actual settings.

These "risk assessments" consider results from a variety of sources, such as animal studies, and attempt to predict a rate of disease (such as cancer), given a specified exposure. Despite many limitations, these assessments provide a basis upon which to determine public health policy (Kreutzer and Arneson 1995).

When communicating risk information to the public, scientists have discovered that the 'actual' risk may have little or no relationship to the "perceived" risk. In some cases, the public greatly overestimates the risk and demands costly and difficult interventions. In other cases, the public may greatly underestimate the risk, and ignore recommendations that might have a substantial impact on their health. Considerable research has been conducted to determine how people perceive risk. More important than technical information are the origin, uncertainty, and familiarity with the risk. Table 11-4 lists some of the determinants of risk perception (Covello 1995).

Risk Communication

Risk communication strategies attempt to bring the perceived risk into line with the actual risk so that the resulting policies are reasonable. Covello defines it more simply as "the exchange of information among interested parties about the nature, magnitude, significance, and control of risk" (Covello 1995). The National Research Council (Maibach and Holtgrave 1995) defines risk communication as "an interactive process of exchange of information and opinion among individuals, groups, and institutions. It involves multiple messages about the nature of risk and other messages, not strictly about risk, that express concerns, opinions, or reactions to risk messages or to legal and institutional arrangements for risk management."

According to Covello (1995), there are three fundamental principles that underlie risk communication:

- *Perceptions are realities:* That which is perceived as real, even if untrue, is real to the person and real in its consequences.
- *The goal is to establish trust and credibility:* When trust and credibility are low, the communicating organization or individual should focus more on actions and communication that enhance trust and credibility and less on the transfer of technical information and facts.
- *Effective risk communication is a skill:* It requires a great deal of knowledge, preparation, and practice.

An important tool used in communicating risk information to the public is "comparative risk assessment." The idea is to put the unknown risk in context by expressing it in comparison with previously quantified risks, such as smoking, driving, or being struck by lightning. Risk comparisons are used when statistical data alone—such as the absolute risk of developing cancer if

Table 11-4. Factors Important in Risk Perception and Evaluation

Factors	Conditions Associated With Increased Public Concern	Conditions Associated With Decreased Public Concern
Familiarity	Unfamiliar	Familiar
Personal control	Uncontrollable	Controllable
Exposure	Involuntary	Voluntary
Media attention	Much media attention	Little media attention
Personal risk	Individual personally at risk	Individual not personally at risk

Source: Covello (1995).

exposed to a certain chemical—are not understood by the public. The theory is that the public will be able to make a more informed assessment of the "importance" of the unknown risk.

Recently, laws have been enacted to formalize the role of risk analysis in policy-making (Johnson and Slovic 1994). Despite the increasingly common practice of comparative risk assessment, however, risk communication specialists warn of a number of limitations. Finkel (1995) suggests that the uncertainty of estimates should be noted when making risk comparisons. For example, the claim was made that aflatoxin contamination of peanut butter was "18 times worse" than the Alar contamination of apple juice. Using a Monte Carlo simulation, Finkel showed that the actual risk estimate was a range—between nearly 400:1 in favor of aflatoxin to nearly 40:1 in the opposite direction. This uncertainty in the health risk may increase perceived risk among the public (Johnson and Slovic 1994).

Freaudenberg and Rursch (1994) noted that there has been little quantitative evidence available on the actual behavioral consequences of risk comparison efforts. When asking college students about their acceptance of an incinerator in their neighborhood (the unknown risk), he demonstrated that the use of comparative risks actually *decreased* support for the incinerator, compared to a simplified statistical summary. He concludes that the perception of risk of a new technology may have less to do with the absolute risk and more to do with citizens' levels of trust in government and industrial actors.

Risk communication research has undergone an evolution over the past 20 years. Fischhoff (1995) prepared an excellent summary of the developmental stages in risk management and communication. Early strategies focused on communicating actual risk information. To increase understanding of these technical data, risk comparisons were used to show people that they have accepted similar risk in the past. More recent strategies focus on developing trust and engaging the public as partners in the decision-making process. Today, most specialists in risk communication draw from all of these stages.

Social Marketing

Increasingly, public health practitioners have turned to formal health communication programs to prevent morbidity and premature mortality (Sutton et al. 1995). These programs have drawn from decades of research and writing on health communication theories, models, and practices. Each discipline offers a different perspective on consumers and the strategies needed to reach them (US Dept of Health and Human Services [US DHHS] 1992). For example, *social marketing* practice considers the perceptions and perceived needs of the target audience as an essential element of planning. *Health education* models involve an exploration of the components of behavioral intention that will influence an individual's willingness to act. *Mass communication* theories help explain factors that influence message transmission between the source and the target audience and the expected effects.

In this section, social marketing will be described (Brehony et al. 1984; Maibach and Holtgrave 1995), which is only one of the many strategies used in formal health communication programs. First articulated by Philip Kotler, this strategy illustrates a fundamental premise of all communications strategies—that is, a thorough understanding of the needs and perceptions of the target audience. The program's components focus on the product, price, place, and promotion.

Product

What is the program trying to communicate to the public? In communicating epidemiologic information to the public, the product is most often information. For example, epidemiologic studies demonstrated that high blood pressure was an important risk factor for stroke and that controlling blood pressure with medication substantial reduced the risk of stroke. Thus, the National High Blood Pressure Program was established to disseminate this information (i.e., the product) and increase the proportion of hypertensives whose blood pressure was under control (Brehony et al. 1984).

Price

What must the consumer give up in order to receive the program's benefits? When communicating epidemiologic information to the public, the "price" may be intangible (e.g., changes in beliefs or habits) or tangible (e.g., money, time, or travel). Kotler quotes Adam Smith as saying: "The real price of everything, what everything really costs to the man who wants to acquire it, is the toil and trouble of acquiring it" (Brehony et al. 1984). For example, informing women about the risk of alcohol and breast cancer may have the "price" of a change in current drinking habits. An additional cost might be the worry about exposure to alcohol in the past, or, if behavior does not change, worry about current alcohol consumption.

Place

What channel does the program use to reach the target audience? The "place" refers to the medium or channel that is used to communicate the information. The selection of the channel depends upon the type of information being communicated and the target audience. For example, information about the health and economic costs of smoking needs to be communicated to employers and policy-makers. Widespread coverage by the news media may be an appropriate channel, but a more directed strategy would be to publish the information in business journals or present it at a legislative hearing.

Promotion

How is the information promoted? What appeals are used to increase the chances that the public will hear, and act on the information? Promotion is a form of communication that encompasses all the tools of the marketing mix, whose major role is persuasive communication (Kotler 1975). Promotional tools include advertising, publicity, personal contact, and incentives (Frederiksen et al. 1984). The promotion of health information differs from commercial products in several ways. Epidemiologists cannot change the product (information) simply to increase its appeal to the consumer. Whereas companies have resources to promote commercial products, few health promotion or epidemiology programs have resources to promote information.

There are many other communication models, such as behavioral intentions, communication for persuasion, diffusion of innovation, PRECEDE, and consumer-based health strategies (US DHSS 1992; Sutton et al. 1995), that can be used to communicate epidemiologic information. Describing the details, strengths, and limitations of each of these approaches is beyond the scope of this chapter. However, common to all models is the importance of a thorough understanding of the needs and perceptions of the target audience. In addition, a careful planning process, such as that developed by the National Cancer Institute, will increase the likelihood of any campaign achieving its intended objectives (US DHHS 1992).

Media Advocacy

Media advocacy is a specialized type of health communication program. It is defined as the strategic use of mass media to advance a social or public policy

(US DHHS 1989). Media advocacy is similar to the health communication strategies described above, with several distinct features. First, it focuses on promoting a specific health policy, and second, it does so by exploiting the media's interest in health issues. Thus, it is promoted as a strategy to communicate health information to the public, without having to conduct an expensive educational campaign.

Media advocacy is not simply media relations—the "traditional" press work of establishing and maintaining media contacts, providing them with accurate and helpful information to support news and feature stories, and communicating media relations to ensure coverage of a particular issue. In contrast, media advocacy uses a range of media and advocacy strategies to define the problem and stimulate broad-based coverage (Wallack 1993). Media advocacy attempts to reframe and shape public discussion to increase support for and to advance healthy public policies.

The impact of policies on the public's health has become increasingly evident over the past decades. For example, a goal might be to increase the use of screening mammography among women. Early campaigns focused on educating women about the value of mammography in detecting breast cancer early. However, few insurance companies reimbursed for this service, and thus physicians were reluctant to recommend one, since women often found the cost a barrier. Thus, the public health campaign shifted its focus from directly promoting mammographs to promoting a policy that mandates insurance reimbursement for screening mammograms. As a result, many states have now enacted laws that mandate that insurance policies cover screening mammograms.

Social, economic, and legal policies have been found to play a critical role in countless other health issues. For example, enacting tough drunk driving laws have reduced alcohol-related motor vehicle injuries. Increasing the price of cigarettes through excise taxes has reduced per capita consumption and youth smoking rates. These community initiatives have provided solid evidence that local groups can gain access to the media, reframe issues to focus on policy, and advance community initiatives for policy change (Wallack 1993).

Wallack has described five steps as necessary in using media advocacy to advance public health policies:

- Establish what the group's policy goal is—what do you want to happen?
- Decide who the target audience is—to whom do you want to speak?
- Frame your issue and construct your message.
- Construct an overall media advocacy plan.
- Evaluate the impact of what you did.

Notice that this strategy differs from the steps used in communicating public health surveillance information in one important way—it starts out with a health policy objective. Whereas traditional public health surveillance communicates the information that is routinely reported to the agency, media advocacy might use the surveillance information to advance a policy objective.

Using science to advance health policy issues is an important role for the practicing epidemiologist. However, there is a fine line between the creative presentation of epidemiologic data to support a health policy, and the misinterpretation, misuse, or distortion of data to support a health policy. A recent study, conducted by researchers at the Centers for Disease Control, brought this issue to the public's eye.

A recent study demonstrated that 2.5% of adults reported an estimated 123 million episodes of being alcohol-impaired during in 1993 (Liu et al. 1997). This corresponds to 655 episodes of alcohol-impaired driving for each 1,000 adults, and 1,623 episodes per 1,000 adults 18–20 years of age. The authors concluded that alcohol-impaired driving is common—even among underage adults. Based on this study, the authors advocated a public policy by stating, "We hope that these results will support expanded efforts to reduce drinking."

Challenging the use of a scientific study to support public policy, Richard Berman, general counsel for the American Beverage Institute, wrote an editorial entitled "Quasi-scientific Journal Article reeks of Advocacy" (*Wisconsin State Journal* 1997). He challenged the study's findings about the number of alcohol-impaired drivers, and stated, "If that were true, I'd drive a tank. But the driving panic is a fabricated scare, ranking right up there with Alar and the belief that cellular phones cause brain cancer . . . . This may sound like science to some, but it smells like 100-proof advocacy to me."

This example illustrates the challenge of media advocacy and the use of epidemiology to support public health policy. It is important that practicing epidemiologists participate in the public debate about the meaning and implications of epidemiologic research. At the same time, one must recognize the distinction between scientific fact and public opinion. The further one deviates from the science in the name of advocacy, the greater the risk of loosing credibility as an unbiased and independent scientist.

Summary

Translating epidemiologic research into public health practice requires that information be communicated effectively to a wide variety of nontechnical audiences. Strategies to communicate health information range from often chaotic media coverage of published research to well-organized national public education campaigns. The strategies described above provide a brief introduction to this complex and evolving field. The challenge for the practicing epidemiologist is to use these strategies to effectively communicate important health information to ultimately improve the public's health.

CASE STUDIES

Disseminating Public Health Surveillance Information: Trends in Breast Cancer Mortality

Background

In order to reduce the mortality from breast cancer, a public health campaign in Wisconsin over the past decade has promoted the use of mammography for early breast cancer detection (Zvara 1991). An analysis of health data in Wisconsin has revealed the following: (1) The number of women who received mammography each year increased from 31,000 in 1980 to 517,000 in 1993 (Lantz et al. 1990, 1995); (2) the proportion of breast cancer cases that were diagnosed in an early (localized) stage increased from 50% in 1980 to 69% in 1994 (Wisconsin Division of Health 1996); and (3) the age-adjusted breast cancer mortality rates increased approximately 8% from 1980 to 1990 (34.3 to 36.9 deaths/100,000 women), but declined by about 9% from 1990 to 1994 (to 33.4 deaths/100,000 women) (Remington et al. 1995).

Key Questions

1. How should these data be interpreted?

The data presented above suggest that (1) more women are having regular mammography, (2) breast cancer is being detected at an earlier stage, and (3) mortality rates are declining. A single communication objective might be to convey that breast cancer mortality rates are declining as a result of increased use of mammography in Wisconsin. These data do not prove that mammography reduces breast cancer mortality. Rather, they are consistent with previous well-designed studies that have demonstrated such a benefit.

Public health departments are a credible source of information and health reports are often covered by the press. However, it is often helpful to frame the issue creatively. For example, a 9% decline in an age-adjusted death rate is rather complex. This same information could be translated into a number of lives "saved" if the death rates of the past decade had continued into the 1990s. This way, the report could state that about 200 *fewer* breast cancer deaths occurred during 1992–1994—a likely result of increases in the use of mammography during the past several years (Remington et al. 1995). The ability to frame the issue as "new" or "important" information may make the difference between a story that is widely covered in the media and one that doesn't even get printed.

2. What is the desired impact of the information?

Many times surveillance data are routinely reported to "inform those who need to know." This information is reassuring because it shows, for the first time in a state, that breast cancer mortality is beginning to decline. This information may encourage health care providers to regularly recommend mammography for their patients. In addition, this information may be used to encourage women to have a mammogram, given the demonstrated public health impact. A women's health advocate may use this information to promote a specific health policy, such as a bill to mandate insurance coverage for mammography in the state.

3. What is the target audience?

Once the objective of reporting the information has been determined, the target audience can be identified. Many times, the objective is simply to increase awareness of a health issue in a community. If this is the case, public health agencies may decide that the general public is the target audience. If the communication objective is more specific and related to a health policy (such as funding a program to provide mammography for uninsured women), the audience might be a community advocacy group or local politicians.

4. What communications medium should be used?

As before, the selection of the communication medium depends upon what target audience is selected. If the target audience is the general public, then the health department might issue a press release. However, if the audience is more specific (such as policy-makers) then other communication strategies must be used, such as a direct mailing or a special meeting.

Implications for Practice

Disseminating surveillance information is a core function of public health. Epidemiologists can lead this effort by conducting the analyses and effectively communicating the results to those who need to know. The final step in the process is the application of the surveillance findings to disease prevention and health promotion programs or policies.

Media Advocacy: Smoking as a Pediatric Disease

Background.

Each year, state health departments throughout the United States conduct telephone surveys of the health habits of approximately 1,800 adults in the state as part of the CDC Behavioral Risk Factor Surveillance System (Remington et al. 1988). These surveys ask questions about preventive health practices, and the major risk factors for chronic diseases and injuries, such as cigarette smoking, alcohol use, and exercise. In 1995, Wisconsin added a question that asked smokers, "About how old were you when you smoked your first whole cigarette?" The results from this survey are presented in Table 11-5.

Table 11-5. Percent of Adults who Began Smoking as Children[a], Wisconsin, 1995

Current age	Percent Who Tried First Cigarette as a Child		Percent Who Became a Regular Smoker as a Child	
	Men	Women	Men	Women
25–34	83%	84%	61%	63%
35–44	79%	66%	61%	63%
45–64	67%	57%	45%	24%
65 +	68%	39%	26%	12%

[a]Children 17 years of age and younger. From the 1995 Behavioral Risk Factor Survey, Wisconsin Division of Health.

Key Questions

1. What do these data say about smoking?

Most smokers try their first cigarette and become regular smokers as children. In Wisconsin, 83% of young adults (25–34 years) tried their first cigarette and 62% became regular smokers under the age of 18. The percentage who began smoking as children has increased dramatically over the last 50 years. In 1995, and in response to similar national data, Dr. David Kessler characterized smoking as a "pediatric disease" (Kessler et al. 1996).

2. What is the effect of calling smoking a "pediatric disease"?

Calling smoking a "pediatric disease" is an example of framing the issue creatively. That is, it presents information that was widely known in a new and interesting way. This approach has several benefits. First, calling smoking a "disease," emphasizes the importance of nicotine addiction. The tobacco industry claim that smoking is an adult choice has been used to oppose previous regulatory efforts. As a disease, smoking is able to be compared to other diseases, such as cancer and heart disease. The term "pediatric" focuses on youth and provides an image of innocence and the need for protection. It musters the support of an entire community of health care that has not traditionally worked on the smoking issue. Finally, and most importantly, the term "pediatric disease" summarizes years of complicated research in a short, easy-to-understand "sound bite." This creates opportunities to bring this issue to the attention of the media, public, and policy-makers.

3. What are the policy implications of defining smoking as a pediatric disease?

In August 1996, the Food and Drug Administration (FDA) issued a regulation restricting the sale and distribution of cigarettes and smokeless tobacco products to children and adolescents (Kessler et al. 1996). This rule will reduce children's access to tobacco products by requiring age verification and by banning vending machines, self-service displays, free samples, and the sale of single cigarettes. In addition, the rule will limit appeal of tobacco products by limiting billboard advertising, permitting black-and-white text-only advertising in publications with significant youth readership, and prohibiting brand-name promotional giveaways and sponsorship (Annas 1996).

Implications for Practice

Epidemiologic information, such as the age of onset of smoking, has profound pubic health implications. However, this information is of little value if it is not communicated effectively and used to shape public health policies and programs.

SUGGESTED READINGS

American Cancer Society. ASSIST. A Guide to Working with the Media. 1993: No. 2013.

Frederiksen LW, Solomon LJ, Brehony KA, eds. Marketing Health Behavior. Principles, Techniques, and Applications. New York: Plenum Press; 1984.

Making health communications work. A Planner's Guide. U.S. Department of Health and Human Service. National Institutes of Health. NIH Publication April, 1992: No. 92-1493.

Gregg M. Communicating Epidemiologic Findings. In: Gregg M, ed. Field Epidemiology. New York, NY: Oxford University Press: 1996.

Riegelman RK, Hirsch RP. Studying a Study and Testing a Test: How to Read the Health Science Literature. Third Edition. Boston MA: Little Brown; 1996.

Tufte ER. The Visual Display of Quantitative Information. Box 430, Cheshire, CT: Graphics Press; 1987.

REFERENCES

American Medical Association. JAMA instructions for authors. JAMA 1997;277:74–78.

Angell M, Kassirer JP. Clinical research—what should the public believe? New Engl J Med 1994;331:189–190.

Annas GJ. Cowboys, camels, and the First Amendment—the FDA's restrictions on tobacco advertising. New Engl J Med 1996;335:1779–1183.

Barefoot JC, Dahlstrom WG, Williams RB Jr. Hostility, CHD incidence, and total mortality: a 25-year follow-up study of 255 physicians. Psychosom Med 1983;45:59–63

Brehony KA, Frederikson LW, Solomon LJ. Marketing principles and behavioral medicine. In: Frederiksen LW, Solomon LJ, Brehony KA, eds. Marketing Health Behavior. Principles, Techniques, and Applications. New York: Plenum Press; 1984: 3–22.

Cancer and Steroid Hormone Study Group. Oral contraceptive use and the risk of breast cancer. NEJM 1986;315:405–411.

Chassin MR, Hannan EL, DeBuono BA. Benefits and hazards of reporting medical outcomes publicly. N Eng J Med 1996;334:394–398.

Covello VT. Risk perception and communication. Rev Can Sante Publique 1995;86:78–82.

Cwikel JG. After epidemiologic research: what next? Community action for health promotion. Public Health Rev 1994;22:375–394.

Epidemiology. Guidelines for Contributors. 1997 Jan;8(1).

Falck F, Ricci A, Wolff MS, Godbold J, Deckers P. Pesticides and polychlorinated biphenyl residues in human breast lipids and their relation to breast cancer. Arch Environ Health 1992;47:143–146.

Feinstein AR, Horwitz RI, Spitzer WO, Battista RN. Coffee and pancreatic cancer. The problems of etiologic research and epidemiologic case-control research. JAMA 1981;246:957–960.

Finkel AM. Toward less misleading comparisons of uncertain risks: the example of aflatoxin and Alar. Environ Health Perspect 1995;103:376–385.

Fischhoff B. Risk perception and communication unplugged: twenty years of process. Risk Anal 1995;15:137–145.

Fischhoff B, Bostrum A, Quadrel MJ. Risk perception and communication. Annu Rev Public Health 1993;14:183–203.

Freaudenburg WR, Rursch JA. The risks of 'putting the numbers in context': a cautionary tale. Risk Anal 1994;14:949–958.

Frederiksen LW, Solomon LJ, Brehony KA, eds. Marketing Health Behavior. Principles, Techniques, and Applications. New York: Plenum Press; 1984.

Goodman R, Remington PL. Disseminating surveillance information. In: Teutsch SM, Churchill RE, eds. Principles and Practice of Public Health Surveillance. New York: Oxford University Press; 1993.

Gregg M. Communicating epidemiologic findings. In: Gregg M, ed. Field Epidemiology. New York, NY: Oxford University Press; 1996.

Halpin TJ, Holtzhauer FJ, Campbell RJ, et al. Reye's syndrome and medication use. JAMA 1982;248:687–691.

Haynes RB, Mulrow CD, Huth EJ, Altman DG, Gardner MJ. More informative abstracts revisited. Ann Intern Med 1990;113:69–76.

Iglehart JK. The National Committee for Quality Assurance. New Eng J Med 1996;335:995–999.

Institute of Medicine. Committee for the Study of the Future of Public Health. The Future of Public Health. Washington, DC: National Academy press;1988.

Johnson BB, Slovic P. Improving risk communication and risk management: legislated solutions or legislated disasters? Risk Anal 1994;14:905–906.

Kaufman DW, Miller DR, Rosenberg L, et al. Noncontraceptive estrogen use and risk of breast cancer. JAMA 1984;252:63–67.

Kessler DA, Witt AM, Barnett PS, et al. The Food and Drug Administrations regulation of tobacco products. New Engl J Med 1996;335:988–994.

Kreutzer R, Arneson C. The scientific assessment and public perception of risk. Curr Issues Public Health 1995;1:102–104.

Krieger N, Wolff MS, Hiatt RA, Rivera M, Vogelman J, Orentreich N. Breast cancer and serum organochlorines: a prospective study among white, black, and Asian women. J Ntl Cancer Inst 1994;86:589–599.

Lantz P, Bunge M, Remington PL. Trends in mammography in Wisconsin, 1980–1989. Wis Med J 1990;89:281–282.

Lantz P, Bunge M, Cautley E, Phillips JL, Remington PL. Mammography use—Wisconsin, 1980–1993. Morb Mortal Wkly Rep 1995;44:754–757.

Levy BS. Communicating public health: a top 10 list. Nation Health 1997;1:2.

Liu S, Siegel PZ, Brewer RD, Mokdad AH, Sleet DA, Serdula M. Prevalence of alcohol-impaired driving. Results from a national self-reported survey of health behaviors. JAMA 1997;277(2):122–125.

Maibach E, Holtgrave DR. Advances in public health communication. Annu Rev Public Health 1995;16:219–238.

MacMahon B, Yen S, Trichopoulos D, Warren K, Nardi G. Coffee and cancer of the pancreas. New Engl J Med 1981;304:630–633.

Miller DR, et al. Breast cancer before age 45 and oral contraceptive use: new findings. New Engl J Med 1989;129:269–280.

Moss ME, Remington PL, Peterson DE. The costs of smoking in Wisconsin: a silent epidemic. Wis Med J 1990;89(11):646,648,651.

Nelkin D. Selling science: how the press covers science and technology. In: Communicating Science to the Public. Ciba Foundation Conference. Chichester, NY:John Wiley, 1987.

Omenn GS, Goodman GE, Thornquist MD, et al. Effects of a combination of beta carotene and vitamin A on lung cancer and cardiovascular disease. New Eng J Med 1996;334:1150–1155.

New England Journal of Medicine. Instructions to authors. N Engl J Med 1996;335(23):1784.

Palmersheim K, Remington P. Trends in breast cancer mortality for blacks and whites in Wisconsin and the United States, 1979–1992. Wis Med J 1996; 95:245–247.

Remington PL, Rowley D, McGee H, Hall WN, Monto AS. Decreasing trends in Reye syndrome and aspirin use in Michigan, 1979 to 1984. Pediatrics 1986; 77(1):93–98.

Remington PL, Smith MY, Williamson DF, Anda RF, Gentry EM, Hogelin GC.

Design, characteristics, and usefulness of state-based risk factor surveillance 1981–1986. Public Health Rep 1988;103(4):366–375.

Remington PL, Fiore M. Trends in lung cancer mortality in Wisconsin. Wis Med J 1989;88:34,36,38.

Remington PL, Goodman R. Chronic disease surveillance. In: Brownson RC, Remington PL, Davis JR, eds. Chronic Disease Epidemiology and Control. Washington, DC: American Public Health Association; 1993.

Remington P, Schell W, Hoffman K, Fox J, Stephenson-Vine L. Breast cancer mortality rates decline in Wisconsin women. Wis Med J 1995;94(10):551–553.

Riegelman RK, Hirsch RP. Studying a Study and Testing a Test: How to Read the Health Science Literature. Third Edition. Boston, MA: Little Brown;1996.

Roper W. Health communication takes on new dimensions at CDC. Public Health Rep 1993;108:179–183.

Shekelle RB, et al. The MRFIT behavior pattern study. AJE 1985;122:559–570

Slovic P. Perception of risk. Science 1987;236:280–285.

Starko KM, Ray CG, Dominguez LB, et al. Reye's syndrome and salicylate use. Pediatrics 1980;66:859–864.

Steinberg KK, Thacker SB, Smith J, et al. A meta-analysis of the effect of estrogen replacement therapy on the risk of breast cancer. JAMA 1991;265:1985–1990.

Sutton SM, Balch GI, LeFebvre RC. Strategic questions for consumer-based health communications. Public Health Rep 1995;110:725–733.

Taubes G. Epidemiology faces its limits. Science 1995;269:164–169.

Thacker SB, Berkelman RL. Public health surveillance in the United States. Epidemiol Rev 1988;10:164–190.

Tufte ER. The visual display of quantitative information. Box 430, Cheshire, CT: Graphics Press; 1987.

US Dept of Health and Human Services. Media Strategies for Smoking Control: Guidelines. Washington, DC: NIH Publication #89-3013; 1989.

US Dept of Health and Human Services. Making Health Communication Programs Work. A Planner's Guide. Office of Cancer Communications, National Cancer Institute, National Institute of Health, Public Health Service, U.S. Department of Health and Human Services. Washington, DC: NIH Publication #92-1493; April 1992.

Waldman RJ, Hall WN, McGee H, et al. Aspirin use as a risk factor for Reye's syndrome. JAMA 1982;247:3089–3094.

Wallack L, Dorfman L, Jernigan D, Themba M. Media Advocacy and Public Health. Power for Prevention. Newbury Park, CA: Sage; 1993.

Wilkes MS, Kravitz RL. Medical research and the media. Attitudes toward public dissemination of research. JAMA 1992;268:999–1003.

Willett WC, Ascherio A. Trans fatty acids: are the effects only marginal? Am J Public Health 1994;84:722–724.

Wisconsin Division of Health. Cancer in Wisconsin, 1994. Madison, WI:Wisconsin Department of Health and Family Services; 1996.

Wisconsin State Journal 1997.

Wynder EL. Invited commentary: response to Science article: "epidemiology faces its limits." Am J Epidemiol 1996;143:747–749.

Zvara JA, Anderson DE, Remington PL, Anderson H. Data-based cancer control programs: a public health response. Wis Med J 1991;90(5):235–236.

12

Epidemiology and Health Policy

ROSS C. BROWNSON

Health policies, in the form of laws, regulations, and organizational practices, have a substantial impact on the health and well-being of the population. Policies can influence one or more of the following: (1) modifiable causes of disease, (2) early detection of disease in asymptomatic persons, (3) disease treatment in persons with symptomatic disease, and (4) rehabilitation and recovery. Formulation of health policies often depends on scientific, economic, social, and political forces (Terris 1980; Ibrahim 1985; Milio 1986; McKinlay 1993).

The influences of epidemiology on health policies are diverse and bidirectional. Epidemiologic studies are essential in the evaluation of new risk factors, therapeutic drugs, medical devices, and screening modalities. Results of these studies and public health surveillance data have been used frequently to inform health professionals, the public, and policy makers about the need for new or different health policies. This process is the translation of epidemiologic research into public health action. Conversely, health policies can have large impacts on the discipline of epidemiology and epidemiologic research (e.g., funding priorities or stringent confidentiality provisions).

Ideally, health policy-making should be based on weighing of societal risks and benefits, with a realistic model balancing special interests and divergent values through a political process (Fox 1977; Rothman and Poole 1985). Rational models of health policy formation are based on scientific inputs, systematic policy development, and comprehensive evaluation—yet are often not utilized in "real world" practice (Bots and Hulshof 1995; Brownson et al. 1997a). Health policy-making depends largely on a process of priority setting—public health and health care resources are limited and epidemiology can provide a reasonable basis for informing health priorities. Health policy development is seldom a straightforward, systematic process. Rather, it is a blend of science, politics, and sound judgment. The complexity of the process is embodied in the science of policy analysis and contains various categories and goals (Table 12-1).

Table 12-1. Seven Categories and Goals of Policy Analysis

Category	Goal/Definition
Policy content	To explain how a particular policy emerges and is implemented
Policy process	To analyze the stages through which issues pass and the influence of different factors
Information for policy-making	To marshal data from a variety of sources to assist policy-makers in reaching decisions
Process advocacy	To improve the nature of the policy-making system
Policy advocacy	To press specific options and ideas, individually and as a group
Policy outputs	To understand the results of policies in the context of social, economic, and other factors
Evaluation studies	To analyze the impacts of different policies on the population

Sources: Hogwood and Gunn (1981); Ham and Hill (1984); Orosz (1994).

It is unrealistic to expect that health policy making will be based solely on what epidemiologic science indicates. In discussing challenges facing epidemiology, it has been noted (Gordis 1988) that linking the science of epidemiology with the policy-making process is among the most challenging of public health issues. This challenge stems in part from the realization that epidemiology has been highly successful in identifying the large risk factors (e.g., smoking and lung cancer) yet is sometimes unable to clearly measure smaller, more subtle individual risks (e.g., diet and breast cancer) that may, nonetheless, have large impacts at the population level. Even when epidemiologic results are clear and consistent, there are multiple interpretations and multiple policy options (Yankauer 1984).

Health and Social Considerations

Health is a complex and multidimensional concept that is related to a variety of physical, mental, and social factors (World Health Organization 1948; Aday 1994). Physical and mental health indicators tend to focus on the individual level, whereas social factors involve the larger context of society (e.g., health policies) (Aday 1994) (Figure 12-1). A broad vision of health and prevention recognizes the importance of individual risk factors (e.g., addiction to nicotine) and personal responsibility for health, environmental factors (e.g., air pollution), and social factors including housing, transportation, employment, civil rights, economic justice, and communications (Beauchamp 1976; Tesh 1981; Aday 1994). Similarly, health policy decisions are

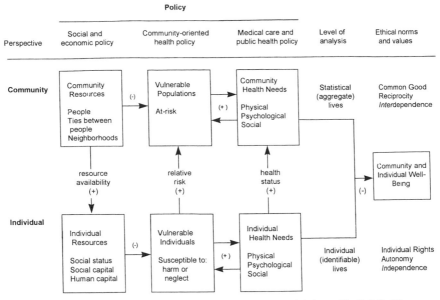

Figure 12-1. Framework for studying vulnerable populations; *Source:* Aday (1994)

influenced by the ethical and ideological frameworks of society (Shannon 1995). The importance of social factors in determining health is related to the philosophical basis for public health—i.e., applying scientific knowledge to achieve social justice (Foege 1993), including the concept of health as a human right (Susser 1993). Public health is ultimately and essentially an ethical enterprise committed to the notion that all persons are entitled to protection from hazards and to minimization of risks of death and disability (Beauchamp 1976).

As noted earlier, the impacts of epidemiology on health policies are extremely broad; thus, comprehensive coverage is not possible in a single chapter. It is possible, however, to discuss several important areas, including: underlying definitions; goals, impacts, and settings; epidemiologic tools, processes, and professional roles; and the community approach and practice guidelines for health policy development.

Definitions

Policies are "those laws, regulations, formal and informal rules and understandings that are adopted on a collective basis to guide individual and collective behavior" (Schmid et al. 1995). In this chapter, a *health policy* is defined broadly to include policies that address prevention on a population basis as well as those influencing health care utilization and quality.

Policies tend to alter or control the legal, social, economic, and physical environment (Cheadle et al. 1992) and are supported by the notion that individuals are strongly influenced by the sociopolitical and cultural environment in which they act. Health policies can be divided into two general areas: legislation/regulation and organizational policy (Cheadle et al. 1992). Legislation or regulation involves formal policies written into law by the appropriate governing bodies (e.g., nutrition guidelines enacted by a government or regulatory policies to limit exposure to occupational chemicals). Organizational policies are those implemented by specific establishments such as schools, health departments, managed care organizations, and health insurance companies. For example, a business may be persuaded of the benefits of worksite health promotion programs, including their cost-effectiveness (Stokols et al. 1995; Pelletier 1996) and therefore may implement policies to encourage exercise, nonsmoking, and other healthy behaviors.

Various definitions of the core functions of public health (Institute of Medicine 1988; Roper et al. 1992; Oberle et al. 1994) recognize the importance of the health policy development process. A common rubric involves assessment, policy development, and assurance (Institute of Medicine 1988). *Assessment* refers to the concept of community diagnosis, including the tools of public health surveillance and epidemiologic research to determine health effects and health hazards. Using the results of assessment as a basis, *policy development* is the process by which society makes decisions about health problems through planning, goal setting, policy leadership and advocacy, and provision of public information. Stated differently, policy development is the "means by which problem identification, technical knowledge of possible solutions, and societal values set a course of action" (Institute of Medicine 1988). *Assurance* is the guarantor function of public health to ensure that health services and legislative mandates are met according to agreed upon goals.

Core functions of public health likely differ based on the location and size of health agency, and roles continue to evolve as the health care system changes. Traditional public health, particularly at the local level, has centered largely on delivery of individual services, such as provision of immunizations or prenatal care. The need for a greater focus on the overall community, focusing on policy initiatives, has been noted (Schmid et al. 1995) and may be a more effective means of utilizing limited public health resources. Policies are likely to have both direct and subtle effects on the health of the population (Brownson et al. 1997a). Direct effects tend to be more measurable and may include risk factor prevalence, disease incidence or prevalence, disability, and mortality. More subtle effects may occur prior to outcome changes. These include changes in social norms, attitudes toward health, or health-care-seeking behavior (Milio 1986). In addition, as health reform efforts progress at the state and local levels, managed health care is stimulating new partnerships between traditional public health and private health care providers (Baker et al. 1994), which may in turn provide a greater emphasis on improving health policies in the overall community.

Goals and Impacts of Health Policies

The overall goals of health policies are usually to enhance disease prevention efforts and improve health care access by achieving specific health objectives (US Dept of Health and Human Services [US DHHS] 1990). For example, the Ottawa Charter (Ottawa Working Group on Health Promotion in Developing Countries 1986) developed goal statements in five areas: building healthy public policy, creating supportive environments, strengthening community action, developing personal skills, and reorienting health service. In the United States, numerous public health objectives (US DHHS 1990) are directly related to policy implementation and evaluation. Within *Healthy People 2000*, three overarching goals aim to (1) increase the span of healthy life for Americans, (2) reduce health disparities among Americans, and (3) achieve access to preventive services for all Americans. Each of these three goals is strongly influenced by health policies. Policy-related issues are addressed as "Services and Protection Objectives" and include items such as ensuring that all states have comprehensive clean-indoor-air laws and increasing the proportion of work sites that offer physical activity programs (US DHHS 1990).

Health policies are most sound when they are based on high-quality scientific evidence. This has occurred in many instances. For example, through numerous randomized clinical trials, consistent evidence has emerged on the benefits of mammography screening among women ages 50 years and older (Harris et al. 1992). This has led to consistent guidelines from at least 12 organizations and professional groups that promote mammography screening in women (Volkers 1994).

Less frequently, policies are advanced that may not be based on careful scientific consideration. For example, the 1975 campaign to immunize the American population against the swine flu was advanced without adequate consideration of the scientific evidence (Ibrahim 1985). Even though the policy was halted shortly after implementation, it led to substantial legal liability for the US government because of the potential link between swine flu vaccination and Guillain-Barré syndrome (Christoffel and Teret 1991). More recently, the ban on silicone breast implants in the United States and related jury awards in class-action settlements have been criticized as being based on sparse epidemiologic evidence (Angell 1996).

Health policies in each the four major areas outlined below can reduce the burden of disease and disability in the population. These four areas are selected to illustrate the impacts of health policies and are not intended as an exhaustive review.

Controlling Environmental and Occupational Hazards

Epidemiologic studies have been successful in identifying many risk factors in environmental and occupational settings. Effects are both acute and chronic, including a wide range of health conditions such as cancer, adverse reproductive effects, and chronic lung diseases. A variety of established and potential risk factors have been evaluated:

- Chemicals such as pesticides, benzene, vinyl chloride
- Ionizing radiation such as X-rays and radon
- Electric and magnetic fields from high-tension power lines
- Dusts such as coal dust and silica dust
- Allergens and molds such as pollen and animal fur

A few examples illustrate the linkage between epidemiologic evidence and public health action. Strong observational evidence has shown that low-level lead exposure can lead to decreased intellectual performance in school-age children (Schwartz 1994). This and other research on the health effects of lead exposure led to a ban on leaded gasoline in the United States. It also has fostered official "action levels" (e.g., 250 (μg/l in the United Kingdom) and "levels of concern" (e.g., 100 (μg/l in the United States) for blood lead concentrations.

Silicosis is a chronic lung disease that most often develops among workers involved in the dry drilling or grinding of rock with a high silica content (Goldring et al. 1993). Silicosis is nine times more common in men than in women. Guidelines known as "permissible exposure limits" have been established by the US Occupational Safety and Health Administration and the Mine Safety and Health Administration. These guidelines have led to improvements in the levels of work-related exposure to silica dust (US DHHS 1994).

Reducing Behavioral Risk Factors

Epidemiologic studies have been successful in identifying and quantifying modifiable, "behavioral" risk factors (e.g., cigarette smoking, lack of physical activity, sexual practices, illicit drug use, lack of screening utilization) for many diseases. These risk factors can be considered "voluntary" since, for the most part, they relate to individual practices, habits, and addictions. Virtually all of these factors have been the subject of health policies to lower disease risk and alter the overall social environment (Brownson et al. 1995; Glanz et al. 1995; King et al. 1995). A few brief examples illustrate the use of policy changes to reduce risk of morbidity.

Environmental tobacco smoke (ETS) has been shown to be a cause of lung cancer in nonsmokers through approximately 35 epidemiologic studies (US Environmental Protection Agency [US EPA] 1993). Based on these data, federal, state, and local governments in the United States and other countries have enacted policies to limit or prohibit smoking in workplaces and other public places. These policies have not only protected the health of non-smokers but have also resulted in other possible benefits including increased cessation rates among smokers and cost savings to employers (Brownson et al. in 1997b).

Over the past few decades, the health benefits of physical activity have been well documented through epidemiologic studies (US DHHS 1996). Physical inactivity is increasingly recognized as a major risk factor for coronary heart disease and is also a risk factor for a variety of other chronic diseases including colon cancer, non-insulin-dependent diabetes, and osteoporosis (US DHHS 1996). Policy changes show promise in reducing physical inactivity (King et al. 1995). Organizational policies in the workplace can influence physical activity without passage of any type of law or regulation. For example, employers can enact policies that encourage walking during coffee breaks or can provide on-site exercise facilities.

Regulating Drugs and Medical Devices

The successful treatment of existing diseases and conditions can be strongly affected by the licensing and regulation of new drugs, medical devices, and medical procedures. Therapeutic drugs and medical procedures can often be evaluated by the most powerful of epidemiologic methods, the random allocation, double-blind, clinical trial (Lilienfeld and Stolley 1994). This is a direct application of an experimental design in the clinical setting that can provide convincing evidence regarding the efficacy of new medical technologies.

Table 12-2 illustrates several recent examples of consumer products, chemicals, and substances that have been the subject of varying degrees of regulatory control. In the United States, the first major federal law governing therapeutic drugs was enacted in 1906, giving the Food and Drug Administration (FDA) the authority to approve new drugs (Merrill 1994). The drug regulatory system requires FDA approval for every important step in the product development process. An extensive review process is designed to ensure that a new drug is safe and effective. In recent decades, concerns over

Table 12-2. Examples of Current and Recent Regulatory Actions
Regarding Consumer Products, Chemicals, and Substances

Action Taken	Substance
Banned or rejected	Rely tampons, silicone breast implants
Limited	Chloramphenicol, nitrates
Monitored	Oral contraceptives, chemotherapy, radiation
Evaluated	Coffee, saccharin, sodium
None (irrationally)	Asbestos, tobacco, alcohol

Source: Modan (1984).

the time for drug approval expressed by advocates and scientists have led to streamlined processes for new drugs for treatment of cancer and AIDS. The FDA has initiated several procedures that allow experimental drugs to be available to seriously ill patients earlier in the drug development cycle (Johnson 1989). These drugs are approved for use by FDA 2.5 to three times faster than other drugs.

Improving the Delivery and Quality of Health Care

As discussed in Chapter 1, dramatic changes are occurring in the delivery of health care in the United States and elsewhere. Epidemiologic studies can provide a scientific basis for evaluating the multiple factors that are responsible for health care costs, quality, value, and effectiveness (Wennberg et al. 1980; Shannon 1995).

A reformed health care system can be based on three mutually reinforcing components (Omenn 1994; Gordon et al. 1996):

- Social, economic, and regulatory policies that promote healthy behaviors, reduce hazardous exposures, and promote healthy standards of living, including access to medical care
- Essential community-based public health services: monitoring health status indicators; educating the public about health risks and promoting healthy behaviors; and reducing risks from air, water, food, consumer products, workplace and recreational hazards
- Clinical preventive services: immunizations, screening tests, and counseling by physicians and other health professionals

The linkage between epidemiology and health care access and quality can be illustrated in the growth of Medicaid managed care in the United States. Medicaid is jointly funded by the federal and state governments and is the nation's principal way of providing medical and long-term care to people with low incomes. Several state programs have applied for and received federal approval for state-wide managed care demonstration projects for Medicaid recipients. Studies are beginning to systematically evaluate the effects of the enrollment of Medicaid beneficiaries in managed care. For example, a recent study of New York Medicaid managed care showed significantly higher odds of satisfaction among managed-care enrollees and a significantly higher chance of having a usual source of health care (Sisk et al. 1996).

Settings for Health Policy-Making

Governmental

Governmental health policies are established through laws and regulations. Laws are passed by legislative bodies, usually by a majority of votes among the particular body. Regulations are commonly established by the executive branch of government, often with legislative input (but not oversight). For example, a state legislature might pass a law mandating statewide cancer reporting from all hospitals and outpatient clinics. The state health department may then be charged with establishing regulations that set out the specific details of reporting (e.g., case definitions, timeliness of reporting, data confidentiality protections). In general, regulations are easier to establish and amend than are laws.

A legitimate debate concerning health policy is where the "locus of control" should reside. Some argue that US health policies should be primarily national in focus (Beauchamp 1976); others suggest the focus should be more at the state and local level. Over the past 30 years, increasing responsibility for health policies has been placed in the hand of state and local governments (WK Kellogg 1996). Presently, the climate in the US Congress is for even further "devolution" of federal mandates (e.g., health care, welfare, environmental issues) to the state and local levels (WK Kellogg 1996).

One of the constraints to successful health policy making in the United States is that governmental responsibility in health is divided among several agencies at the local, state, and federal levels, with a resulting involvement of multiple decision-makers (Institute of Medicine 1988). Therefore, responsibility and accountability can be diffuse and delays and conflicts are inevitable. A criticism of health policy-making in the public health sector is that government agencies tend to respond to the issue of the moment rather than benefiting from careful assessment of existing knowledge, establishing priorities based on data, and allocating resources according to objective criteria (Institute of Medicine 1988).

In the United States, five federal agencies have been charged with primary authority to regulate activities and substances that pose acute and chronic health risks: the Environmental Protection Agency, the Food and Drug Administration, the Occupational Safety and Health Administration, the Consumer Product Safety Commission, and the Health Care Financing Administration. Governmental bodies at the state and local levels with a significant potential to affect health policies include state legislatures, state and local health agencies, county boards of health, and city councils.

Nongovernmental

Private Sector Influences. Individuals and private companies play important roles in determining health policies. Individuals can exert influence in a democratic and pluralistic society by voting or by becoming an advocate for a certain health issue or policy. Producers and providers of health care play important roles in shaping health policies by attempting to influence public opinion and by influencing elected officials. Accreditation policies in health care can also have strong effects on health policies. These policies, affecting hospitals and nursing homes, health maintenance organizations, and medical schools, are adopted by private organization but often receive official government sanction. For example, the federal Health Care Financing Administration confers "deemed status" on accredited hospitals for the purposes of granting participation in the Medicaid and Medicare programs.

In many situations, private companies have implemented health policies to benefit their workers, to serve their customers, and to control costs. Excellent examples are present in the area of worksite health promotion. In the United States, more than 110 million workers are employed and corporations pay 30–40% of the national health expenditures (Stokols et al. 1995). Based on a 1992 national survey, 81% of companies with 50 or more employees offer at least one health promotion activity (US DHHS 1993). Based on a comprehensive body of evaluation studies, worksite health promotion programs have been shown to be cost-effective (Pelletier 1996; Stokols et al. 1995). Numerous worksite interventions focus on changes in health policies such as banning smoking at the worksite, requiring the use of safety belts in all company-sponsored trips, and allowing employees flex time or work time to exercise (US DHHS 1993; Stokols et al. 1995).

Communities. Many informal policies can be implemented in a community without changes in official laws or regulations. Often, these actions lead to changes in social norms that are "de facto" policies. For example, a community might unite to implement its own neighborhood watch program. If such a program is successfully implemented, it can lead to changing social norms that discourage crime and hence reduce the risk of violence to community residents. More complete discussion of related issues is provided in a later section: "Community Development to Impact Health Policies."

Epidemiologic Tools, Processes, and Professional Roles

Epidemiologists and health policy-makers have a variety of "tools" at their disposal that can help inform the policy development process. Many practitioners may not have the title of "epidemiologist" yet often make valuable use of these tools. Some of these involve epidemiologic methods; others involve processes in which epidemiologists can help inform policy-making. It is important to note that many of the tools and processes in the following section are overlapping and are not mutually exclusive.

Public Health Surveillance

Public health surveillance systems are components of evaluation, and they have several key characteristics (discussed in detail in Chapter 4). These include the collection, analysis, and interpretation of health data essential to the planning, implementation, and evaluation of public health practice (Thacker and Berkelman 1988). These activities must be closely integrated with the timely dissemination of data to the appropriate audience(s).

Policy initiatives have not commonly been the focus of surveillance systems; however, when implemented properly, policy surveillance systems can be an enormous asset for the policy development process. For example, the National Cancer Institute's State Cancer Legislative Database (National Cancer Institute 1994) tracks various cancer-related state legislation and is a valuable tool for researchers examining policy initiatives. As noted in Figure 12-2, the frequency of state mammography laws requiring private insurance coverage has increased sharply. Systematic evaluation processes can be established for linkage with policy surveillance systems (e.g., assessing the strength of state laws on youth access to tobacco) (Alciati et al. in review). In addition, policy effects can be evaluated by linking policy surveillance systems with other systems that measure risk factor or disease outcomes.

Risk Assessment

As noted in Chapter 5, quantitative risk assessment provides the scientific basis for regulating toxic exposures (Hertz-Picciotto 1995). Risk assessment is the process of determining risks to health attributable to environmental or other hazards (World Health Organization 1989). Four key steps in risk assessment are hazard identification, risk characterization, exposure assessment, and risk estimation (World Health Organization 1989). Risk assessment has been described as a "bridge" between science and policy-making (Hertz-Picciotto 1995). There has been considerable debate over the US risk

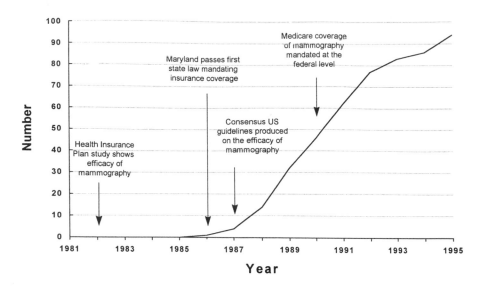

*Includes the District of Columbia
(Source: el Arculli R. State Cancer Legislative Database Program.
Unpublished data Bethesda, MD: National Cancer Institute; July 1996)

Figure 12-2. Cumulative number of state* mammography laws and amendments requiring third-party coverage, United States, 1983–1995

assessment policies, and the most widely recognized difficulties in risk assessment are due to extrapolation-related uncertainties (Sexton et al. 1995).

Epidemiologic studies offer the most relevant data for the assessment of human health risks due to low-level exposures to environmental agents (Hertz-Picciotto 1995). Despite difficulties, through an established process (described in detail in Chapter 5), expert scientific input is provided to agencies that regulate environmental or occupational exposures.

Assessing the Health of the "Community"

Community health assessment, a linkage between epidemiology, behavioral science, and other disciplines, relies on data to determine a community's major health problems and the factors influencing these problems. In general it relies on existing data sets (e.g., data from the census, mortality, disease registries, behavioral risk factor surveys) to give a cross-sectional "snapshot" of the community. Data are typically analyzed for descriptive variables within a defined geographic area (e.g., a zip code, a county) to inform health planning and priority setting. Frequently these data are communicated to policy makers and are used as the basis for new or refined health policies at the local level.

Several planning models rely on community health assessment to inform the process. Two examples are the Planned Approach to Community Health (PATCH) (Centers for Disease Control [CDC] 1992a) and the Assessment Protocol for Excellence in Public Health (APEX/PH) (National Association of County Health Officials 1991). PATCH was developed by the CDC and consists of five phases: (1) mobilizing the community, (2) collecting and organizing data, (3) choosing health priorities and target groups, (4) choosing and conducting health promotion interventions, and (5) evaluating the process and interventions (CDC 1992a). APEX/PH was designed to help local health agencies in assessing and improving their own organizations and in working with the community in improving community health status (Oberle et al. 1994). Epidemiologic data helps to inform the community assessment portion of APEX/PH through health status data and perceptions of various health issues.

Cost-Effectiveness and Cost-Benefit Analysis

Cost-effectiveness and cost-benefit are similar analytic techniques that allow a comparison of the economic efficiencies of various health care and preventive technologies (see Chapter 9). Cost-effectiveness compares the net monetary costs of a preventive intervention with some measure of health outcome (e.g., years of life saved). Cost-benefit is assessed in the same way, except that health outcomes are converted to monetary units, allowing comparison of the monies paid for an intervention with the monies saved (CDC 1994). Measurement of the cost-effectiveness and cost-benefit of health policies can present difficulties. In many cases, it is difficult, if not impossible, to adequately weigh costs (or benefits) that are not easily quantified (Warner 1995). For example, in regulating smoking, how does one quantify the value of a non-smoking employee's desire to work in a smoke-free environment or the value of a smoker's loss of ability to smoke anywhere in a work site (Warner 1995).

Cost-effectiveness analysis is the most commonly conducted economic analysis for health programs (CDC 1994). It is especially useful when the goal is to identify the most cost-effective prevention strategy among a number of options.

Meta-Analysis and Weight of the Evidence Synthesis

Over the past two decades, meta-analysis has been increasingly used to synthesize the findings of multiple research studies. The key contribution of meta-analysis has been to provide a systematic, replicable, and objective method of integrating the findings of individual studies (Glass 1976; Slavin 1995). Meta-analysis is discussed in Chapters 2 and 5.

Another approach to synthesizing multiple research studies is "best evidence" or "weight of the evidence" synthesis (US EPA 1986; Slavin 1995). In this approach, the systematic literature review techniques of meta-analysis are combined with detailed critical analysis of study issues and characteristics. In the area of health policy, much of the focus has been on determining the carcinogenicity of chemicals and substances in humans. For example, the EPA has developed guidelines for assessing the weight of the evidence based on (1) characterization of the evidence from human studies and from animal studies individually, (2) combination of the characterizations of these two types of data into an indication of the overall weight of the evidence for human carcinogenicity, and (3) evaluation of all supporting information to determine if the overall weight of the evidence should be modified (US EPA 1986). As noted in Chapter 5, a variety of evidence from epidemiologic studies is taken into account to form a five-tier classification scheme for carcinogenicity:

- *Group A:* carcinogenic to humans
- *Group B:* probably carcinogenic to humans
- *Group C:* possibly carcinogenic to humans
- *Group D:* not classifiable as to human carcinogenicity
- *Group E:* evidence of noncarcinogenicity for humans

One of the most important aspects of a classification scheme such as this is that it takes into account the uncertainty in risk assessment and synthesis of evidence by providing varying degrees of certainty.

Expert Panels and Expert Review

Virtually every government agency, in both executive and legislative branches, utilizes expert panels or expert review when examining epidemiologic studies and their relevance to health policies. The main goal of expert panels is to provide peer review—i.e., using scientific experts to review the quality of the science and scientific interpretations that underlie health policy decisions. When conducted well, peer review can provide an important set of checks and balances for the regulatory process (The Presidential/Congressional Commission on Risk Assessment and Risk Management 1997). The expert review process can have a number of variations but tends to have the following common properties:

- Experts are sought in epidemiology and related disciplines (e.g., medicine, biomedical sciences, biostatistics).
- Panels typically consist of eight to 15 members and meet in person to review scientific data.
- Written guidance is provided to panel members.
- Panel members should not have financial or professional conflicts of interest.

• Draft findings from expert panels are frequently released for public review and comment prior to final recommendations.

One of the successful outcomes of expert panels has been the production of guidelines for public health and medical care. A recent example is the publication of the second edition of the *Guide to Clinical Preventive Services* (US Preventive Services Task Force 1996). This document is a careful review of the scientific evidence for and against hundreds of preventive services (e.g., childhood immunizations, tobacco cessation counseling). Its production was overseen by a 10-member expert advisory committee.

The Role of the Epidemiologist in Health Policy-Making

Epidemiologists have numerous opportunities for influencing the development, implementation, and evaluation of health policies. An epidemiologist may affect health policy by conducting and disseminating their own research, commenting on others' research to the media or in other public settings, serving on advisory groups that make policy recommendations (expert panels), serving as an expert witness in litigation, testifying before a policy-making body (e.g., city council or state legislature), or working with a health-related coalition to achieve policy objectives. It is well established that epidemiologists can play important roles in informing health policy development and in the absence of their involvement, less qualified individuals are likely to interpret epidemiologic studies for policy makers (Foxman 1989). There also has been debate in the scientific literature over whether research articles should include public health policy recommendations (Rothman 1993; Teret 1993).

To encourage a more active role for epidemiologists in the health policy-making process, guidance has been provided to: (1) organize affected parties and the voluntary sector to collaborate with government, (2) activate citizens to become active in issues that affect their health, (3) communicate responsibly regarding health hazards, and (4) join forces with other professionals to achieve these ends (Cwikel 1994).

Given the multiple opportunities, there are differing views on the level to which epidemiologists should be involved in the health policy making process. Largely, the differences focus on the role of epidemiologists as *advocates* (i.e., those who make public recommendations).

There are two major areas in which epidemiologists can play advocacy roles. The first is in influencing overall epidemiologic and scientific research policies. These may involve funding for a certain research area (e.g., research on HIV/AIDS) or more complete inclusion of certain population subgroups (e.g., women, racial/ethnic minorities) in epidemiologic research. Some have reasoned forcefully that scientists *must* be involved in this process:

There are those who believe that scientists should stay out of politics. This is not a luxury we have; in truth, it is a luxury we have never had. Each of us needs to be a partisan for science, to embrace a partisanship born of hope for the future. It is not partisanship based on party ideology but on concern over the possibility that the work of generations that has put us in the forefront of world science and technology could be undone in a few budget cycles. It is a personal partisanship based on conviction, and such partisanship is the moral calling of every citizen in a democracy. (John H. Gibbons, director, White House Office of Science and Technology Policy—from Woolley, 1995)

The second major area, a more direct interface between epidemiology and health policy, involves recommending or advocating for specific health policies that are supported by epidemiologic research. An epidemiologist considering his or her role as a policy advocate should be aware of several potential pitfalls. Epidemiologists who take a public stance on a given health policy issue face the possibility of real or perceived loss of objectivity that may adversely affect their research on the same topic (Poole and Rothman 1990). For example, taking a public stand on a specific issue could potentially result in an epidemiologist being less willing to test certain hypotheses, conduct particular analyses, or publish certain results (Poole and Rothman 1990). Another area of consideration in epidemiology and policy advocacy is time intensiveness. Active involvement in the policy making process can be extremely time consuming, particularly when assuming a leadership role (e.g., chairperson of a health coalition). These activities may take time away from other professional pursuits that are valued in academic or health care settings (i.e., writing grants, conducting research, publishing results, administrative duties).

It is also important to recognize the importance and complexity of health policy analysis (Poole and Rothman 1990). This established discipline takes many factors into account including health risks, economics, civil liberties, and political forces (Table 12-1) (Ham and Hill 1984; Doron 1992; Hendrick and Nachmias 1992; Orosz 1994). The findings of epidemiologic research are only *one* of the scientific inputs into health policy analysis (Fox 1977; Stein 1977). Short of conducting full policy analyses, epidemiologists should carefully consider the specificity of health policy recommendations when they summarize their research. For example, it may be entirely appropriate to conclude a scientific paper or presentation with the recommendation: "action should be taken to address this public health problem." It may be less advisable to describe the *specific* public health action that should be taken (Charles Poole, personal communication, August 1996), particularly when considering a "new" epidemiologic association that has not been the subject of multiple, rigorous investigation.

The role of epidemiologists in promoting health policies has been reviewed in three sets of ethics guidelines (Weed 1994). In spite of their diversity, the guidelines appear to accept advocacy as a legitimate professional role for epidemiologists (Weed 1994). However, some guidelines caution regarding the difficulty in separating roles when an epidemiologist acts as both a scientist and an advocate (Beauchamp et al. 1991). Savitz et al. (1990) have described the "thoughtful advocate" as one who "acknowledges uncertainties, anticipates policy option consequences, and balances consequences of intervention versus no intervention." When an epidemiologist advocates for a health policy in a reasoned, dispassionate, and evidence-based manner, threats to objectivity are lessened.

The differing level of involvement in health policy development and advocacy likely varies according to the organizational location of an epidemiologist (i.e., practitioner versus academic). Epidemiologists in a practice setting such as a state or local public health agency are probably less likely to conduct analytic research yet may be closer to the policy-making process. Academic epidemiologists are likely to have more day-to-day involvement in research, yet are probably more distant from health policy development. Academic epidemiologists may add "objective" credibility to the process. Frequent interaction between epidemiologists in practice and academic settings is likely to inform the policy-making process and help refine the involvement in policy advocacy.

The questions surrounding the role of the epidemiologist in health policy development, particularly in policy advocacy, are complicated and lack easy solutions. It is likely an area in which sweeping pronouncements are not suitable; epidemiologists should exercise their own individual judgment after careful consideration of potential positive and negative consequences.

The Community Approach and Practice Guidelines for Health Policy Development

As epidemiologic findings are translated into health policies, the process becomes both an art and a science. Successful policy development and implementation involves many disciplines and audiences, including epidemiologists, behavioral scientists, public information and media specialists, policy analysts, and policy makers. The translation of epidemiology into health policy has been outlined in different frameworks (Figures 12-3 and 12-4). While none of these fits every situation, they do provide some basis for rational decision-making regarding health policies. This section provides a brief background on community approaches to health policy development and describes a framework for practitioners.

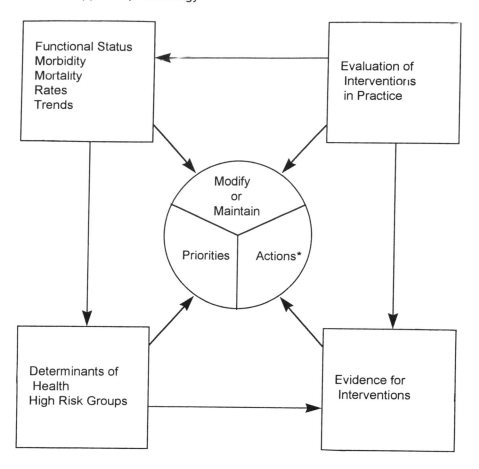

*legislative, regulatory, programmatic

Figure 12-3. Intersections of epidemiology and public policy, from development of health-related information to action and evaluation; *Source:* Shapiro (1991)

Community Development to Impact Health Policies

Community action may hold the greatest potential for changing health policies (Green and Raebum 1990; Fawcett et al. 1993). In the community orientation to health, well-being is determined not only by individual risk factors but also by overall health policies that affect risks for diseases and injuries (Fawcett et al. 1993).

Coalition Building. Community coalitions are formed to refine policy content and to engender support among policy-makers and the general public. A coalition is a group of people and/or organizations working together for a common goal. An effective coalition has the power to influence policy much beyond the influence of any single member group. In successful coalition building, special attention is given to recruiting coalition member organizations that can provide accurate and timely epidemiologic data, directly communicate with policy-makers, access the media, mobilize grassroots support, and generate fiscal resources. Individual coalition members often bring unique abilities. For example, some coalition constituent organizations may be precluded from direct involvement in lobbying or media advocacy (e.g., public health agencies)—other coalition members may not have such constraints. If a coalition is engaged in a legislative campaign, obtaining the services of a recognized lobbyist also may be necessary, depending on the lobbying strength of the organizations opposing the health policy.

It is accepted that community coalitions progress through dynamic stages that include mobilization, establishing structures, building capacity, planning for action, implementation, refinement, and institutionalization (Florin and Stevenson 1993). Attributes and processes of successful coalition building are discussed in more detail elsewhere (Bracht and Kingsbury 1990; Davis et

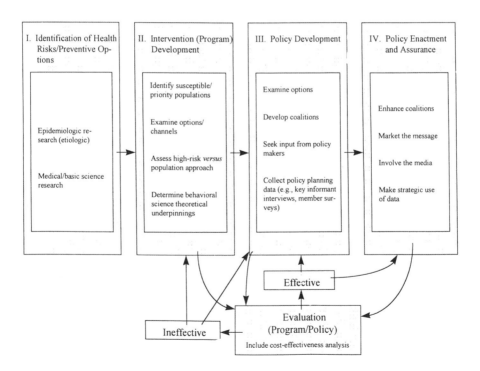

Figure 12-4. Four-stage framework for public health policy development and evaluation; *Source:* Brownson et al. (1997a)

al. 1993; Florin and Stevenson 1993; Davis and Brownson 1994). Increasingly, electronic communication systems to inform coalition building and decision-making are available on the Internet or through dial-in computer modem (e.g., AIDSNet or SCARCNet (Smoking Control Advocacy Resource Center Network) (American Public Health Association 1996).

Coalition formation is frequently but not always necessary for policy enactment. Sometimes, support from a key individual within a legislative body (e.g., a committee chair) may be sufficient for passage of a health policy. Similarly, organizational policies (e.g., implementing a worksite health promotion program) may be enacted by a single individual (often the CEO of the company).

Behavioral Science Models. A few common behavioral models that are used in community development to impact policies are briefly discussed. Most successful community efforts use multiple behavioral models to accomplish their goals. Many of these are multivariable models postulating that behavior is influenced by personal factors, including cognitions, as well as environmental influences. They stress the importance of people's ability to regulate their own behavior by setting goals, monitoring progress toward their goals, and actively intervening in their social or physical environments to support these goals.

One commonly used "top-down" approach is social planning: Expert planners are responsible for problem solving, building linkages, setting goals, and designing plans to reach goals (Rothman and Tropman 1987). The locality development model, a "bottom-up" approach, uses broad citizen involvement in setting goals and taking action in the community (Rothman and Tropman 1987). Another theory applicable in health policy development is the diffusion of innovation theory (Rogers 1983). Diffusion has been described as "the process by which an innovation is communicated through certain channels over time among the members of the social system" (Rogers 1983). Such modifications provide support for healthy lifestyles through multiple intervention channels (e.g., media, worksites, health care settings). The "stage theory of innovation" suggests that innovations such as new ideas or practices are diffused in discrete stages that can be successfully applied to community-based interventions.

Stepwise Guidelines for Practice Settings

As noted earlier in this chapter and elsewhere (Williams-Crowe and Aultman 1994; Robert Wood Johnson Foundation 1995), public health agencies are frequently reacting to a public health crisis rather than proactively planning for health policy changes. While some public health policy-making will remain reactive due simply to the nature of the process, a strong understanding of epidemiologic principles can inform the process and may lead to more effective health policy-making. This section describes an eight-step process that may be useful for the health practitioner. While there is considerable overlap between steps and the framework is not linear, it can provide a basis for actively informing health policy-making based on science and data.

As described elsewhere in this chapter, policy analysis is a science in itself. The involvement of an experienced health policy analyst (or an epidemiologist trained in policy analysis) is essential. In the steps outlined below, the input of policy analysis expertise is especially critical in "option selection" and "priority setting."

In addition to individual expertise needed in health policy development, organizational factors appear to predict success in the health policy arena. For example, a recent content analysis of state public health agencies found five key areas that predicted health policy capacity:

1. A well-organized agency including an effective organizational structure and central liaison responsibilities
2. Talented staff
3. Clear communications between the public health agency and policy makers
4. Effective negotiation skills
5. Active participation (Williams-Crowe and Aultman 1994)

1. Literature Review and Synthesis. Since health policy decisions should not generally be based on a single epidemiologic study or even a few studies, a public health practitioner should begin by conducting a comprehensive literature search of the topic of interest. A search of relevant topics can be accomplished through scientific databases such as MEDLINE, databases on program and policy descriptions (e.g., the CDC's Combined Health Information Database), and a variety of databases on the World Wide Web (e.g., WONDER [Friede et al. 1993] CDC 1997). The initial literature search should generally focus on review articles and/or meta-analyses. The basic principles of meta-analysis are discussed in Chapter 2. It may also be useful to contact an expert who has conducted research in the area of interest or has a strong working knowledge of relevant research. Such experts are often present in larger public health agencies, health care organizations, the federal government, and academic institutions.

2. Local Problem Orientation. After review of analytic studies, it is often useful to orient local data by descriptive categories of person, place, and time with basic epidemiologic tools such as rates and risks. For example, review of the epidemiologic literature might suggest that seatbelt use is shown to reduce automobile-related injuries and health care costs. Data by state or region might show the demographic subgroup(s) most affected by automobile injuries (e.g., young, rural males) and whether rates are changing over time. Many data sets are available from public health agencies including information on mortality, disease and injury registries, risk factors, and hospital discharges (see Chapter 3). Increasingly, these data sets are available on the World Wide Web (e.g., CDC 1997). Even when data are readily available, a policy-maker or budget analyst often wants an immediate answer and time for careful analysis is limited.

3. Option Selection. In the next step, a variety of health policy options should be examined. The list of options can be developed from a variety of sources. The initial review of the scientific literature can sometimes highlight various health policy options. More often, expert panels or professional associations provide health policy recommendations on a variety of issues. Simply stating the pros and cons of each policy option is an important input in this step. The process of option setting should also take into account the appropriate level for health policy enactment. For example, an isolated local public health problem (e.g., toxic emissions from a local factory) might be dealt with most effectively at the local level. Alternatively, a problem that has state or national implications (e.g., eliminating tobacco sales to minors) might be more appropriate for state or federal action. It can be particularly important to understand the sociopolitical forces at work in this step. For example, if one was addressing the preceding issue of toxic emissions from a factory, the economic impact of cleanup or closure must be weighed alongside the health risk.

It is usually beneficial to involve health policy-makers in the early deliberations regarding selection of policy options. Supportive policy-makers can frequently provide advice regarding timing of policy initiatives, methods for "framing" the issue, strategies for identifying sponsors, and ways to develop support among the general public. During policy assessment, several additional "environmental" conditions outlined by Milio (1987) should be considered: how and by whom the policy should be implemented, success indicators (sources of evaluation), and if necessary, how the policy should be reformulated. During this phase, public opinion data can be extremely beneficial. Such data may include cross-sectional surveys. For example, one might poll the voting public to measure support for a public health issue (e.g., raising the alcohol excise tax). Additional planning data may include key informant interviews or coalition member surveys (Florin and Stevenson 1993).

In determining the appropriate health policy, health professionals and policy-makers may need to determine whether a "high-risk" or "population-based" strategy is most appropriate. The high-risk approach tends to identify susceptible individuals and offers them individual prevention technologies (Rose 1985). The population-based strategy seeks to lower the mean level of risk factors in the population, in part through alterations in social norms of behavior (Rose 1985). The "policy-makers' paradox" has been described as the notion that effectiveness of a particular public health intervention may be demonstrated among persons at high risk for disease, yet population-wide interventions may have the biggest impact among those at low to moderate risk (Brown et al. 1992).

4. Priority Setting. After a set of policy options has been developed, priorities among the options are developed. Appropriate priority setting relies on a number of factors including the costs and cost-effectiveness of various options (see Chapter 9), the perceived level of public support for the issue, the perceived level of political support for the issue, and the consensus of health officials and advocates who will be largely responsible for garnering support for the policy. Many of the epidemiologic "tools" that are discussed earlier in this chapter are useful in setting priorities among multiple options.

During the priority-setting phase, it is critical that coalitions and public health organizations clearly define their policy-related goals. While this may appear straightforward, one of the most common reasons for failure to achieve the desired health policy outcome is the lack of clear goals and action steps necessary to achieve these goals.

5. Informing the Public. There are two major ways to advocate for a health policy. The first is for the scientist or practitioner to advocate as an individual citizen. The second is to raise awareness and motivation for advocacy among the public. For enactment of most health policies in a democratic society, it is essential to have an informed and supportive public. Since it is well established that the public obtains most information about health through mass media (Chananie 1993), strategies to increase visibility for a health policy issue through the media are key.

As discussed in Chapter 11, one method to increase visibility for a health policy issue among the public is media advocacy, which is the strategic use of the mass media to promote public policy initiatives, that is, making sure that the story gets told from the public health point of view (US DHHS 1989a; Wallack et al. 1993). Media advocacy can be accomplished in three steps: setting the agenda, shaping the debate, and advancing the policy (Wallack et al. 1993). Several strategies are recommended in dealing with the media, including cultivating relationships with journalists so they know they have a credible and reliable source; creating news with news conferences, news releases, or polling data; linking local stories with breaking national news; and using paid advertising (Wallack and Dorfman 1996). Identifying and training a local spokesperson (e.g., a celebrity or community leader) will enhance the chances for widespread coverage of health issues.

The effective use of data, or "creative epidemiology," is crucial in communicating information to the media. Creative epidemiology is simply a method of making data interesting to the media and the general public. It blends the science of the researcher with the creativity of the advocate (US DHHS 1989a). For example, the tobacco industry spent over $6 billion to advertise and promote tobacco products in 1993. A more meaningful presentation might translate this as spending $190 per second. Techniques in communicating epidemiologic information are discussed in more detail in Chapter 11.

6. Informing Policy-Makers. It is important for the practitioner to understand the process differences in decision making in the epidemiologic versus political environments (Table 12-3). Frequently in epidemiology and medicine, decisions are made by one person or a small number of persons. Conversely, in the political system, many decisions are made by consensus (Sederburg 1992). For example, in the US Congress there are 435 representatives and 100 senators and legislation is passed by a simple majority of votes (i.e., 218 representatives and 51 senators).

A top priority of a scientist is to remain objective and to base decisions on a well evaluated body of evidence. Policy-makers, in turn, are influenced by many different constituent groups and may base decisions on other criteria. At times, the role of epidemiologic data in the policy-making process may be limited, given the impact of special interest groups and the divergent values of the political process (Foxman 1989).

When informing policy makers, practitioners should recall the well-known quote from former House Speaker Tip O'Neill: "All politics is local." A strength of a broad-based health coalition is that local experts can build credibility and can assist in educating their elected officials on particular health policy issues. Another important consideration in establishing contact

Table 12-3. Comparison Between Epidemiologic and Political Decision-Making Processes

Epidemiologic Process: Rational Decision Making	Political Process: Intuitive Decision Making
Identify problem	Identify problem
Develop options	Place in context
Analyze options	Use judgment
Implement policy	Assess reaction
Evaluate effect	Prepare for next crisis

Source: Sederburg (1992).

with elected officials is the use of short summaries and fact sheets. The majority of policy makers will not read detailed scientific reports. Therefore, brief fact sheets (no more than one-page, front and back) are essential. Five key aspects of communicating epidemiologic and surveillance information to policy makers have been outlined (Sederburg 1992): (1) Make data understandable by condensing them to a few key points, (2) use outside expertise such as experts in the field who are also constituents, (3) learn about the political process, (4) use the media to influence public opinion, and (5) understand that social attitudes change slowly and political change is incremental.

7. Evaluating the Process. Despite the recognized importance of policy making to the overall health of the population, relatively little attention has been paid to research on policy implementation, including evaluation of the factors predicting successful health policy enactment and implementation. Such an evaluation tends to focus on the process and includes questions on the "hows" and "whys" of health policy development.

This type of qualitative evaluation frequently can serve as a useful complement to quantitative evaluation (Steckler et al. 1992). Qualitative evaluation tends to be case-oriented with more subjective measures, whereas quantitative evaluation is generally population focused with more objective measures (Steckler et al. 1992). One might ask the following questions when conducting a process evaluation of a health policy:

1. What key factors benefited enactment of the policy?
2. What key factors impeded enactment of the policy?
3. How effectively is the policy being implemented?
4. Why are some persons not abiding by the policy?
5. Why is the public unaware of a certain policy?
6. How can support for a policy be increased among elected officials?

A qualitative evaluation of a given policy might include key informant surveys with policy makers, focus groups with the public and elected officials, and case studies of successful or unsuccessful policy implementation.

8. Evaluating the Impacts and Outcomes. In addition to evaluation of the process of policy enactment and implementation, impact and outcome evaluation of a health policy is important. Typically, this involves quantitative evaluation and includes systematic monitoring to determine whether the policy change has the predicted effect (Shapiro 1991; Brownson et al. 1997a). For example, legislative or organizational policies may go into effect, providing free or reduced cost mammography screening for women of certain ages. Some of the questions typically posed in an outcome evaluation would include:

1. Is the rate of mammography screening increasing?
2. Is the stage at which breast cancer is diagnosed changing over time?
3. Is the rate of mammography screening increasing at similar rates in sub-groups of women (e.g., low-income women, racial/ethnic groups)?
4. If so, can the increase be attributed to the new health policy?
5. What are the costs and benefits of the new policy?
6. Would similar effects be expected in other populations and locations?

Evaluation of the effects of health policies can be complex—true experimental conditions are not possible, many factors must be taken into account, and it may take years for policy effects to be observed. When conducting health policy evaluation, practitioners should carefully consider issues of validity and reliability. Validity seeks to determine whether observed effects can be attributed to the policy (i.e., internal validity) and whether these effects can be generalized to other populations (i.e., external validity) (Rossi and Freeman 1993; Fink 1993). Reliability corresponds to whether repeated measurement of policy effects shows consistent results (Rossi and Freeman 1993; Fink 1993).

Barriers to Effective Use of Epidemiology in Health Policy Development

There are a number of barriers to successful and appropriate use of epidemiology and other scientific inputs in policy development and implementation (Terris 1980). This section briefly highlights several of the most important barriers.

Failure to Recognize the Importance of Prevention

Despite the enormous resources that are spent on health care, the United States and most other countries spend relatively little on prevention. For example, of the total US health care budget, only about 3% is allocated to prevention (CDC 1992b; Roemer 1995). The changing health care system has the potential to place a higher priority on prevention due to the focus on capitated payment and the integration of health care services into large corporate organizations (Gordon et al. 1996). Increasingly, much of the information concerning prevention priorities is being supplemented with cost-effectiveness data. In many cases, interventions in primary and secondary prevention are more cost-effective than many established medical treatments (Tengs et al. 1995). Among the most cost-effective interventions are smoking prevention, childhood immunizations, environmental lead reduction, and fluoridation of public water supplies (Gordon et al. 1996). As prevention effectiveness is measured in the future, it must account for years and quality of life gained, rather than only economic savings (Roemer 1995).

Unwillingness to Accept the Validity of Epidemiologic Evidence

Scientific proof is seldom, if ever, absolute. Epidemiologic evidence about disease etiology and intervention effectiveness is subject to potential methodologic limitations (see Chapter 2). History shows that clinicians can be unwilling to accept the validity of epidemiologic discoveries (Terris 1980). Some researchers (e.g., Feinstein 1988), have raised a litany of criticisms of epidemiology. These mainly focus on methodologic limitations and overinterpretation of epidemiologic data by the public. Careful review of the evidence suggests that many of these criticisms are unfounded (Savitz et al. 1990). Proper use of epidemiologic data in formulation of health policies should take into account the costs and benefits of intervention, while weighing the uncertainties in causal inference and the imperfect decision rules (Savitz et al. 1990).

The Power of Vested Interests

Health policy formulation involves a political process and at times can be difficult because it may challenge some very important and powerful interests in society (Beauchamp 1976). In the early 1900s, the chemical and lead industries distorted epidemiologic data that revealed health hazards among workers (Watterson 1994; Weindling 1985). More recently, the tobacco and asbestos industries have been noted to exclude or suppress epidemiologic and toxicologic data to mask the health hazards associated with use of their products (Watterson 1994; Glantz et al. 1995). Research studies sometimes invite vigorous attack because of their huge financial implications (Deyo et. al. 1997).

Isolation From the Political Process

As discussed in earlier sections, epidemiologists are sometimes isolated from the political process. This can be both an advantage and a disadvantage. The beneficial aspect is that epidemiologists can retain their complete objectivity without fear of political influences. Conversely, lack of scientific involvement among policy-makers may mean that the ignorant or those with vested private interests potentially wield undue influence.

Timing

Epidemiologic studies are not always conducted at the right time to influence policy decisions (Foltz 1986; Foxman 1989). Epidemiologic research tends to progress in a deliberate, although not always predictable pace. Several steps are needed before a research project is begun: a research question is developed, a team of researchers is identified, funding sources are investigated, a grant application is written and submitted, and funding is obtained (often after rewriting and resubmitting the application). Frequently, epidemiologic research projects take 3–6 years to complete and as many as 8–10 years may pass from the time of the initial question to dissemination of findings. In most cases, timing for the policy-making process is entirely different. Public officials are usually elected every 2–6 years and are often dealing with hundreds of policy issues in a single year. By the time that epidemiologic research findings are sufficient to support policy changes, the political and social climates may not be receptive.

Lack of a Focus on Evaluation

Others (Tugwell et al. 1985; Brownson et al. 1997a) have highlighted the need for a systematic evaluation framework when examining the impact of epidemiology on health policies. In some cases, health care procedures or interventions (e.g., reimbursement for diagnostic tests or treatments) have been supported by policy for years, yet may not be a high current priority if held to the same evaluation standards as many new technologies (Borst-Eilers 1996).

Differing Perceptions of Voluntary and Involuntary Risks

Individuals react differently to health risks that are imposed voluntarily (e.g., lack of physical activity) compared with those acquired involuntarily, often as the result of advancing technology (e.g., a nuclear power plant) (Starr and Whipple 1980). In general, individuals and society have been more willing to accept voluntary risks than involuntary risks. The methods for quantitative risk assessment outlined in Chapter 5 can lead to a more rational basis for risk evaluation. Despite the availability of increasingly sophisticated methods, it is challenging to apply quantitative risk assessment procedures to voluntary and involuntary risks when the process becomes both scientific and political (Starr and Whipple 1980).

Summary

This chapter has highlighted several of the major ways in which epidemiology can influence health policies. Just as the opportunities for scientifically based health policy development are vast, the challenges in translating epidemiologic discoveries into rational health policies are sizable.

One of the continuing challenges for epidemiologists and policy-makers is to determine when scientific evidence is sufficient for public health action. In most cases, epidemiologic studies cannot demonstrate causality with absolute certainty (Hill 1965; Susser 1977). This demarcation is seldom distinct and requires careful consideration of evidence as well as assessment of costs and benefits of policy options (see Chapter 9). The difficulty in determining scientific certainty was aptly summarized by A.B. Hill (1965):

> All scientific work is incomplete—whether it be observational or experimental. All scientific work is liable to be upset or modified by advancing knowledge. That does not confer upon us a freedom to ignore the knowledge we already have, or to postpone the action that it appears to demand at a given time.

In some cases (e.g., smoking and lung cancer, aspirin and Reye syndrome), waiting for absolute scientific certainty would mean delaying action that would be costly to the health of the public (Savitz et al. 1990).

For successful translation of epidemiologic discoveries into public health action, partnerships between health agencies and universities are ideal vehicles for success because each entity brings unique abilities to the table. Health agencies generally have greater access to populations at risk and have more experience working at the community level. University researchers can add epidemiologic and evaluation expertise that may be lacking in some public health agencies and health care organizations.

Educators should consider a stronger emphasis on the interrelationships between epidemiology and health policies. Training in epidemiology currently focuses on epidemiologic methods. There is little focus on how the science of epidemiology is translated into effective health care policy. As schools of public health and medicine review and enhance their curricula and internship placements, new emphasis is needed to enhance understanding of epidemiologic inputs into health policy development.

In summary, the use of epidemiology in shaping health policies is increasing (Foege 1984; Ibrahim 1985). As methods in epidemiology continue to improve, the opportunities to enhance epidemiologic influences on health policy development will draw heavily on the issues highlighted elsewhere in this book. Epidemiology can provide an important basis for many health policies; however, health policy development is complicated and should not be based solely on epidemiologic data. Epidemiologic findings always have

some degree of uncertainty, and the development of a health policy is dependent on many social, cultural, and economic factors.

CASE STUDIES

AIDS Policy: The Roles of Health Professionals and Schools of Public Health

Background

Five cases of *Pneumocystis carinii* pneumonia (in Los Angeles, in 1981) signaled the
beginning of the acquired immune deficiency syndrome (AIDS) epidemic caused by
the human immunodeficiency virus (HIV). As the worldwide scope of the HIV/AIDS
epidemic became apparent, so did the social and political implications of the disease.
Because a primary mode of transmission of AIDS was through anogenital intercourse
in homosexual men, the disease was sometimes called the "gay plague." This term
emphasized the social, political, and medical aspects of HIV/AIDS (Fee and Krieger
1993).

Against this backdrop, two events occurred in 1986 that further showed the sociopolitical aspects of AIDS. The US Justice Department ruled that section 504 of the
Rehabilitation Act of 1973 did not protect employees from discrimination based on the
fear that they might spread AIDS at work, regardless of whether the fear was "rational
or irrational from a medical perspective." At the same time, the California proposition
64, the LaRouche "Prevent AIDS Now" initiative, qualified for the November ballot
(Krieger and Lashof 1988).

These incidents led the School of Public Health at the University of California at
Berkeley to initiate a protest of the Justice Department ruling from all 23 schools of
public health. In addition, the school expanded efforts, and with California's three
other schools of public health, undertook a policy analysis of proposition 64. This
analysis exposed the false claims regarding casual transmission of AIDS and served to
educate the electorate on the issue (Krieger and Lashof 1988).

Key Questions

1. What should be the role of individual health professionals, schools of public
health, and other health-related institutions in health advocacy?

Krieger and Lashof (1988) concluded that public health professionals, both as
individuals and as members of the profession, have a responsibility not only to educate, but to advocate those policies that best represent the public's interest, based on
their own scientific knowledge, judgment, and values. As noted earlier in this chapter,
it is important for a scientist to maintain a reasoned and evidence-based stance when
entering into advocacy. In the case of widespread health threats such as AIDS, it is not
a matter of *whether*, but *which* health policies will be developed (Krieger and Lashof
1988). If public health professionals refrain from advocacy, uninformed health policies
are more likely.

3. How can health professionals best educate the public on the scientific basis for
health policies?

As stated earlier in this chapter and in Chapter 11, a variety of methods or "channels" can be used to educate the public on health issues. A broad-based coalition can

be a distinct asset. In addition, the print and electronic media are important vehicles for education on public health issues.

4. How can health policy analysis be used to support public health?

The policy analysis of proposition 64 identified five main areas of public health liability, suggesting that it would (1) foster inaccurate beliefs on the transmission of HIV/AIDS, (2) deny jobs and health insurance to people who pose no threat to the general public's health, (3) force those who suspect they are infected with the AIDS virus to avoid using health services, (4) hamper necessary and critical research regarding transmission, and (5) waste state funds on coercive intervention programs (Krieger and Lashof 1988). These five points emphasized proposition 64's negative effects on public health.

Implications for Practice

As a result of the policy analysis and widespread educating on and organizing against proposition 64, the measure was defeated on November 4, 1986, by more than a two-to-one margin. The lessons learned from this example can be applied to other contemporary public health issues.

Tobacco Excise Taxes and Health Promotion (Proposition 99)

Background

Due to the overwhelming epidemiologic evidence that smoking is a major public health problem in the United States and California and to the need for strengthened public health efforts to control tobacco, California voters passed an earmarked tobacco excise tax in 1988 (Bal et al. 1990). Known as "proposition 99," this effort has been a national and international model that illustrates the interface between epidemiology, health policy, and health promotion. It raised the excise tax on cigarettes by 25 cents per pack and placed an initial tax of 42 cents on other tobacco products, with the rate on other tobacco products adjusted annually by the State Board of Equalization (Bal et al. 1990; Breslow and Johnson 1993). This revenue was used to fund (1) healthcare services for the medically indigent; (2) statewide antitobacco health education efforts in schools and communities; (3) public resources; and (4) research on tobacco-related disease (Breslow and Johnson 1993). This effort launched one of the most intensive and aggressive public health interventions ever undertaken (Elder et al. 1996).

Key Questions

1. How can epidemiologic and survey data be used to support health policy initiatives such as proposition 99?

A variety of different types of epidemiologic data can be instrumental in supporting policy initiatives such as proposition 99. These data can include decades of research and thousands of epidemiologic studies that have established cigarette smoking as the "single most important preventable cause of premature death" (US DHHS 1989b). Economic studies show that increased tobacco taxes are an important tool for decreasing tobacco consumption (Sweanor et al. 1992). Finally, polling data generally show high voter support for significant increases in tobacco taxes (Sweanor et al. 1992).

2. What are the constraints, both in government and in the private sector, on passage of such a policy measure?

Legislators are often unwilling to institute large increases in tobacco taxes. Therefore, voter-initiated campaigns such as proposition 99 are sometimes the only viable mechanisms for increasing the tax on tobacco products. A strong coalition is vital to the success of policy initiatives such as proposition 99.

3. How would one evaluate the effects of a state-wide tobacco tax on smoking initiation and prevalence?

An array of data sets can be used to evaluate the effects of a tobacco tax. Surveys of youths and adults can allow calculation of rates of smoking initiation and prevalence. Tax records and census statistics can provide data on per capita cigarette consumption. A difficulty in the evaluation of a large-scale intervention such as proposition 99 is the lack of a comparison group.

4. What are the effects of the California initiative on cigarette sales and smoking behavior?

The California tobacco excise tax sharply accelerated the drop in both sales of cigarettes and in smoking. Other factors may also have been involved (e.g., the general economic downturn). Per capita cigarette sales have declined 41% between 1988 and 1994. There has been a 28% decline in smoking prevalence between 1988 and 1993 (California Dept of Health Services 1996). This is double the expected decline based on the 1974–1987 trend.

5. Can changes be attributed to any particular aspect of the initiative?

In addition to the tax itself, the state's paid advertising campaign against tobacco use and the state-wide tobacco control activities also appear to have contributed to this decline (Breslow and Johnson 1993; Glantz 1993). A great proportion of smokers who quit attribute their action to media influence. It is noteworthy that the tobacco industry directed a major effort at stopping the media campaign (Breslow and Johnson 1993).

Implications for Practice

The California experience is an example of a policy measure that will have a positive effect on the health of the population. In addition to reducing smoking prevalence, the California campaign has stimulated grassroots health promotion efforts. For example, local communities throughout the state substantially increased the number of antitobacco coalitions focusing on local policies such as clean indoor air ordinances and removal of vending machines; a greater attention is now being paid to prevention and cessation, especially among racial/ethnic minorities; collaboration between health and education agencies has been enhanced; and there has been an increase in technical assistance and evaluation. Proposition 99 has also stimulated innovative tobacco use research.

SUGGESTED READINGS

Brown EY, Viscoli CM, Horwitz RI. Preventive health strategies and the policy makers' paradox. Ann Intern Med 1992;116:593–597.

Brownson RC, Newschaffer CJ, Ali-Abarghoui F. Policy research for disease prevention; challenges and practical recommendations. Am J Public Health 1997; 87:735–739.

Foege WH. Uses of epidemiology in the development of health policy. Public Health Rep 1984;99:233–236.

Ibrahim MA. Epidemiology and Health Policy. Rockville, MD: Aspen; 1985.

Milio N. Promoting Health Through Public Policy. Ottawa, Ontario: Canadian Public Health Association; 1986.

Shapiro S. Epidemiology and public policy. Am J Epidemiol 1991;134:1057–1061.

Terris M. Epidemiology as a guide to health policy. Annu Rev Public Health 1980;1:323–344.

Warner KE. Public policy issues. In: Greenwald P, Kramer BS, Weed DL, eds. Cancer Prevention and Control. New York: Marcel Dekker; 1995:451–472.

REFERENCES

Aday LA. Health status of vulnerable populations. Annu Rev Public Health 1994;15:487–509.

Alciati MH, Frosh M, Green SB, et al. An evaluation of state laws on youth access to tobacco in the United States. Am J Public Health (in review).

American Public Health Association. Harnessing information superhighway does wonders for public health advocacy. Nation Health; 1996:14.

Angell M. Science on Trial. The Clash of Medical Evidence and the Law in the Breast Implant Case. New York: W.W. Norton; 1996.

Baker EL, Melton RJ, Stange PV, et al. Health reform and the health of the public: forging community health partnerships. JAMA 1994;272:1276–1282.

Bal DG, Kizer KW, Felten PG, Mozar HN, Niemeyer D. Reducing tobacco consumption in California: development of a statewide anti-tobacco use campaign. JAMA 1990;264:1570–1574.

Beauchamp DE. Public health as social justice. Inquiry 1976;13:3–14.

Beauchamp TL, Cook RR, Fayerweather WE, et al. Ethical guidelines for epidemiologists. J Clin Epidemiol 1991;44(Suppl):151S–169S.

Borst-Eilers E. Perspectives on epidemiology in Europe. Int J Epidemiol 1996;25:469–473.

Bots PWG, Hulshof JAM. Applying multi-criteria group decision support to health policy formulation. Presented at the ISDSS Conference in Hong Kong, June 23–24, 1995.

Bracht N, Kingsbury L. Community organization principles in health promotion. A five-stage model. In: Bracht N, ed. Health Promotion at the Community Level. Newbury Park, CA: Sage; 1990:66–88.

Breslow L, Johnson M. California's Proposition 99 on tobacco, and its impact. Annu Rev Public Health 1993;14:585–604.

Brown EY, Viscoli CM, Horwitz RI. Preventive health strategies and the policy makers' paradox. Ann Int Med 1992;116:593–597.

Brownson RC, Koffman DM, Novotny TE, Hughes RG, Eriksen MP. Environmental and policy interventions to control tobacco use and prevent cardiovascular disease. Health Educ Q 1995;22:478–498.

Brownson RC, Newschaffer CJ, Ali-Abarghoui F. Policy research for disease prevention: challenges and practical recommendations. Am J Public Health 1997a;87:735–739.

Brownson RC, Eriksen MP, Davis RM, Warner KE. Environmental tobacco smoke: health effects and policies to reduce exposure. Annu Rev Public Health 1997b; 18:163–185.

California Department of Health Services. Toward Tobacco Free California. Mastering the Challenges 1995–1997. Sacramento, CA: California Department of Health Services; 1996.

Centers for Disease Control. Planned Approach to Community Health (PATCH): Program Description. Atlanta, GA: US Public Health Service, Centers for Disease Control; 1992a.

Centers for Disease Control. Estimated national spending on prevention—United States, 1988. Morb Mortal Wkly Rep 1992b;41:529–531.

Centers for Disease Control and Prevention. A Practical Guide to Prevention Effectiveness: Decision and Economic Analyses. Atlanta, GA: Centers for Disease Control and Prevention; 1994.

Centers for Disease Control and Prevention. CDC Wonder home page. [on-line]. 1997. Available: http://wonder.cdc.gov

Chananie D. The American Public's Understanding of Biomedical Sciences. Paper presented at the 1993 International Congress for the Public Understanding of Science and Technology. Brussels: Commission of the European Communities; 1993.

Cheadle A, Wagner E, Koepsell T, Kristal A, Patrick D. Environmental indicators: a tool of evaluating community-based health-promotion programs. Am J Prev Med 1992;8:345–350.

Christoffel T, Teret SP. Epidemiology and the law: courts and confidence intervals. Am J Public Health 1991;81:1661–1666.

Cwikel JG. After epidemiological research: what next? Community action for health promotion. Public Health Rev 1994;22:375–394.

Davis JR, Brownson RC. A policy for clean indoor air in Missouri: history and lessons learned. St. Louis Univ Public Law Rev 1994;13:749–762.

Davis JR, Schwartz R, Wheeler F, Lancaster RB. Intervention methods for chronic disease control. In: Brownson RC, Remington PL, Davis JR, eds. Chronic Disease Epidemiology and Control. Washington, DC: American Public Health Association; 1993:51–81.

Deyo RA, Psaty BM, Simon G, Wagner EH, Omenn GS. The messenger under attack—intimidation of researchers by special-interest groups, New Engl J Med 1997;336:1176–1180.

Doron G. Policy sciences: the state of the discipline. Policy Studies Rev 1992;11:303–309.

Elder JP, Edwards CC, Conway TL, et al. Independent evaluation of the California tobacco education program. Public Health Rep 1996;111:353–358.

Fawcett SB, Paine AL, Francisco VT, Vliet M. Promoting health through community development. In: Glenwick DS, Jason LA, eds. Promoting Health and Mental Health in Children, Youth, and Families. New York: Springer; 1993:233–255.

Fee E, Krieger N. Thinking and rethinking AIDS: implications for health policy. Int J Health Services 1993;23:323–346.

Feinstein AR. Scientific standards in epidemiologic studies of the menace of daily life. Science 1988;242:1257–1263.

Fink A. Evaluation Fundamentals. Guiding Health Programs, Research, and Policy. Newbury Park, CA: Sage; 1993.

Florin P, Stevenson J. Identifying training and technical assistance needs in community coalitions: a developmental approach. Health Educ Res 1993;8:417–432.

Foege WH. Uses of epidemiology in the development of health policy. Public Health Rep 1984;99:233–236.

Foege WH. Preventive medicine and public health. JAMA 1993;270:251–252.

Foltz A-M. Epidemiology and health policy: science and its limits. J Ambulatory Care Manage 1986;9:75–87.

Fox PD. The American point of view. Int J Epidemiol 1977;6:197–198.

Foxman B. Epidemiologists and public health policy. J Clin Epidemiol 1989;42:1107–1109.

Friede A, Reid JA, Ory HW. CDC WONDER: a comprehensive on-line public health information system of the Centers for Disease Control and Prevention. Am J Public Health 1993;83:1289–1294.

Glantz SA. Changes in cigarette consumption, prices, and tobacco industry revenues associated with California's Proposition 99. Tobacco Control 1993;2:311–314.

Glantz SA, Barnes DE, Bero L, Hanauer P, Slade J. Looking through a keyhole at the tobacco industry. The Brown and Williamson doucments. JAMA 1995;274:219–224.

Glanz K, Lankenau B, Foerster S, Temple S, Mullis R, Schmid T. Environmental and policy approaches to cardiovascular disease prevention through nutrition: opportunities for state and local action. Health Educ Q 1995;22:512–527.

Glass GV. Primary, secondary and meta-analysis of research. Educ Res 1976;5:3–8.

Goldring JM, James DS, Anderson HA. Chronic lung diseases. In: Brownson RC, Remington PL, Davis JR, eds. Chronic Disease Epidemiology and Control. Washington, DC: American Public Health Association; 1993:169–197.

Gordis L. Challenges to epidemiology in the next decade. Am J Epidemiol 1988;128:1–9.

Gordon RL, Baker EL, Roper WL, Omenn GS. Prevention and the reforming U.S. health care system: changing roles and responsibilities for public health. Annu Rev Public Health 1996;17:489–509.

Green LW, Raeburn J. Contemporary developments in health promotion. Definitions and challenges. In: Bracht N, ed. Health Promotion at the Community Level. Newbury Park, CA: Sage; 1990:29–44.

Ham C, Hill M. The Policy Process in the Modern Capitalist State. New York: St. Martin's Press; 1984.

Harris JR, Lippman ME, Veronesi U, Willett W. Breast cancer (first of three parts). New Engl J Med 1992;327:319–327.

Hendrick RM, Nachmias D. The policy sciences: the challenge of complexity. Policy Studies Rev 1992;11:310–328.

Hertz-Picciotto I. Epidemiology and quantitative risk assessment: a bridge from science to policy. Am J Public Health 1995;85:484–491.

Hill AB. The environment and disease: association or causation? Proc R Soc Med 1965;58:295–300.

Hogwood BW, Gunn LA. The Policy Orientation. University of Strathclyde, Centre for the Study of Public Policy; 1981.

Ibrahim MA. Epidemiology and Health Policy. Rockville, MD: Aspen; 1985.

Institute of Medicine. Committee for the Study of the Future of Public Health. The Future of Public Health. Washington, DC: National Academy Press; 1988.

Johnson J. Drug approval: "too cautious"? Congressional Res Serv Rev 1989; March:21.

King AC, Jeffery RW, Fidinger F, Dusenbury L, Provence S, Hedlund SA, Spangler K. Environmental and policy approaches to cardiovascular disease prevention through physical activity: issues and opportunities. Health Educ Q 1995;22:499–511.

Krieger N, Lashof JC. AIDS, policy analysis, and the electorate: the role of schools of public health. Am J Public Health 1988;78:411–415.

Lilienfeld DE, Stolley PD. Foundations of Epidemiology. Third Edition. New York: Oxford University Press; 1994.

McKinlay JB. The promotion of health through planned sociopolitical change: challenges for research and policy. Soc Sci Med 1993;36:109–117.

Merrill RA. Regulation of drugs and devices: an evolution. Health Affairs 1994; Summer:47–69.

Milio N. Promoting Health Through Public Policy. Ottawa, Ontario: Canadian Public Health Association; 1986.

Milio N. Making healthy public policy; developing the science by learning the art: an ecological framework for policy studies. Health Promotion 1987;2:7–28.

Modan B. Epidemiology and health policy: prevention initiatives, resource allocation, regulation, and control. Public Health Rep 1984;99:228–233.

National Association of County Health Officials. Assessment Protocol for Excellence in Public Health (APEX/PH). Washington, DC: National Association of County Health Officials; 1991.

National Cancer Institute. State Cancer Legislative Database Program. Bethesda, MD: Division of Cancer Prevention and Control; August, 1994.

Oberle MW, Baker EL, Magenheim MJ. Healthy people 2000 and community health planning. Annu Rev Public Health 1994;15:259–275.

Omenn GS. Prevention: Benefits, Costs, and Savings. Washington, DC: Partnership for Prevention; 1994.

Orosz E. The impact of social science research on health policy. Soc Sci Med 1994;39:1287–1293.

Ottawa Working Group on Health Promotion in Developing Countries. Health promotion in developing countries. The report of a workgroup. Health Promotion 1986;1:461–462.

Pelletier KR. A reveiw and analysis of the health and cost-effective outcome studies of comprehensive health promotion and disease prevention programs at the worksite: 1993–1995 update. Am J Health Promotion 1996;10:380–388.

Poole C, Rothman KJ. Epidemiologic science and public health policy [letter]. J Clin Epidemiol 1990;10:1270.

Robert Wood Johnson Foundation. Transforming Public Health: A Concept Paper to Guide Program Activity. Princeton, NJ: Robert Wood Johnson Foundation; November 28, 1995.

Roemer MI. Commentary: prevention in diverse health systems. Am J Prev Med 1995;11:351–353.

Rogers EM. Diffusion of Innovation. Third Edition. New York: Free Press; 1983.

Roper WL, Baker EL, Dyal WW, Nicola RM. Strengthening the public health system. Public Health Rep 1992;107:609–615.

Rose G. Sick individuals and sick populations. Int J Epidemiol 1985;14:32–38.

Rossi PH, Freeman HE. Evaluation. A Systematic Approach. Newbury Park, NJ: Sage; 1993.

Rothman J, Tropman JE. Models of community organization and macropractice perspectives: their mixing and phasing. In: Cox FM, Erlich J, Rothman J, Tropman JE, eds. Strategies of Community Organization: Mcaro Practice. Itasca, IL: Peacock; 1987:3–25.

Rothman KJ. Policy recommendations in epidemiology research papers. Epidemiol 1993;4:94–95.

Rothman KJ, Poole C. Science and policy making. Am J Public Health 1985;75:340–341.

Savitz DA, Greenland S, Stolley PD, Kelsey JL. Scientific standards of criticism: a reaction to "Scientific Standards in Epidemiologic Studies of the Menace of Daily Life," by A.R. Feinstein. Epidemiol 1990;1:78–83.

Schmid TL, Pratt M, Howze E. Policy as intervention: environmental and policy approaches to the prevention of cardiovascular disease. Am J Public Health 1995;85:1207–1211.

Schwartz J. Low-level lead exposure and children's IQ: a meta-analysis and search for a threshold. Environ Res 1994;65:42–55.

Sederburg WA. Perspectives of the legislator: allocating resources. Morb Mortal Wkly Rep 1992:41(Suppl):37–48.

Sexton K, Reiter L, Zenick H. Research to strengthen the scientific basis for health risk assessment: a survey of the context and rationale for mechanistically based methods and models. Toxicology 1995;102:3–20.

Shannon IR. Epidemiology and the public policy process. In: Oleske DM, ed. Epidemiology and the Delivery of Health Care Services. New York: Plenum Press; 1995:187–203.

Shapiro S. Epidemiology and public policy. Am J Epidemiol 1991;134:1057–1061.

Sisk JE, Gorman SA, Reisinger AL, Glied SA, DuMouchel WH, Hynes MM. Evaluation of Medicaid managed care. Satisfaction, access, and use. JAMA 1996;276:50–55.

Slavin RE. Best evidence synthesis: an intelligent alternative to meta-analysis. J Clin Epidemiol 1995;48:9–18.

Starr G, Whipple C. Risks of risk decisions. Science 1980;208:1114–1119.

Steckler A, McLeroy KR, Goodman RM, Bird ST, McCormick L. Toward integrating qualitative and quantitative methods: an introduction. Health Educ Q 1992;19:1–8.

Stein H. Epidemiology and health policy. Int J Epidemiol 1977;6:198–200.

Stokols D, Pelletier KR, Fielding JE. Integration of medical care and worksite health promotion. JAMA 1995;273:1136–1142.

Susser M. Judgement and causal inference: criteria in epidemiologic studies. Am J Epidemiol 1977;105:1–15.

Susser M. Health as a human right: an epidemiologist's perspective on the public health. Am J Public Health 1993;83:418–426.

Sweanor D, Ballin S, Corcoran RD, et al. Report of the Tobacco Policy Research Study Group on tobacco pricing and taxation in the United States. Tobacco Control 1992;1(Suppl):S31–S36.

Tengs TO, Adams ME, Pliskin JS, et al. Five-hundred life-saving interventions and their cost-effectiveness. Risk Anal 1995;15:369–390.

Teret S. So what? Epidemiology 1993;4:93–94.

Terris M. Epidemiology as a guide to health policy. Annu Rev Public Health 1980;1:323–344.

Tesh S. Disease causality and politics. J Health Polit Policy Law. 1981;6:369–380.

Thacker SB, Berkelman RL. Public health surveillance in the United States. Epidemiol Rev 1988;10:164–190.

The Presidential/Congressional Commission on Risk Assessment and Risk Management. Framework for Environmental Health Risk Management. Final Report, Volume 1. Washington, DC: The Presidential/Congressional Commission on Risk Assessment and Risk Management; 1997.

Tugwell P, Bennett KJ, Sackett DL, Hayes RB. The measurement iterative loop: a framework for the critical appraisal of need, benefits and costs of health interventions. J Chron Dis 1985;38:339–351.

US Dept of Health and Human Services. Media Strategies for Smoking Control: Guidelines (NIH Publication No. 89-3013). Washington, DC: US Government Printing Office, 1989a.

US Dept of Health and Human Services. Reducing the Health Consequences of Smoking—25 Years of Progress: A Report of the Surgeon General. Rockville, MD: US Dept of Health and Human Services, Public Health Service, Centers for Disease Control, Center for Chronic Disease Prevention and Health Promotion, Office on Smoking and Health; DHHS publication (CDC) 89-8411; 1989b

US Dept of Health and Human Services. Healthy People 2000: National Health Promotion and Disease Prevention. Washington, DC: US Government Printing Office; No. 017-001-00473-1; 1990.

US Dept of Health and Human Services. 1992 National Survey of Worksite Health Promotion Activities. Washington, DC: US Dept of Health and Human Services, Office of Disease Prevention and Health Promotion; 1993.

US Dept of Health and Human Services. For a Healthy Nation. Returns on Investment in Public Health. Washington, DC: US Dept of Health and Human Services, Public Health Service; 1994.

US Dept of Health and Human Services. Physical Activity and Health: A Report of the Surgeon General. Atlanta, GA: US Dept of Health and Human Services, Centers for Disease Control and Prevention; 1996.

US Environmental Protection Agency. Guidelines for carcinogenic risk assessment. Federal Register 1986;51:33992–34003.

US Preventive Services Task Force. Guide to Clinical Preventive Services. Second Edition. Baltimore, MD: Williams & Wilkins; 1996.

Volkers N. NCI replaces guidelines with statement of evidence. J Natl Cancer Inst 1994;86:14–15.

Wallack L, Dorfman L, Jernigan D, Themba M. Media Advocacy and Public Health. Power for Prevention. Newbury Park, CA: Sage; 1993.

Wallack L, Dorfman L. Media advocacy: a strategy for advancing policy and promoting health. Health Educ Q 1996;23:293–317.

Warner KE. Public policy issues. In: Greenwald P, Kramer BS, Weed DL, eds. Cancer Prevention and Control. New York: Marcel Dekker; 1995:451–472.

Watterson A. Whither lay epidemiology in UK public health policy and practice? Some reflections on occupational and environmental health opportunities. J Public Health Med 1994;16:270–274.

Weed DL. Science, ethics guidelines, and advocacy in epidemiology. Ann Epidemiol 1994;4:166–171.

Weindling P, ed. The Social History of Occupational Health. London: Croom Helm; 1985.

Wennberg JE, Bunker JP, Barnes B. The need for assessing the outcome of common medical practices. Annu Rev Public Health 1980;1:277–295.

Williams-Crowe SM, Aultman TV. State health agencies and the legislative policy process. Public Health Rep 1994;109:361–367.

WK Kellogg. Communicating with Policy Makers. Module Two. Battle Creek, MI: W.K. Kellogg Foundation; 1996.

Woolley M. What are you waiting for? J Women Health 1995;4:457–458.

World Health Organization. Constitution of the World Health Organization. In: Handbook of Basic Documents. Geneva: WHO; 1948.

World Health Organization. Assessment and Management of Environmental Health Hazards. Geneva: WHO/PEP/89.6; 1989.

Yankauer A. Science and social policy. Am J Public Health 1984;74:1148–1149.

Index